Multilingual Aspects of Signed Language Communication and Disorder

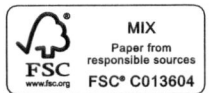

COMMUNICATION DISORDERS ACROSS LANGUAGES
Series Editors: Dr Nicole Müller and Dr Martin Ball, *University of Louisiana at Lafayette, USA*

While the majority of work in communication disorders has focused on English, there has been a growing trend in recent years for the publication of information on languages other than English. However, much of this is scattered through a large number of journals in the field of speech pathology/ communication disorders, and therefore not always readily available to the practitioner, researcher and student. It is the aim of this series to bring together into book form surveys of existing studies on specific languages, together with new materials for the language(s) in question. We also have launched a series of companion volumes dedicated to issues related to the cross-linguistic study of communication disorders. The series does not include English (as so much work is readily available), but covers a wide number of other languages (usually separately, though sometimes two or more similar languages may be grouped together where warranted by the amount of published work currently available). We have been able to publish volumes on Finnish, Spanish, Chinese and Turkish, and books on multilingual aspects of stuttering, aphasia and speech disorders, with several others in preparation.

Full details of all the books in this series and of all our other publications can be found on http://www.multilingual-matters.com, or by writing to Multilingual Matters, St Nicholas House, 31–34 High Street, Bristol BS1 2AW, UK.

Multilingual Aspects of Signed Language Communication and Disorder

Edited by
David Quinto-Pozos

MULTILINGUAL MATTERS
Bristol • Buffalo • Toronto

Library of Congress Cataloging in Publication Data
Multilingual Aspects of Signed Language Communication and Disorder/Edited by David
Quinto-Pozos.
Communication Disorders across Languages: 11
Includes bibliographical references and index.
1. Sign language. 2. Multilingual communication. 3. Communicative disorders. I.
Quinto-Pozos, David, editor of compilation. II. Series: Communication disorders across
languages.
P117.M85 2014
419–dc23 2013034247

British Library Cataloguing in Publication Data
A catalogue entry for this book is available from the British Library.

ISBN-13: 978-1-78309-130-0 (hbk)
ISBN-13: 978-1-78309-129-4 (pbk)

Multilingual Matters
UK: St Nicholas House, 31–34 High Street, Bristol BS1 2AW, UK.
USA: UTP, 2250 Military Road, Tonawanda, NY 14150, USA.
Canada: UTP, 5201 Dufferin Street, North York, Ontario M3H 5T8, Canada.

The policy of Multilingual Matters/Channel View Publications is to use papers that are
natural, renewable and recyclable products, made from wood grown in sustainable for-
ests. In the manufacturing process of our books, and to further support our policy, preference is given to printers that have FSC and PEFC Chain of Custody certification. The FSC
and/or PEFC logos will appear on those books where full certification has been granted
to the printer concerned.

Typeset by Techset Composition India (P) Ltd., Bangalore and Chennai, India.
Printed and bound by CPI Group (UK) Ltd, Croydon, CR0 4YY

Contents

Contributors

Joanna Atkinson is a Clinical Research Fellow at Deafness Cognition and Language Research Centre, UCL, London. She is also a certified clinical psychologist with additional qualifications in applied clinical neuropsychology. Her research includes: the impact of neurological conditions such as stroke, dementia and autism on BSL; schizophrenia, psychosis and voice-hallucinations in deaf people; and the clinical assessment of acquired and developmental neurological conditions in Deaf BSL users. Jo works as an Honorary Clinical Psychologist providing cognitive assessment of Deaf BSL users at the Cognitive Disorders Clinic, National Hospital for Neurology and Neurosurgery in London.

Anne Baker is professor emeritus of linguistics and sign linguistics at the University of Amsterdam. She does research on variation in language acquisition, developmental and acquired language disorders, and explores the relationship between cognition and language. She has published widely on the acquisition of sign languages, in particular on Sign Language of the Netherlands (NGT).

Deborah Chen Pichler is Associate Professor in Linguistics at Gallaudet University. Since 2002, she has taught courses on first and second language acquisition (of both signed and spoken languages) and generative syntax. Her research interests focus on L1 acquisition of ASL and English by Deaf children of Deaf families (both with and without cochlear implants) and hearing children of Deaf families (bimodal bilingual children or kodas), as well as L2 acquisition of ASL by hearing adults. She also has a strong interest in the use of technology in teaching, particularly in Deaf classrooms.

Marielle Fieret has a Bachelor's degree in sign linguistics (University of Amsterdam). Her Bachelor's thesis was about the influence of dementia on the language of deaf sign language users. Currently she is following a Masters program in applied linguistics with the specialization of Dutch as a second language.

Tobias Haug studied sign language linguistics at Hamburg University and Deaf education at Boston University, where he received his masters in 1998. In 2009 he earned his PhD in sign languages with the specialization on sign language assessment at Hamburg University. From 2000 to 2004 he worked as a sign language interpreter and researcher. Since 2004 he has been the programme director and lecturer in the sign language interpreter programme in Zurich, Switzerland. One of his main research interests is sign language development and assessment for different target groups (L1 and L2 learner) in connection with computer-assisted language testing. Since 2002 he has hosted a website on sign language tests.

Peter C. Hauser, PhD, is a deaf clinical neuropsychologist and an associate professor in the Department of American Sign Language and Interpreter Education at the National Technical Institute for the Deaf at Rochester Institute of Technology in Rochester, NY, USA. He is on the Executive Team of the National Science Foundation Science of Learning Center on Visual Language and Visual Learning. His laboratory develops sign language assessment instruments and consults with other countries on how to develop similar tests.

Ros Herman is a speech and language therapist and Reader in Communication and Deafness at City University, London. Her research interests include language acquisition in British Sign Language (BSL) and communication interventions and literacy development. Ros works closely with colleagues at the Deafness, Cognition and Language Research Centre, where she is a Research Associate. Ros runs a sign language assessment outreach service at City University's on-site clinic, offering clinical assessments of communication in BSL and reading to deaf children and adults.

Jimmy Lee, MS, CCC-SLP, first worked with kodas as a graduate student in the Gallaudet University Hearing and Speech Center (GUHSC). He returned to working with kodas as a clinical educator in the GUHSC. For many years, Mr Lee conducted and refined speech and language evaluations and the interpretation of the findings/results. He also conducted language stimulation groups working with kodas and their families to promote lifelong, fully bilingual, bimodal communicators. During these years, he was a staunch advocate for kodas and a cultural broker between public schools and Deaf families. He has published and presented many of his observations.

Susan C. Levine received her BA from Simmons College in Mathematics, Psychology, and Education and her PhD from MIT in Psychology. Upon graduating she joined the faculty at the University of Chicago, where she is the Rebecca Anne Boylan Professor in Education and Society in the Department of Psychology. She is also a member of the Department of Comparative Human Development and the Committee on Education at

Chicago. Her research focuses on the role of input variations on young children's language, numerical and spatial development. As part of a collaborative longitudinal language project, she is studying the relation of early language and gestural input in the home to the development of children's language, literacy, and mathematical skills, both in typically developing children and children with pre- or perinatal brain injury. Her studies range from basic laboratory investigations of children's cognitive development and learning to naturalistic studies of how children learn at home and at school. Her work also examines socio-emotional factors that may impact children's learning, including the anxieties and stereotypes of teachers, parents, and children themselves.

Diane Lillo-Martin is Board of Trustees Distinguished Professor in Linguistics and Director of the Cognitive Science Program at the University of Connecticut. She is also a senior research scientist at Haskins Laboratories. She has been conducting research on the structure and acquisition of sign languages since her graduate training at the University of California, San Diego and the Salk Institute. Her current research focus is on the development of bimodal bilingualism and ASL acquisition by Deaf children; she is also working on developing sign language corpora, and she continues to have an interest in theoretical studies of ASL morphology and syntax.

Wolfgang Mann received his PhD in Special Education from the University of California, Berkeley. Since then, he has worked as researcher/part-time lecturer in the Division of Language and Communication Science at City University London and at the Deafness Cognition and Language Research Centre (DCAL) at University College London (UCL). Dr Mann's areas of interest include language development and language difficulties in deaf children as well as (sign) language assessment. He is currently a Marie Curie Research Fellow, studying deaf children's response to dynamic assessment procedures within a language-learning context, as part of a collaborative project with the University of Texas at Austin.

Chloë R. Marshall, PhD, is Reader in Psychology and Human Development at the Institute of Education, University of London, where she is Programme Leader for the Masters in Special and Inclusive Education. Her research investigates typical and atypical language acquisition in hearing and deaf children, with a focus on specific language impairment and dyslexia.

Kathryn Mason is a psychology graduate with a masters degree in psychological research methods. Before starting her PhD at UCL, Kathryn worked with deaf children in schools in the UK and Hong Kong, and as a researcher at the Deafness Cognition and Language Research Centre and City University, London. Her research interests include language impairment in deaf signing children, sign language acquisition and the development of executive function in deaf children.

Richard P. Meier received his doctorate in linguistics from the University of California San Diego in 1982. After postdoctoral work in psychology at the University of Illinois and at Stanford, he joined the Department of Linguistics of the University of Texas at Austin in 1986; he has been department chair since 2006. Beginning with his dissertation work, he has been particularly interested in the questions of whether and how language modality (that is, the transmission channel in which a language is produced and perceived) interacts with the structure and acquisition of language.

Gary Morgan is Professor of Psychology at City University, London and deputy director of the Deafness, Cognition and Language Centre at UCL. He has worked on the acquisition of BSL, cognitive development of deaf children, and gesture and language disorder. Together with Bencie Woll he is the editor of *Directions in Sign Language Acquisition* (2002, John Benjamins), and with Eleni Orfanidou and Bencie Woll he is an editor of *Methods in Sign Language Research* (forthcoming 2014, Wiley-Blackwell).

David Quinto-Pozos, PhD, is a signed language linguist and an Assistant Professor in the Department of Linguistics at the University of Texas, Austin, TX. He is an affiliated researcher at the National Science Foundation Science of Learning Center on Visual Language and Visual Learning. In addition to his research on developmental signed language disorders, David's current work includes projects on the interaction of language and gesture and trilingual (Spanish–English–ASL) interpreting. David has also written about signed language contact and language teaching. He is also a certified ASL–English interpreter and President of *Mano a Mano*, a national organization for trilingual (Spanish–English–ASL) interpreters.

Kate Rowley graduated in Deaf studies before completing an MA in linguistics. She worked as a researcher before embarking on her PhD at University College London. She has carried out research into: language impairments in sign language; the development of sign language assessments; semantic and phonological organisation in BSL; and changing languages and identities in the British Deaf community.

Aaron Shield earned his doctorate in linguistics at the University of Texas at Austin in 2010. His dissertation examining the effects of autism spectrum disorders on the acquisition of American Sign Language (ASL) by deaf children won the Outstanding Dissertation Award at the University of Texas at Austin. After a postdoctoral research fellowship in psychology at the University of Chicago, in 2011 he became a postdoctoral research fellow in psychology at Boston University, where he is further investigating the effects of autism on ASL acquisition in deaf children. His research seeks to probe the relationship between language and non-linguistic social cognition, especially theory of mind, perspective taking and the development of the concepts of self and other.

Jenny L. Singleton, PhD, is an educational psychologist and a Full Professor at the School of Psychology at Georgia Institute of Technology, Atlanta, GA, USA. She is a collaborating scientist with the National Science Foundation Science of Learning Center on Visual Language and Visual Learning. Her laboratory focuses on how deaf infants and toddlers learn from their environments, particularly in activities that involve joint attention. She has published scholarly work on sign-based specific language impairment and sign language assessment.

Patricia Spanjer studied sign linguistics at the University of Amsterdam. She completed a Bachelor's thesis on the topic of language symptoms of dementia in an older signing population. Prior to that she created her own company and has advised the public sector for more than 10 years.

Martha E. Tyrone is an assistant professor in the Department of Communication Sciences and Disorders at Long Island University – Brooklyn, and a senior research scientist at Haskins Laboratories. She has studied the phonetics of typical and atypical signing in ASL and BSL, with an emphasis on neuromotor disorders in adults. Her current research focuses on quantitative measures of sign language production, with the ultimate goal of developing measures of accent, cross-linguistic variation and language deficits in the sign modality.

Beppie van den Bogaerde is Professor of NGT [Sign Language of the Netherlands] at the University of Amsterdam, and Professor of Deaf Studies at the Utrecht University of Applied Sciences, the Netherlands. Her main focus on research is on L1 and L2 acquisition of NGT, on issues in the Deaf community, and on interpreting studies. She is also involved in the UUAS Bachelor and Master program for teacher/interpreter NGT, and curriculum development. Recently she has been working on developing language descriptors for different levels (CEFR) in L2 acquisition for signed languages, in an international context.

Geoff Whitebread began his study of sign language stuttering for his Honors thesis at Gallaudet University. He graduated with a Bachelor's degree in psychology and a Master's in linguistics. Geoff is continuing his graduate studies at The George Washington University in political science and teaches in the Honors Program at Gallaudet University.

Bencie Woll is Professor of Sign Language and Deaf Studies at University College London and Director of the Deafness Cognition and Language Research Centre. Her research interests embrace a wide range of topics related to sign language, including the linguistics of BSL and other sign languages; the history and sociolinguistics of BSL and the Deaf community; the development of spoken and signed language in young children; sign language and the brain; and developmental and acquired sign language impairments.

Foreword

While writing a book on children with specific language impairment (SLI), I once stated that the prevalence of this disorder should be approximately 7% in children who are acquiring a sign language. This estimate was based on the fact that the prevalence figure for hearing children with SLI – the only children with SLI studied at that point – was 7.4%. Although the sentence flowed easily from my fingertips to the keyboard at the time, I realized only later that I was making an important assumption in offering the 7% estimate. My statement assumed that the cause of SLI is unrelated to auditory perception, even though some accounts prominent in the literature at the time argued to the contrary. I still believe that deficits in auditory perception are not a principal cause of SLI. But what if such deficits account for some smaller proportion of cases of SLI? The implications are twofold: first, of course, it might mean that the prevalence of this disorder is not 7% in children acquiring sign language, as auditory perception is unlikely to serve as a factor in these cases. Less obviously, it suggests that, in the sign language learning population, too, there may be modality-specific sources of language impairment, just as auditory perception problems might cause SLI in a select number of hearing children. These are important questions, and the current volume provides a wonderful start in trying to answer them.

Of course, the issue is not limited to SLI. It applies to other communication disorders as well. For each of several communication disorders, there may be common neurological, motor and linguistic processes that are responsible for the deficit in speaking and signing individuals alike. However, there may well be processes more affected by limitations in one modality than the other. It will be important for researchers to discover the proper mix, for this will not only benefit individuals having difficulty with sign language but will also provide scientists with a deeper understanding of the communication disorders themselves. The diversity of communication disorders covered in this volume will give readers an excellent appreciation for how these factors may interact.

My original comment about the prevalence of SLI in the signing population also glossed over the logistical challenges in pursuing such a question.

In my previous writings on the obstacles in diagnosing SLI in children acquiring very diverse spoken languages, I have pointed out how the culture surrounding the child must be the first consideration. Diagnosis depends not only on a child's relative standing among peers but also on whether members of the child's society view the symptoms as problematic. Competent individuals and proper tools for assessing the condition are also critical. A strong sense of what the typical child can say or understand at each age is also of the utmost importance. It is probably clear that these observations can apply equally well if we replace 'diagnosing SLI in children acquiring diverse spoken languages' with 'diagnosing a communication disorder in sign language users'. The issues are similar, including the need to develop norms on the language milestones of children who are developing sign language in typical fashion.

I am pleased to see that all of these considerations – and many more – are discussed in the present volume. The authors provide many insights into the complexities of communication disorders in the signing population, and their contributions reveal a level of sophistication that is quite remarkable for such a young field of study. This is a ground-breaking volume and I have learned much from reading it.

Laurence B. Leonard

Preface

This book is intended to serve as a resource for language and development researchers, students who are learning about language and development, and school professionals (e.g. speech and language therapists, school psychologists, teachers) who are interested in a signed language user's linguistic and cognitive abilities. Research on users of signed language is not new, yet there exist many questions about atypicality with respect to production and comprehension of signed language – for children and adults. This collection brings together work on various aspects of signed language, and it considers various profiles of a signed language user: deaf and/or hard of hearing, hearing, childhood, adolescent, adult, geriatric, cognitively intact and impaired, and motorically typical and impaired. The work that is represented in this book spans multiple research labs (including various countries and signed languages), and it approaches language and communication from a variety of theoretical frameworks. Yet, the various works are united by a central theme of aiming to understand the language and development of signed language users throughout their lifespan, whereby gaining a wealth of knowledge about signed language structure, processing, acquisition, and use by bilinguals.

The book is divided into several parts, which contain writings by established researchers in their fields and junior investigators who are breaking ground in areas of inquiry that have received little attention over the years. Part 1 covers developmental language disorders and Part 2 addresses fluency disorders, neurogenics and acquired communication disorders. Both of these first parts focus on deaf and hard of hearing users of signed language. As a complement to the first two parts of the book, Part 3 presents the case of hearing children who are raised in signing households. Together, the three parts cover much ground with respect to common populations of signed language users throughout the world.

The book is both multilingual from the points of view of covering different signed languages and also recognizing that signed language users are typically bilingual. Data from different signed languages (American Sign Language, British Sign Language, Sign Language of the Netherlands) are presented, and various works highlight the bilingual nature of signed language users – whether one is referring to sign–speech bilingualism or sign–print bilingualism.

Many people have contributed to making this book possible, and I wish to express my gratitude. The National Science Foundation Science of Learning Center based at Gallaudet University, Visual Language and Visual Learning (VL2), has supported some of my own work on the topic of atypical sign language acquisition (Grant # SBE-0541953), and this has influenced the creation of this book greatly. The chapter authors and their research programs are of the utmost importance, and I thank them for their drive to learn more about their areas of inquiry. The book has also benefited from rigorous reviews that were undertaken by various experts in their respective fields. Among the reviewers are the following: Jo Atkinson (University College London), Courtney Byrd (University of Texas at Austin), Brent Gregg (University of Central Arkansas), Mary Pat Moeller (Boystown National Teaching Hospital), Thomas Marquardt (University of Texas at Austin), Ronice Müller de Quadros (Universidade Federal de Santa Catarina), Jenny Singleton (Georgia Institute of Technology), Bencie Woll (University College, London), and others who have chosen to remain anonymous. I would also like to express my gratitude to Larry Leonard for his willingness to review the manuscript draft and provide a Foreword for the book. I also thank the series editors (Nicole Müller and Martin Ball) for envisioning such a volume within a larger series on multilingual communication disorders and the Multilingual Matters staff who have worked through the production process with me. Manuel, my partner, has provided much encouragement throughout the process of working on this book, and I thank him for his undying support. I am also indebted to my Deaf friends and colleagues for sharing their beautiful and complex signed languages with me and for allowing me to investigate various aspects of those languages. I appreciate professionals at schools for the deaf, parents of deaf children, and signing deaf children who have participated in studies with the goal of advancing research in this area. My hope is that this book will contribute to the work that needs to be done.

David Quinto-Pozos
Austin, TX, USA

1   Considering Communication Disorders and Differences in the Signed Language Modality

David Quinto-Pozos

Introduction

Over five decades of inquiry into signed languages have allowed language and communication researchers to expand what is known about structural variation and human language, patterns of language learning, and the cognitive processing of language by children and adults. Surprisingly, comparatively little work during this same period has focused on signed language communication disorders even though there are likely thousands of signed language users (including school-aged children[1]) throughout the world who possess some type of signed language deficit. Perhaps one reason for the lack of research on this topic lies in a major challenge faced by researchers. Specifically, there is much variation among deaf signers with respect to whether they have language input from models who are fluent in a signed language; this is true both for first exposure and for regular interaction with native or native-like language users. For many deaf children atypicality has been viewed as simply a developmental phase – something that is expected to 'go away' as they get older. Unfortunately, this view has resulted, at least in some cases, in late identification of linguistic and/or cognitive deficits that could have been addressed earlier. This chapter and this volume are intended to serve as a resource for researchers and clinicians on the topic of signed language communication disorders, and on the question of how disorders of visual language might be considered within the contexts of deaf, hard of hearing and hearing individuals who acquire and use a signed language.

Similarities and Differences Across Modalities

A major question within this area of inquiry is the following: how are signed language communication disorders similar to or different from spoken language communication disorders? Recent writings have also addressed this question (Woll, 2012; Woll & Morgan, 2012). Presumably, we should expect multiple parallels across disorders of signed and spoken languages because of similarities between signed and spoken language structures and between the ways in which both types of languages are acquired by children. However, we might also expect characteristics of each modality to influence the types of communication disorders that appear in signers and speakers; some possible areas of consideration include the linguistic signal, the articulators used for language, and the articulator space. See Table 1.1 for a summary of the comparisons. In this section, sign and speech are compared in order to provide the researcher, the student and the practitioner with a way to consider possibilities for communication disorders in signed languages.

Table 1.1 Similarities and differences between signed and spoken languages

Similarities	Differences
• both possess multiple levels of structure	• signs articulated slower than spoken words
• both possess sub-lexical structure	• potentially more information in visual signal at any point in time
• both demonstrate hemispheric lateralization for language	• larger (paired) primary articulators and articulator space in sign
• both are affected by degradation of tissue in cases of dementia, aphasia and brain insult	• manipulable articulators in sign, not in speech
• both demonstrate similar L1 acquisition milestones for native users	• only partial visual feedback for signer compared with full auditory feedback for speaker
	• signing space used grammatically and topographically
	• partitioned lexicon in sign (core signs, fingerspelling-influenced signs, classifiers), less so in spoken languages
	• comparatively more iconicity in sign

Similarities

Signed languages are natural languages that are structurally similar to spoken languages

For decades, research has shown that signed languages are natural languages that can be described with reference to levels of structure that characterize spoken language such as phonology, morphology, syntax and semantics/pragmatics (see, for example, Brentari, 2012; Emmorey, 2002; Johnston & Schembri, 2007; Klima & Bellugi, 1979; Sandler & Lillo-Martin, 2006; Woll & Sutton-Spence, 1999). For example, lexical signs can be broken down into multiple phonological units with handshape, place of articulation, movement and palm orientation values specifying how a sign is to be articulated.[2] Linguistic descriptions of signed minimal pairs and performance-based slips of the hand (i.e. errors where target phonological features of a sign are incorrectly produced) provide evidence for the sublexical structure of sign (Hohenberger *et al.*, 2002; Klima & Bellugi, 1979). Many authors have suggested that the movement of a sign is a key feature of signed syllables, although there is less agreement about the internal structure of the signed syllable (see Emmorey, 2007; Jantunen & Takkinen, 2010; Wilbur & Allen, 1991; Wilbur & Petersen, 1997). Consistent with the sublexical structure of signs, phonological disorders (e.g. Broomfield & Dodd, 2001) may appear in certain signers, with characteristic errors in one or more phonological values within signs (also see Corina, 1998 for paraphasias in adult aphasics). One report of children's deficits with signed phonological structure appears in Quinto-Pozos *et al.* (2011), in which second-hand accounts of deaf children who struggle with movement, place of articulation and palm orientation of signs are described.[3] For that study, the authors interviewed professionals at bilingual (ASL–English) schools for the Deaf about their experiences with native signing deaf children who appear to be struggling with the acquisition of American Sign Language (ASL).

Evidence of struggles with aspects of signed language phonology can be found in the language production of children who have been diagnosed with autism spectrum disorder (ASD). In the current volume, Shield and Meier describe incorrect palm orientation or movement values that are produced by deaf children with ASD. For example, rather than fingerspelling with the palm facing toward an interlocutor, they sometimes have their hand turned toward themselves. This type of error is apparently unattested in typically developing children over the age of 18 months of age. The authors argue that the palm orientation errors during sign production are evidence of impaired perspective-taking abilities for the ASD children. A learner of a signed language must attend to orientation of the palm (i.e. the direction in which the palm is facing) in order to correctly produce a sign, since signs look rather different to the addressee than they do to the signer. Since perspective taking is typically challenging for children with ASD (hearing or deaf), children who are acquiring a signed language may show effects within their linguistic development. The signing space and perspective taking are discussed in more detail in the next section. Shield and Meier also provide an extensive review of pertinent literature on ASD and provide other examples and suggestions of the types of language impairments that might be expected in deaf children who have been diagnosed with ASD. Their work represents some of the first writings on this topic (see also Denmark, 2011; Shield & Meier, 2012).

Neurological evidence for similarities across modalities

Research on brain structures that are crucial for language comprehension and production also suggests that we might expect some similar neurogenic disorders across modalities. There exists much evidence for adult disorders of signed language in the form of case studies of deaf stroke patients who were fluent in signed language before a cerebral insult (American Sign Language: Emmorey et al., 1995; Hickok et al., 1996; Loew et al., 1997; Poizner et al., 1987; British Sign Language: Marshall et al., 2004). These aphasia studies indicate that brain structures commonly used by spoken language are similar to those used by signed language (also see Tyrone, this volume, for additional discussion). As would be expected, signers with damage to left hemisphere networks (in particular the inferior frontal cortex and the temporal lobes) have difficulty with comprehension and/or production of sign, whereas signers who experience damage to the right hemisphere do not have the same language problems.

Neuroimaging studies have also provided evidence for the important role of the right hemisphere in signed language communication. Although some researchers have found no differences between signers and speakers with respect to lateralization of language across modalities (e.g. MacSweeney et al., 2002), others have suggested that there is a greater involvement of the right hemisphere for sign over speech (Neville et al., 1998; Newman et al., 2002).[4] With respect to production, signed language *classifiers* have been shown to recruit the use of the right hemisphere.[5] In particular, the placement and movement of classifier constructions have been shown to engage bilateral networks (Emmorey et al., 2005, 2013), and some studies even suggest that classifiers and lexical signs engage different hemispheres during production (Hickok et al., 2009). The use of right hemisphere networks for aspects of signed language production and comprehension supports the premise that the right hemisphere can play a key role in some aspects of language, although there are also many similarities across modalities with respect to the networks that are engaged.

The degradation of brain tissue and function that results in dementia (for example as an accompaniment to Parkinson's or Alzheimer's diseases) can also be the source of atypical or impaired signed language abilities. An early report describing patterns of signing in Parkinson's patients appears in Kegl and Poizner (1998); the authors also analyze the techniques that are used by interlocutors to compensate for the Parkinson's patient's lack of appropriate attention during signing and less-than-clear articulation (i.e. maximization of distinction in linguistic contrasts by the interlocutors). In a recent study, Falchook et al. (2012) described the case of a deaf individual with Alzheimer's disease and her challenges with the production and comprehension of finger-spelling and grammatically complex sentences. The signer was also reported to exhibit impaired episodic memory, signs of anomia, an ideomotor apraxia and characteristics of a visual-spatial dysfunction. Cases such as these have provided evidence that dementia affects signed language abilities in deaf signers, as would be expected.

Additional cases of dementia and its effect on signed language use are described in the chapter in the present volume from Spanjer, Fieret and Baker. These authors describe various types of atypical language production that are evident in data from four older deaf users of Sign Language of the Netherlands (NGT) who are suffering from symptoms of dementia. In particular, they identify language problems that tend also to plague hearing users of spoken language with dementia, such as word finding difficulties, grammatical errors and inappropriate (i.e. pragmatically odd) responses. Additionally, they carefully consider the bilingual status of those patients (NGT and Dutch) and why that aspect of language learning must be considered when addressing the linguistic abilities of deaf patients with dementia. The work of Spanjer and colleagues is particularly important because it considers the language and communication abilities of multiple signers and also considers the data from a bilingual perspective.

Similarities concerning childhood acquisition of language

Signed languages are acquired by native-signing deaf children following a timeline that largely parallels the acquisition of spoken language by hearing children (Baker & Woll, 2008; Bonvillian *et al.*, 1983; Newport & Meier, 1985; Petitto, 1987). Because of similarities in acquisition across the two modalities, we might also expect children to exhibit developmental signed language disorders paralleling at least some of those that have been identified and studied for spoken language. Symptoms of those disorders might be language delay, language processing deficits and issues concerning language and memory (see Schwartz, 2009 for an overview of child spoken-language disorders). Additionally, we might expect to find cases of specific language impairment (SLI) in children acquiring a signed language (e.g. see Mason *et al.*, 2010; Morgan *et al.*, 2006; Quinto-Pozos *et al.*, in preparation), since SLI is a disorder of language comprehension and/or production that manifests in otherwise typically developing children (Leonard, 1998).

A chapter in this volume on deaf children acquiring British Sign Language (BSL) provides evidence for SLI in deaf signing children. The collective work of Herman and colleagues is notable because it represents the first set of in-depth studies that have considered communication disorders in signed languages. In their chapter for this volume, Herman, Rowley, Marshall, Mason, Atkinson, Woll and Morgan describe the main components of their several-years study of atypically developing deaf children in the United Kingdom. They detail a survey methodology that they have used for the identification of atypically developing children and they describe the tests of BSL comprehension and production that they administered. An overall claim from multiple studies conducted by members of that team is that signed language disorders are to be expected in a fraction of the population matching the proportion of children expected to have SLI in the acquisition of English, or approximately 7% of deaf children (Herman *et al.*, this volume; Mason *et al.*, 2010). The sign disorders resemble delays in language acquisition rather than idiosyncratic examples of language production, not unlike hearing children's spoken language disorders. Without a doubt, the BSL researchers have been pioneers in this area of developmental research on communication disorder in sign.

Differences

One might also expect a subset of signed language disorders to differ from spoken language disorders because of key differences between sign and speech. The modalities differ with respect to the signal in which language is encoded (e.g. auditory versus visual) and with respect to the articulators and articulatory space used for producing and comprehending language. There are also linguistic features of signed languages that might result in unique characteristics of at least some signed language disorders. In particular, it could be argued that signed languages appear different from spoken language with respect to characteristics of vocabulary items and how those items may be structured in the mental lexicon. The consideration of vocabulary items and related grammatical processes (e.g. a verb sign and its manner of inflecting for person and number) requires a discussion of iconicity and gestural resources and how those features of communication might influence signed language structures.

Differences in the linguistic/communicative signals

Since signed languages are typically perceived by the eyes rather than the ears (except in the case of tactually produced and perceived signed language, which is used by many individuals who are deaf and blind; see Quinto-Pozos, 2002), it may be useful to highlight a few key differences between the auditory and visual signals. Light travels much faster than sound does, and the speed of light at small distances appears instantaneous to humans (see Brentari, 2002 for a discussion). Meier (2002) points out that for sign, the source of the signal (i.e. light) is external to the signer, whereas for speech the sound is generated within the speaker (also see Tyrone, 2007 for a discussion).[6] Meier also suggests that the visual signal has the capacity to capture a greater amount of information than the auditory signal can relay within the speech stream. This phenomenon can be exemplified by appealing to the concept of bandwidth as it applies to auditory versus video recordings; a 60-second audio file requires much less memory for storage than a 60-second video file does. It has been suggested that bandwidth differences could support an advantage in vision for vertical processing (i.e. processing simultaneously occurring information), but not in horizontal processing (i.e. sequential information) across time (Brentari, 2002; Emmorey, 2007).

One question to consider is how characteristics of the signal might influence the ways in which language is processed. Presumably, the processing of sequential information is of particular importance for spoken language because sounds are strung together to form words, and multiple words are arranged in sequence to create a sentence. The importance of sequence has been captured within theories of perceptual processing and language impairment. For example, the Auditory Processing Deficit (APD) hypothesis has been suggested to account for language deficits of hearing children (see Tallal & Benasich, 2002 for a review). The APD hypothesis claims that the speed at which phonetic elements in the speech signal must be processed is too rapid for children who struggle with temporal processing; this causes a notable percentage of otherwise typically developing children to exhibit developmental language impairment. Tallal's approach reflects the premise that children with language disorder can be characterized by a general slowing of processing vis-à-vis typically developing children (Tallal & Benasich, 2002). Whether the temporal characteristics of the visual signal could result in processing difficulties that are specific to signed languages is unclear.

The processing of sequential information is requisite in sign, as in the processing of phonological sequences in signs (e.g. handshape or place of articulation changes) or syntax. However, the processing of simultaneous information is equally important for signed language because of the typical linguistic structures of visual-gestural language. In sign, the synchronous use of manual and non-manual articulators allows for the creation of multiple simultaneously produced morphemes with information appearing on the hands and face; sometimes movement of the torso and body are also significant. For example, a lexical verb in ASL such as DRIVE is produced with the hands, modification of the verb with quickly repeating path movements adds a simultaneously articulated aspectual morpheme, and an additional adverbial modifier is communicated by postures of the lips and mouth area that encode information about the manner (e.g. carefully, haphazardly, etc.) in which the driving was conducted. Thus, linguistic and emotive facial expressions – in addition to manual articulations – are part of the signal to be deciphered by a viewer of sign. There is clearly much occurring simultaneously in sign. Spoken languages also allow for multiple simultaneously produced morphemes (e.g. a lexical item produced with grammatical tone), although spoken languages generally prefer concatenative morphology, with strings of affixes being the typical realization of morphological processes (Fernald & Napoli, 2000; Aronoff et al., 2005).

The perception and processing of multiple layers of signed information simultaneously has been described in terms of parallel or vertical processing (Brentari, 2002; Emmorey, 2007), and this difference in comparison to spoken language is notable. Interestingly, the results of psycholinguistic experiments that employ gating tasks to examine sign recognition have shown that signs are identified more quickly than spoken words are (Emmorey & Corina, 1990;

Grosjean, 1981), and handshape, place of articulation and palm orientation are identified at the same time, whereas movement information is available later (see Emmorey, 2007 for a discussion of this two-stage process of sign identification). In addition, research on tip-of-tongue states (i.e. when a speaker or signer is having difficulty retrieving a word form even though they feel confident that they know the word) shows that the amount of phonological information that is retrieved simultaneously by signers is significant: signers are often able to remember up to three of the phonological features (e.g. handshape, place of articulation, palm orientation) of a sign, even though the sign itself could not be remembered (Thompson *et al.*, 2005). These studies add support for the hypothesis that vertical processing is a psychologically valid concept. Whether or not the processing of multiple simultaneously produced meaning units has an effect on children who are at risk for a developmental language disorder is an important question for researchers interested in signed language communication disorder. A main question to consider is whether some deaf signers might have difficulties managing the simultaneous processing that is required for comprehending and remembering important aspects of the visual signal.

One aspect of signed languages is notable for its sequential structure, and it provides evidence that horizontal processing is also important in signed language. *Fingerspelling* can be described as the manual production of letters of a written language alphabet. In ASL, the fingerspelling of English words constitutes approximately 5–20% of the lexical items in various types of language use (Morford & MacFarlane, 2003; Padden & Gunsauls, 2003); this includes the use of fingerspelling for proper nouns, for words that do not have single signs as equivalents, and for discourse-related purposes. There are also instances when fingerspelling is used in spite of the existence of a semantically similar sign, although some commonly fingerspelled items undergo linguistic processes that allow them to resemble signs phonologically (Battison, 1978; Brentari & Padden, 2001; Cormier *et al.*, 2008). Fingerspelling is articulated quickly in comparison to lexical signs. Fingerspelling rate generally ranges between three and eight letters per second, or approximately 125–250 ms per letter (see Quinto-Pozos, 2010; Zakia & Haber, 1971). This speed is comparable to ranges of syllable rate in spoken languages (see Dolata *et al.*, 2008; Verhoeven *et al.*, 2004), although not to common speaking rates of individual phonemes of words. Wilbur and Nolan (1986) suggest that syllable rates in ASL and English are comparable. Because of these rate characteristics of fingerspelling, it appears to be notably different from lexical signs, which raises the possibility that it may be processed in unique ways. The processing of fingerspelling also requires bilingual skills since fingerspelling represents the spelling of words from the ambient spoken/written language. Bilingualism is discussed later in this chapter.

Work on visual and auditory memory suggests that differences in the signal across modalities influence short-term memory performance. With respect to sequential memory tasks, it has been shown that fewer sequentially viewed elements in the visual signal (digits or letters) are typically remembered when compared to sequences of elements that are perceived and processed via audition: on average, approximately five sequential elements for sign versus seven for speech (Boutla *et al.*, 2004; Emmorey & Wilson, 2004; Wilson *et al.*, 1997). This generalization holds true whether digits or phonologically balanced letters are considered (Bavelier *et al.*, 2006). Importantly, the cause of the difference is not the ability to hear, but rather lies in constraints of visual sequential memory. Hearing bilinguals who are native users of both English and ASL perform differentially based on the modality in which they are tested (Boutla *et al.*, 2004). Emmorey (2007), in appealing to Baddeley (1986) and his model of working memory, suggests that memory capacity in sign may be limited by articulation rate. Presumably, this is because signs are, on average, longer in duration than words and therefore may occupy relatively more space in working memory.[7] Short-term memory differences across the modalities could presumably contribute to language disorders in different ways in spoken versus signed languages. At the very least, these differences should be considered since memory deficits have been implicated in many studies as a main factor in childhood language disorders (see Schwartz, 2010 for a review).

Another notable difference between sign and speech regards the extent to which the communicative signal produced by the sender is available to that person through sensory feedback (also see Tyrone, this volume). In speech, auditory feedback allows for a speaker to attend to their output and revise their language production appropriately. In sign, the language user often visually perceives her hands only peripherally, with some signs being largely out of the limits of vision (e.g. the ASL sign HORSE articulated with thumb contact on the temple), although the manual articulators do become a focus of attention in some cases (e.g. in classifier signs and for purposeful focus on a sign's articulation).[8] It has been suggested that signers do not use visual feedback as a comprehension-based monitor, but rather as a guide to help modulate how much of the signing space they are using for articulation (Emmorey *et al.*, 2009). In addition to visual or auditory feedback, both signers and speakers do typically possess kinesthetic feedback from the articulators, and it may be the case that such feedback – along with tactile feedback involving the manual articulators – takes on a more important role in signing when visual feedback is limited.

Signal feedback is an important topic for communication disorders. As one example of this importance, auditory feedback during speech production has been suggested as a contributing factor in fluency disorders (e.g. stuttering) of speech (Civier *et al.*, 2010; Marist & Hutton, 1957; Neilson & Neilson, 1987; Nudelman *et al.*, 1989). The argument is that a speaker exhibits more disfluencies when she is receiving auditory feedback than when she is not. In light of this work, it would be very useful to explore signed language fluency, with a focus on stuttering in signed language. It could be argued that the difference in visual feedback for sign might mitigate the prevalence of stuttering disfluencies in the visual-gestural modality.[9]

In the present volume, Whitebread discusses so-called stuttering in signed language. In doing so, he reviews past studies on the topic and discusses the rates of prevalence of stuttering that have been reported for deaf and hard of hearing school-aged children. By comparing the reported rates of stuttering in the deaf populations to prevalence and incidence rates for hearing children who use spoken language, Whitebread is able to highlight the importance of considering signed stuttering for theories of spoken language disfluencies that highlight auditory feedback. The author also provides a summary of the characteristics of signed stuttering that have been reported in older studies versus those that are commonly used to categorize types of spoken language disfluencies. In concert with other writings in this volume, Whitebread also considers the role of bilingualism, or the (occasional) use of speech by deaf signers, and its possible effect on sign disfluencies. This chapter synthesizes information about fluency in sign with a focus on stuttering that has not been presented elsewhere.

Differences in the articulators and the spaces they traverse

It is clear that there are differences in the articulators between languages across modalities (see Meier, 2002 and Tyrone, this volume, for additional comparisons), and these differences could have an effect on some of the language and communication disorders that arise within each modality. Signed languages capitalize on the use of two comparably large manual articulators (i.e. the hands) that exhibit a series of visible movements and static postures in the articulatory space during the production of signs. As noted in the previous section, the manual articulators are complemented – sometimes obligatorily – by multiple non-manual articulators (e.g. the torso, head, eyegaze and facial features) for meaning creation. The articulators are not only visible in sign, they are manipulable; another person can help the signer position the hands and fingers to approximate a target form, which is potentially very useful for assisting the signer when intervention is needed (see Quinto-Pozos et al., 2010 for discussions of so called 'signed language therapy'). Spoken languages, on the other hand, utilize comparably smaller articulators (i.e. the tongue, lips, glottis – along with movement of the mandible) for the production of speech, some of which are not visible (or only partially visible) to the perceiver of language. The articulators of speech are not manipulable by another person as they are in sign. In the case of speech, the mandible has been claimed to serve as the basis for oscillatory movements that, with the articulation of consonant and vowel segments, create syllables in spoken languages (MacNeilage, 1998). In spite of the fact that several researchers argue for the existence of syllables in signed language (as noted earlier), there is little evidence for internal structure to those syllables (see Emmorey, 2007, although see Jantunen & Takkinen, 2010). The lack of a clear internal structure for a signed syllable may be a function of signed languages not having a primary dominant oscillator (like the mandible in speech) for the articulation of movement. The extent to which the parsing of the speech stream differs from the parsing of the sign stream because of these fundamental differences in the signal has not been the focus of inquiry, although it might be useful for discussions of signed language communication disorders.

The use of hands for articulators could be a topic of inquiry for researchers who work on language fluency, the patterns of deficits that typically affect one's ability to articulate phonemes and phonological patterns effectively, and the intervention strategies that are employed by clinicians. As one example, it would be useful to examine limb apraxia to determine if childhood apraxia of speech (a difficulty in making the movements for speech) would have a parallel in the signed modality. Interestingly, signed language is sometimes used in interventions with hearing children who have apraxia of speech.

One of the chapters in the present volume focuses on sign production and neural pathologies that might have an effect on the articulation of signs. In particular, Tyrone reviews studies of sign production in ASL and BSL with a focus on various motor disorders including limb apraxia, Parkinson's disease, cerebellar ataxia and progressive supranuclear palsy. She proposes that examples of *sign dysarthria*, such as deficits in articulatory coordination, can be found in sign – just as in speech – because of the coordinated and complex movements that are involved in the production of signs. In addition, Tyrone suggests that different movement disorders appear to disrupt sign production in different ways, and those disorders can be dissociated from linguistic disorders that affect movement in a sign. Her conclusion based on the literature is that, broadly speaking, motor disorders have similar effects on the production of signed and spoken language. Her writings provide an important link between discussions of motor abilities and motor impairments across linguistic modalities.

With respect to articulator space, there are clear differences across communication modalities. The articulators of speech are bounded by a comparably smaller articulatory space (i.e. the oral cavity) than that which is used by signed language articulators. The *signing space* has been described as '... a highly restricted space defined by the top of the head, the waist and the reach of the arms from side to side (with elbows bent)' (Klima & Bellugi, 1979: 51). A common argument is that it requires more time for the hands to traverse the articulatory space during the production of a sign than it does for the tongue to move around in the much smaller oral cavity. This difference could account for data that suggest that ASL requires, on average, approximately twice the length of time to articulate a sign than that which is typically needed to utter a spoken English word (Bellugi & Fischer, 1972; Klima & Bellugi, 1979).[10] This may also be true of other signed languages, although it is not clear if some typologically distinct spoken languages (e.g. polysynthetic languages with long words that contain multiple morphemes) would be more similar to a signed language in this aspect of timing. As one example, Hwang (2011) has shown that Korean, an agglutinative language, can be characterized as being closer to ASL in its rate of production of words, yet it is less similar when considering syllable or morpheme rates. In spite of the word-versus-sign difference, it has been reported that a measure of propositions per second (i.e. meaningful sentences) in ASL is similar to similar propositions in English. In could be the case that these motoric differences in the rate of movement of articulators might result in at least some different instantiations of communication disorder across modalities, although more research is needed in this area of inquiry.

Many researchers suggest that the signing space is multifunctional, and it is regularly used to indicate grammatical distinctions, location information for entities, and the depictive bodily actions of a signer. In some cases, the various uses overlap. It is clear that the signing space functions differently from how the oral cavity does. This raises the question of whether aspects of these functions could lead to differences across modalities with respect to language and communication disorders. A brief review of some writings about the signing space follows.

Various authors have suggested that the *signing space* can be considered to function in multiple ways (e.g. see Emmorey, 2002; Perniss, 2012). *Shared space* is the use of the signing space in ways that take advantage of the immediate environment (e.g. the signer will point to a dog located at its side to refer to that particular dog). *Abstract space* (also known as *grammatical* space) has been described as utilizing loci in the signing space to establish – via manual pointing, eyegaze, or direction of movement/placement of a sign – locations for referents that serve syntactic functions (e.g. pronouns, subjects or objects in a sentence, etc.). *Topographic space* refers to the use of locations in the signing space to create a map-like depiction of a scene. The signer is using space topographically when she employs *classifiers* to indicate the location, orientation and movement of objects with respect to one another. Finally, *viewer space* is the use of the signing space in a full-scale representation of characters interacting with other characters and the environment. Additionally, a signer can engage topographic space and viewer space simultaneously (e.g. by manually articulating a person classifier while also shifting one's posture and facial expression to portray aspects of a character), which is a complex skill that requires years of development for proper management (Dudis, 2004; Emmorey & Reilly, 1998; Morgan, 2002). Even though spoken language does not engage the articulatory space (i.e. the oral cavity) in the same ways as signed language capitalizes on the space in front of a signer's body, co-speech gestures can be readily compared with a signer's use of topographic space and viewer space (Cormier *et al.*, 2012; Quinto-Pozos & Parrill, submitted).

From a neurological point of view, it is useful to consider how comprehension and production might provide insights about the linguistic processing of the signing space. Neurological evidence for a multi-faceted signing space first appeared in studies of deaf signing aphasics, which were mentioned earlier. Poizner *et al.* (1987) showed that adult signers who suffered strokes to the right hemisphere also possessed deficits in spatial skills that affected their communication. They argued for a dissociation between syntactic and topographical spatial skills (also see Emmorey *et al.*, 1995; Hickok *et al.*, 1996), and provided evidence for a dissociation of aspects of viewer space from grammatical space (Loew *et al.*, 1997). Generally, the stroke patients in those studies performed similarly to normal controls on grammatical (i.e. syntactic) use of space; however, they exhibited significant difficulties with topographical uses of the signing space. The patients also performed poorly on non-linguistic tests requiring spatial skills. Studies of normal signers (i.e. non-aphasics) have also shown that the processing of space has some unique properties (e.g. see Capek *et al.*, 2009).

It could be the case that a deficit in visual-spatial skills could cause an otherwise typically developing child to struggle with aspects of signed language that require certain functions of the signing space.[11] For example, if a child fares poorly on tasks such as remembering the location and orientation of objects, then that child might struggle with classifier comprehension and production. The same child might be challenged when giving directions or explaining where something is located. Quinto-Pozos *et al.* (in press) report such a case in their description of a native signing deaf adolescent who struggled with the comprehension and production of topographic and viewer space, but not other aspects of ASL grammar. That child scored in the impaired range on various tests of visual-spatial skills, but she also performed within the average range on a general measure of ASL comprehension and production.

Various types of atypical development could also have an influence on how a child is able to engage visual-spatial skills during the process of language acquisition. As noted in the chapter by Shield and Meier (this volume), deaf children with autism often struggle to produce the correct phonological value for palm orientation for some signs, as the signer must perform a perspective-shift (180°) in order to be able to articulate those signs correctly. It has also been shown that signers who are not exposed to a fully-fledged sign language in their youth do not develop visual-spatial cognition as robustly as those who are exposed to a sign language early (Pyers *et al.*, 2010). Interestingly, non-linguistic visual tasks have also been shown to be difficult for hearing children with language impairment (Windsor *et al.*, 2008). It would be useful to consider possible similarities between visual-spatial skills and language acquisition across signed and spoken language.

A deaf adult signer who struggles with visual processing of the signing space would be particularly unexpected because it has also been shown that normal adult native signers of ASL possess *enhanced* visual-spatial skills – presumably due to their experience with a signed language (Emmorey & Kosslyn, 1996; Emmorey *et al.*, 1993, 1998; Masataka, 1995; McKee, 1987;

Talbot & Haude, 1993, Wilson *et al.*, 1997), and there is some evidence that deaf children also possess enhanced visual-spatial skills (Bellugi *et al.*, 1990). Because of the enhanced visual-spatial skills, it may be difficult to identify impairment in this aspect of language and communication for adult deaf signers.

Differences in vocabulary inventories and grammatical structures

Signed languages, like spoken languages, possess words (i.e. signs) and grammars that govern the way the words are modulated and sequenced with respect to one another. However, it could also be argued that there are notable differences across modalities. Both types of languages contain content words (e.g. nouns and verbs) and function words (e.g. conjunctions, prepositions) although various function words (e.g. prepositions, articles, copula verbs, etc.) appear comparatively less frequently in signed languages. Signers also capitalize on the use of classifier signs for various types of descriptions, which are highly productive and are used regularly within some genres of language use, such as narratives. Signed languages allow for modifications of signs in visually iconic ways for the creation of specific meanings (Klima & Bellugi, 1979), and iconicity figures prominently in the sign modality (Perniss *et al.*, 2010). These characteristics of signed languages should be considered since they might influence the types of deficits that occur for children who struggle with word learning, word modification (e.g. inflectional morphology) and remembering a diverse set of words.

One model of the structure of the signed language lexicon divides lexical items into native and foreign items, the latter exhibiting influence from English via fingerspelling (Brentari & Padden, 2001; Padden, 1998).[12] Vocabulary items that have been influenced by English (via fingerspelling or the use of a handshape that represents a fingerspelled letter) can violate standards of phonological well-formedness characteristic of the native vocabulary.

Another characteristic of the signed language lexicon, according to Brentari and Padden, is that the native lexicon can be divided into core and non-core portions; the core includes signs that are highly stable and standardized in form and meaning, and used frequently in the language, whereas the latter includes classifier signs. Some authors have also suggested that the non-core is heavily influenced by gesture (Cormier *et al.*, 2012). The existence of a partitioned lexicon could have implications for how children acquire a signed language vocabulary and reach milestones of vocabulary development as they develop.[13] With respect to signed languages, it may be that children could show deficits in the development of one aspect of the vocabulary (e.g. the case of a visual-spatial deficit and its effect on the use of topographic space and classifiers), but not in others (e.g. the use of visually iconic nouns).

One feature of signed languages that is particularly prominent is visual iconicity (see Taub, 2001). In Taub's terms, one type of iconicity can be described as 'the shapes of the articulators themselves and using them to encode images of similar shapes' (Taub, 2001: 68). For example, the ASL sign TREE depicts a tree trunk and its branches via the arm and fingers of the hand, respectively. In spoken language, sound-based iconicity appears in onomatopoetic words, although signed languages possess more iconic devices than spoken languages (see Perniss *et al.*, 2010 for a review of iconicity in signed and spoken language).

The literature is mixed with regard to whether there exists a facilitative effect of iconicity with respect to vocabulary learning. Various reports suggest that young deaf children do not use iconicity as a tool for learning signs more quickly (Miller, 1987), for conjugating verb forms appropriately (Meier, 1987), or for learning the form-to-meaning mappings in their language more quickly (Morgan *et al.*, 2008). Iconicity of target forms has been reported not to support more accurate children's productions (Meier *et al.*, 2008). In addition, adults do not appear to use iconicity as a differential way of processing in a semantic priming task (Bosworth & Emmorey, 2010). However, other studies have shown that iconicity can have a facilitative effect. For example, iconicity could contribute to performance on tests administered in sign language (Markham & Justice, 2004), iconicity makes it easier for deaf children to learn new signs (Thompson *et al.*, 2012), iconicity can assist with processing for deaf children (Ormel *et al.*, 2009), and adult L2 learners capitalize on iconicity to remember signs that have been learned (Lieberth & Belille Gamble, 1991). Without a doubt, iconicity is a prevalent feature of signed languages, and the degree to which it influences the way such languages are learned and processed – especially later in development when children can make connections between iconic linguistic forms and the real-word objects and concepts that they symbolize – is worth considering, especially within the larger topic of communication disorder.

Summary of similarities and differences

This section has highlighted some of the similarities and differences between signed and spoken languages in order to allow for the consideration of communication disorders across the two modalities and where different disorders might be predicted to appear in sign. Multiple similarities exist between sign and speech, and evidence has been provided for some similar types of communication disorder in sign, in spite of the differences in the linguistic signal, the articulation of signed languages and the ways in which visual-gestural languages are structured in terms of mental vocabularies. However, differences across modalities are important to consider because they force us to investigate whether signed language communication disorders could reveal unique aspects of processing and memory that are associated with visual-gestural space. More specifically, visual perception and processing and the manual articulation of signs or the production of non-manual-signals – especially those articulations that use the signing space in complex ways – provide good test cases for spoken language theories of communication disorder.

Users of Signed Languages as Default Bilinguals

An important consideration for the investigation of signed communication disorders is that users of signed languages are commonly bilingual or multilingual (Grosjean, 2010), and this raises various questions with respect to the interaction between languages and the overall linguistic development of an individual. This is true whether someone is a hearing child of deaf adults (i.e. a *coda* or *koda;* kid of deaf adults), or a deaf/hard of hearing child. Deaf people are typically exposed to the ambient written language of their region, and in the case of deaf children this often occurs with their early educational experiences. In cases in which a deaf individual possesses sufficient residual hearing or uses an augmentative hearing device to perceive the speech stream (e.g. hearing aid, cochlear implant, etc.), exposure to a spoken language constitutes a part of their linguistic experience. One other important point that has yet to be made is that there is also a visual signal connected with speech (i.e. speechreading), and deaf individuals are exposed to speakers' mouth, lip and jaw movements during their production of speech. The extent to which these visual cues contribute to childhood language acquisition and/or adult learning is, unfortunately, an area that has received very little attention in the developmental literature (see McQuarrie & Parrila, 2009).

Many deaf adults and children are exposed to more than two languages. For example, a growing number of deaf children in the United States are exposed regularly to two different spoken languages (e.g. Spanish in the home and English at school), a signed language (e.g. ASL), and one or two written languages (English and possibly Spanish). Gallaudet Research Institute (GRI) data from 2010 report that 11.4% (or 4409) of deaf and hearing-impaired children throughout the US were raised, at least in part, in homes in which Spanish is the spoken/written language of the home, and that 9.4% (or 3533) came from homes in which multiple languages were used. It is likely that some of the children in the latter category were also receiving Spanish input at home along with input from other languages. In all of these cases it is clear that deaf individuals are not like monolinguals who are exposed primarily to one language via speech and writing.

Multiple questions arise when considering the bilingual status of deaf individuals as it concerns disorders of language and communication, and there is a growing literature on disorders within bilingual speaking communities that can provide guides for how to consider bilingual communities and provide language services for these populations (e.g. see Bedore & Peña, 2008; Kohnert, 2010; Sheng *et al.*, 2012). In general, such studies suggest that bilingual children are able to successfully acquire two (or more) languages as they develop, but their developmental patterns do not always resemble those of monolinguals, such as in areas of vocabulary development, cognitive control and memory performance. In some areas, they outperform their monolingual peers (e.g. cognitive control), whereas in other aspects of development they appear to lag behind (e.g. aspects of vocabulary; see Bialystok, 2009, for a review). What might deaf children who are acquiring more than one language (simultaneously for some, and sequentially for a small minority who might only receive input in a signed language at home from their Deaf family members) teach us about the acquisition of two (or more) languages in spite of possible communication challenges along the way?

Hearing children who simultaneously acquire a signed and a spoken language

Various researchers have described the bilingual acquisition of hearing children who are exposed to a signed and a spoken language from a very early age (e.g. Baker & van den Bogaerde, this volume; Chen Pichler *et al.*, this volume; Kanto *et al.*, 2013; Morgan, 2005; Petitto *et al.*, 2001; Woll & Morgan, 2012). There are, however, fewer descriptions of linguistic deficits within this bilingual population of hearing signers. In a recent report, Woll and Morgan (2012) provide an account of the English and BSL skills and selected aspects of the cognitive abilities of several hearing English-BSL users: twin females with Down syndrome (exposed to BSL by their Deaf parents), a child who was claimed to be mildly autistic and severely apraxic, and a child with Landau–Kleffner syndrome (LKS) who was exposed to BSL at age 13. In the case of the child with LKS, which is an auditory processing disorder involving phonology, English abilities were determined to be impaired, whereas signed language abilities were spared. Thus, as expected, the impairment of rapid processing did not affect the signed language development of the child. In the other cases reported by the authors, language abilities across modalities were comparable, which suggests that similar areas of linguistic structure and processing are affected for some of these bimodal bilinguals – depending on the etiology of the impairment. Each of these cases is different because of the children's unique profiles and the distinct syndromic conditions. In addition to this report, Morgan (2005) provides a brief description of a hearing child with Deaf parents who appears to exhibit language disorders in both English and BSL. Much can be learned about language acquisition from these bimodal bilinguals who demonstrate atypical development.

Other works have looked primarily at typical development among bimodal bilinguals. A report of children who reach their first linguistic milestones at the same ages as bilingual peers who are acquiring two spoken languages (i.e. *unimodal bilinguals*) can be found in Petitto *et al.* (2001). In that study, Petitto and colleagues show that the bilingual children are particularly sophisticated with respect to knowing which of their two languages they should use when addressing different interlocutors, and the authors also describe the language mixing patterns that characterize the bimodal bilinguals versus the unimodal bilinguals. One notable difference is that the bimodal bilinguals are able to mix languages simultaneously because they can sign and use spoken words at the same time, whereas the unimodal bilinguals exhibit sequential patterns of language mixing.

In the present volume, Baker and van den Bogaerde describe their approach for investigating the linguistic development of hearing children who are acquiring NGT and Dutch. As noted with respect to the Petitto *et al.* (2001) study, one unique aspect of this bimodal bilingualism (i.e. spoken-signed language bilingualism) is that the language user can engage in oral and manual articulations simultaneously. This type of language use allows for analyses that look closely at how the two languages interact throughout a child's development. Baker and van den Bogaerde focus on children's *code-blends*, or examples of utterances containing both signed and spoken language material. Along with their linguistic analyses of these children's productions, the authors also consider the influence of factors such as the form of input offered, family environment and social attitudes. The authors suggest that although there are some differences from other unimodal bilingual children, these bimodal bilingual children can usually be considered to be typically developing bilingual children. This work provides important data from NGT and Dutch about the role of bimodal bilingualism in childhood koda signers.

A second chapter in the present volume also takes up the case of hearing children from signing households, although these children, unlike the Dutch-NGT kodas in the Baker and van den Bogaerde chapter, are exposed to ASL and English. Chen Pichler, Lee and Lillo-Martin examine some of the cross-linguistic influences between the languages, and they consider the roles of quantity and quality of input in their analyses. The authors also provide suggestions for maintenance and continued development of ASL based on practices that were followed at the Hearing and Speech Center (HSC) at Gallaudet University. One of the authors was a speech and language therapist at the HSC, and he was involved in the use of dynamic assessment techniques to evaluate the language skills of these bimodal bilingual children. The assessment techniques were designed to provide as comprehensive a picture as possible of a child's developing bilingual competency, with the goal of distinguishing language *disorder* from language *difference* influenced by ASL–English bilingualism. The authors note that bilingual bimodal children in the US vary widely in their English development, and they display characteristics that may be typical for a developing bimodal bilingual, but not particularly common in a unimodal bilingual child. Such differences constitute important areas to investigate through targeted linguistic research.

The acquisition of literacy as a facet of bilingualism

As noted earlier, the development of deaf signing children not only involves a signed language, but also a written form of an ambient spoken language. The investigation of the learning/acquisition of a written language by deaf children can provide valuable information about bilingual development, but it can also provide insight into language processing and, similarly, language and communication disorder. Various studies suggest that deaf children who struggle with reading tasks are at a disadvantage because of deficits in sound-based phonological awareness, a key component of literacy acquisition according to some researchers (e.g. see Musselman, 2000; Perfetti & Sandak, 2000). However, a meta-analysis of phonological awareness studies has shown that phonological coding and phonological awareness are only a mild to moderate predictor of reading ability for deaf children (Mayberry et al., 2010).

Other writings also suggest that a lack of sound-based phonological awareness of the spoken/written language is not necessarily at the heart of the children's struggles (see Clark et al., 2011; Miller & Clark, 2012; Piñar et al., 2011). Instead, other influences have been suggested as contributing to reading ability in deaf children such as the shallowness/depth of the orthography (Kargin et al., 2012) and deficits with structural (i.e. syntactic) knowledge (Miller et al., 2012). Myers et al. (2010) point out that minority status within the deaf community is also a factor that should also be considered with regard to the acquisition of reading.

There are likely a myriad of factors that contribute to deaf children's acquisition of literacy, although multiple authors have suggested that language ability (in a first language, such as a signed language) is an important one to consider. Accordingly, it has been shown that signed language skills correlate with reading ability (Emmorey & Petrich, 2012; Freel et al., 2011; Hermans et al., 2008; Mayberry et al., 2010). This finding is supported by processing studies that provide evidence for activation of the signed language during reading comprehension (Morford et al., 2011). It is likely that fingerspelling plays an important role in the acquisition of literacy since it can provide a child with a connection between aspects of manual language (e.g. handshapes and movements) and the sequences of letters that form the written word. It has been suggested that deaf children acquire fingerspelling in at least two stages: the first is as a holistic unit that represents the entire word or concept, and the second is the understanding of the individual letters that comprise the written word (Padden, 2006). The recent increase in studies of the role of signed languages in the development of literacy for deaf children is promising because it provides us with valuable data about the effects of bilingualism and how the case of deaf children can be considered in a more holistic fashion (i.e. focus is not only placed on the development of literacy or signed language development, but instead both are considered).

Default bilinguals summary

It is important to remember that those individuals who are exposed to signed language – whether they are deaf or hearing – are default bilinguals, and their language development should ideally be considered within that context. The extent to which spoken language will also play an important role in communication differs from individual to individual, although hearing children who are acquiring sign language undergo development of their spoken language skills, too. Since (signed) language ability has been shown to be an important factor for successful acquisition of reading, presumably a signed language disorder could also play a role in the acquisition of literacy.

Deaf Signers and Multiple Disabilities

In many cases, deaf individuals are also challenged by neurological, physical and cognitive deficits that could have a noticeable impact on aspects of their signed language acquisition, including comprehension and production. These cases are important to consider since they provide additional challenges for the researcher, teacher or clinician who is working with an individual suspected of having a linguistic or cognitive disorder. However, they may also provide an interesting viewpoint from which to consider the acquisition and continued maintenance of communication within the visual-gestural modality.

Deaf children and multiple disabilities

Various writings have indicated that a notable percentage of deaf and hard of hearing children have been diagnosed with a disability other than deafness, with estimates ranging as high as 40% (Guardino, 2008; Knoors & Vervload, 2003; Mitchell & Karchmer, 2006; Moores, 2001; van Dijke et al., 2010). Gallaudet Research Institute (GRI) data from 2010–2011 report nearly 34,000 Deaf and hard of hearing students in pre-K through 12th grade in the United States during that academic year, and of that number, approximately 5.3% were reported as having a developmental delay, 8.0% as exhibiting a learning disability, and 5.4% as being diagnosed with attention deficit disorder (ADD)/attention deficit hyperactivity disorder (ADHD). Several of the diagnosed disabilities could presumably have an impact on the acquisition and development of a signed language.

Some cognitive disabilities can be characterized by atypical *Executive Function* resources (e.g. working memory, attention, etc.), and these struggles would presumably present challenges for the robust acquisition of a signed language (Jones & Jones, 2003; Jones et al., 2006). For example, a child with a diagnosis of ADD/ADHD may have difficulties in focusing and/or maintaining their eyegaze in the direction of the signer, which could result, in theory, in the perception of incomplete messages and less-than-robust language input. Unlike spoken language, the signed language signal cannot be perceived if a viewer is not visually attending to the producer of language. Atypical attention could presumably also affect the development of joint attention, which has been shown to be an important strategy for the acquisition of language and general cognitive development (Lieberman *et al.*, 2011, 2013; Visual Language and Visual Learning Science of Learning Center, 2012).

Autism is another cognitive disability that could influence a deaf child's acquisition of a signed language. In the present volume, Shield and Meier describe aspects of the language of deaf children who have been diagnosed with ASD, and they summarize and contextualize previous studies on the topic – including those have focused on children acquiring BSL. As noted earlier, deaf children with ASD might have challenges with visual perspective taking, which could affect aspects of their signed language phonology (i.e., specifically, correct interpretation of the signer's palm orientation for the production of fingerspelling and some signs). Whereas Shield has focused on phonological aspects of the manual articulators for his own work, other studies have looked at the comprehension of facial expressions by deaf children with ASD (Denmark, 2011), since children with autism are often shown to exhibit difficulties with evaluating the mental states of others. Denmark conducted a study of deaf children acquiring BSL. She showed that a sample of 13 deaf childhood signers of BSL who had diagnoses within the autism spectrum range (age range 8.5–18 years) were not impaired with respect to general processing (i.e. comprehension) of facial expressions, although there were some difficulties with the production of affective facial actions in BSL and adverbial (i.e. linguistic) non-manual facial movements that accompany signs.

Motor impairments and deaf signers

Poizner *et al.* (1984) suggest that movement deficits could be considered along linguistic, symbolic and motoric levels, and it could be the case that one level reveals a deficit whereas the others do not. Motor impairments could cause difficulty with signed language production (e.g. see Tyrone, 2007, this volume). As an example, a neuromuscular disease – such as a muscular dystrophy – would likely impair a signer's ability to move her hands/arms freely and quickly through the signing space; this may result in a production disorder. A neurodegenerative condition that affects motor control, such as Parkinson's disease, could also affect signed language production. For example, Brentari *et al.* (1985) describe handshape and movement anomalies that were demonstrated by two deaf users of ASL who had been diagnosed with Parkinson's disease. In comparison with normal controls, the Parkinsonian signers coordinated movements and handshape changes in ways that caused their signing to appear monotonous to observers, as reported by the authors. Brentari and colleagues also noted that the anomalies were likely the result of atypical motor planning. Tyrone and Woll (2008) also focus on the language-articulation effects of Parkinson's on a deaf signer's productions, but their case study concerns the use of BSL. These authors discuss challenges with production that implicate handshape as the phonological parameter that seems the most affected in the Parkinson's patient. In particular, the patient often produced a lax handshape rather than one whose form matched the handshape targets for signs and fingerspelling. As noted earlier, Tyrone's work on motor impairments is also included in the present volume (see also Tyrone, 2007), in which she describes cases of sign dysarthria.

With respect to the linguistic and symbolic levels of processing suggested by Poizner and colleagues, studies of aphasic patients are particularly useful for understanding the ways that movement can be understood within the context of signed language. Specifically, the researchers considered the case of four deaf patients with aphasia and whether their manual abilities could also be characterized in terms of apraxia, a neural disorder of purposive movement. Of the four patients, one showed signs of ideomotor apraxia (i.e. difficulty gesturing to command or imitating gestures), whereas three did not. Their data provide evidence for independence of motor deficits of sign language from those of non-linguistic gesture. In other words, according to Poizner and colleagues, the movements of sign are driven by linguistic processes, whereas that is not necessarily the case for movements of other communicative acts.

Possible connections between non-linguistic motor abilities and signed languages continue to be the focus of study for researchers. For example, Meronen and Ahonen (2008) claim that motor development is an important area of focus when considering deaf children and signed language acquisition. In their study, tests of manual dexterity (serial fingertapping) correlated with tests of ASL skills. This suggests that there is a connection between motor and language skills, which is a hypothesis that merits further work.

Deaf signers and syndromic conditions

Another consideration with respect to deafness and additional disabilities concerns syndromic conditions that are often accompanied by audiological deafness. In particular, what are the cognitive characteristics of the different syndromes and how might those features influence the acquisition and maintenance of a signed language? There are multiple syndromes that co-occur with permanent hearing loss, and the most frequent examples from one report are the following (listed in decreasing order of incidence): Down, Usher, Pierre Robin, Treacher Collins and C.H.A.R.G.E (see Picard, 2004). In some cases, the syndromes are characterized by cognitive deficits (e.g. mental retardation in the case of Down & Pierre Robin) or other sensory deficits (e.g.

blindness in Usher) and that could also have an effect on signed language acquisition. Much can be learned by considering deaf individuals who are audiologically deaf and who have additional conditions that may pose challenges for the acquisition and use of signed language. This is a population of deaf signers that could benefit greatly from research on disorders of signed language communication.

What Types of Signed Language Communication Disorders Might We Expect?

Where might communication disorders in sign appear, based on what we know about the perception, processing and production of signed language? As reported within this chapter, there are some preliminary suggestions based on previously published work (e.g. Herman *et al.*, this volume; Quinto-Pozos *et al.*, this volume), but this section lays out a few additional suggestions. At this early stage in the research on signed language communication disorders, some of the proposals provided here may appear primarily speculative, although the rationale for their inclusion is based on characteristics of the signal and the articulators and articulator space, and the suggested structure of signed language lexicons. The proposed challenges are outlined in Table 1.2, and the suggested benefits of the visual-gestural modality when considering language and communication disorders are outlined in Table 1.3 (see p. 27).

Role of perception and processing

Signed language deficits might be expected in aspects of linguistic processing where visual processing of the signal is arguably more demanding – especially for the language user with specific deficits. For example, since the use of topographic space in signed language involves mental rotation and/or perspective-taking skills, a child or adult who is weak in those types of visual-spatial skills may struggle with full comprehension (and perhaps production) of those constructions. In such cases, the signers' resources for simultaneously processing linguistic information (e.g. handshape, place of articulation, syntactic function, etc.) and visual-spatial information (e.g. appropriate interpretation based on perspective) could be lacking. Such a phenomenon has been attested in several accounts of deaf signers (e.g. Atkinson *et al.*, 2002; Penn *et al.*, 2007; Quinto-Pozos *et al.*, in press; Shield & Meier, 2012, this volume).

A deficit could also presumably arise if an individual struggles with the processing of multiple types of information simultaneously. Since it is the case that various phonological features of a sign's onset are processed quickly and simultaneously (Emmorey, 2007), any disruption in the ability of

Table 1.2 Possible challenges for compromised signed language users

Comprehension	Production
Possible difficulties in processing: • multiple simultaneously realized morphemes • (rapid) fingerspelling • longer sentences or sequences of discrete items • shifts in perspective for comprehending use of topographic and grammatical space	Possible difficulties in production: • multiple simultaneously realized morphemes (difficulty in planning for production) • multiple characters in discourse (difficulty representing differences between signer, signer as narrator, and signer as other character) Difficulty with motor control to produce: • complex movements and challenging postures (depending on particular motor deficit) • multiple coordinated movements that are timed with respect to each other (e.g. path and hand-internal movement combined), including bimanual coordination • fingerspelling at normal rates

an individual to attend to multiple bits of information at the same time could presumably cause a processing deficit that would surface in language comprehension.

Signers who possess particularly slow processing abilities could also be affected, especially with respect to the rapid processing of fingerspelling. As noted earlier, fingerspelling is produced with rapid changes in handshape in sequence, and this is true whether a signed language has a one- or two-handed fingerspelling system. The processing of such forms could be problematic for signers who struggle with processing speed, and there is also likely to be an effect of literacy that accompanies a struggle. If a child (or adult) has poor reading and writing skills, they may likely have poor comprehension of fingerspelling since they will not be able to translate the rapid sequences of fingerspelled letters into lexical items that can be interpreted within context.

In addition, because of sequential memory constraints for visual signals, we might predict that signed language users would struggle to remember all the components of a long string of signs, whereas users of spoken language would presumably perform comparatively better on the task of remembering a string of spoken words of comparable length. If indeed that were the case, a potential signed language deficit might appear for children with less-than-robust memory when presented with sentences (or sentences with lists of items) that are relatively long.

Role of production and processing

It might also be expected that language production would be affected for those individuals with processing deficits with respect to the simultaneous expression of multi-morphemic, simultaneously articulated constructions. For example, some constructions in signed language narratives have been characterized as particularly complex, with the hands depicting entities in space (e.g. via classifiers), the torso and head movement depicting postures of a character within that space, and the face showing emotive and/or linguistic modifications, as appropriate (e.g. see Dudis, 2004; Emmorey & Reilly, 1998; Morgan, 2002). Signers with processing difficulties (i.e. challenges of being able to produce multiple morphemes or perspectives simultaneously) would be predicted to struggle with such constructions because of their complexity (e.g see Penn *et al.* 2007; Morgan *et al.* 2008).

Processing deficits are not the only cause of challenges with deaf signers with respect to production. In some cases, motor movements might be limited or impaired, and this could cause a signer to struggle with correct productions. For example, the production of fingerspelling might be impaired if someone has a deficit in the ability to produce fine motor movements in relatively rapid sequence. Signs that require bimanual coordination could also be challenging for some impaired signers (e.g. see Tyrone *et al.*, 2009). See Tyrone (this volume) for a discussion of various motor impairments and how signers with those impairments might be characterized with respect to phonological features of signing.

An important question to consider with respect to motor issues is whether a deficit can be linked to motor planning (i.e. processing) or motor control/coordination. A deficit in muscular control would presumably be a result of poor motor control or coordination rather than impaired motor planning. There is also the question of how motor abilities correlate with language abilities for signers. As noted earlier, studies have found relationships between the two skills for signers (e.g. Meronen & Ahonen, 2008).

Role of co-occurring cognitive deficits

One would also expect challenges for those signers who have been diagnosed with a neurocognitive condition that would affect an aspect of their cognition that is needed for language acquisition and learning. Earlier it was mentioned that ADHD/ADD might be problematic because it would not allow for optimal attention to the visual signal. This hypothesis seems plausible, although reports of such children are not common in the literature on deafness or ADHD/ADD. Of course, other cognitive deficits could also cause problems with signed language acquisition. For example, a child with a learning disability or a developmental delay could presumably show signs of deficits in their signed language abilities.

Another possibility is that a syndromic condition that affects auditory processing would have an effect on a bimodal bilingual's spoken language development, but not their signed language acquisition. This is exactly the type of case reported in Woll and Morgan (2012), with their case report of Stewart, a hearing individual with LKS.

Researchers from the UK have also reported the case of a deaf adult with Williams syndrome (WS) (Atkinson *et al.*, 2004; Woll & Morgan, 2012). This child fared poorly with respect to her performance on tests of visual-spatial skills, which would be expected of a patient with WS. There have been reports of deficits in spatial aspects of spoken language in hearing patients with WS (Laing & Jarrold, 2007; Landau & Zukowski, 2003), although the BSL case describes visual-spatial challenges associated with the syndromic condition and the processing and use of the signing space in signed language. The deficits affected grammatical and topographical uses of the signing space.

Challenges with the acquisition of literacy skills

A bimodal bilingual child might exhibit difficulties with the acquisition of literacy if indications of a language disorder appear in one of their languages. For example, weak phonological awareness skills (either auditory-based phonology or visual-based phonology) could reflect weakness in some types of metalinguistic skills, and this may have an effect on the acquisition of literacy. A diagnosis of dyslexia for signing children is not uncommon (e.g. Enns & Lafond, 2007; Miller *et al.*, 2012), and the challenge for the investigator or clinician is to determine whether a weakness in reading skill is due to reading-specific challenges or a more fundamental problem in that individual's acquisition of language (either signed or spoken).

Predictions for signed language resistance to some communication disorders

It could also be the case that some types of language and communication disorder are not comparably represented in the signed modality. Presumably, a lack of representation may be influenced by the same characteristics that make the signed modality distinct from the spoken modality such as aspects of the signal and characteristics of the articulators and articulation space. See Table 1.3 for a summary of suggested benefits for signed language users.

Earlier in this chapter it was suggested that reports of so-called signed language stuttering generally propose a much lower prevalence than that which has been reported for users of spoken languages. In the current volume, Whitebread suggests that consideration of signed language stuttering could allow for the critical evaluation of theories that target auditory

Table 1.3 Suggested benefits for compromised signed language users

Comprehension	Production
Beneficial aspects of the signal:	Beneficial aspects of the signal & the articulators:
• iconicity may support comprehension and word learning • slower articulation of signs may result in comparably fewer temporal processing deficits • size and visibility of manual gestures may make signs easier to perceive and recognize	• aspects of sensory feedback and bimanual articulation may result in lower prevalence of some disfluencies in sign (e.g. stuttering) • manipulable articulators may support language learning and communication intervention • slower articulation of signs may result in comparably few motor coordination problems

feedback as one of the primary factors that influence a person's degree of stuttering. Without comparable feedback, signers presumably do not have a similar type of interference from a feedback loop (see the section on visual feedback in sign), and this could mitigate potential fluency issues that would arise. However, there could be other possible reasons for less representation of stuttering among signers. One possibility is that the planning and coordination of bimanual articulation leads to comparably fewer problems with fluency in signed language. This is an area that could use empirical studies to investigate the possibilities.

As noted earlier, the rate at which signs are produced is generally slower than the rate at which spoken words are uttered – seemingly due to the size of the articulators in sign and the fact that they must traverse a larger articulatory space than that for speech. An important question is whether the slower temporal rate of the signed signal (at least for lexical signs, less so for fingerspelling) would lead to fewer deficits that are influenced by the required speed of processing.

Even though there remains considerable debate about whether sign iconicity plays a facilitative role in the learning of new signs and general comprehension of a signed message, iconicity has shown by some studies to be facilitative, and iconic aspects of a signed vocabulary are worth considering. It may be the case that children and adults who are cognitively compromised would benefit from iconicity, although age could presumably be a variable to be considered.

Signs are highly perceptible to the typical viewer, which has been suggested as a possible reason for the degree to which they are recognized by caregivers in the early communication of their deaf children (Newport & Meier, 1985). This degree of perceptibility may provide a benefit to users who present with a deficit that impairs their ability to recognize and process signs.

Over the years there have been many examples of signed languages being used as resources for communication therapy for children and adults with language and communication disorders (see Bonvillian *et al.*, 1981, Seal & Bonvillian, 1997). It would be worthwhile to consider why signed language allows for communication in cases when spoken language production is not successful. It could be that the speech articulators are more difficult to manage in comparison with the signed language articulators, although the comparison might be challenging to make based on different muscular structures and neural processes that manage the motor movements. However, there are aspects of the articulators and articulator space that may be useful when conducting communication intervention via signed language: the rate at which the articulators generally produce signs and the fact that they are manipulable. As noted earlier, signs are articulated more slowly than words are, but the articulation can be slowed down further to assist with language learning and intervention. An intentional slowing of the signal could also be possible in spoken language, but that may result in a distorted message. Because signed articulators are manipulable, a signed language professional can assist a child or adult with the correct articulation of a sign.

Challenges of Working on Signed Language Disorders

There exist various challenges with the task of conducting research on communication disorders within the signed modality, and this has also been suggested by other authors (e.g. Morgan, 2005). One of the primary challenges concerns the availability of instruments for assessing the language and communication of deaf individuals – both children and adults. Unfortunately, it appears as though natural signed language has generally not been considered in past research on communication disorders and approaches to intervention for deaf children and adults. There are also some challenges that are related to characteristics of the population of daily signed language users. Each of these topics is treated within this section.

Availability of assessments

There is clearly a lack of (normed) instruments that focus on language and communication with which to assess signing (both deaf and hearing) individuals. Mann and Haug (this volume) highlight this point in their chapter while providing a context for understanding the types of language and communication assessments that have been available until the present time. The authors note that there are four broad categories of assessments that exist: (1) tests for sign language acquisition; (2) tests for educational purposes; (3) tests for research on linguistic and cognitive development; and (4) tests for adult second language learners. In some cases, a single test might be used for multiple purposes. Critically, Mann and Haug provide a cross-linguistic perspective to the topic of signed language assessment because they perform a broad-based review of instruments that have been created in various countries. This is particularly important for those signed languages that do not have as extensive a history of research. The authors also provide suggestions about how to create tests that are reliable and valid. This could serve as a very useful resource for researchers and clinicians throughout the world.

The vast majority of tests that have been developed for assessing signed language were not designed with the primary purpose of identifying children or adults with language or communication deficits. Such diagnostic instruments are lacking, although there have been recent efforts to change this, such as the creation of a BSL non-word repetition test, with the goal of serving as one measure of deaf signing children's language impairment (Mann & Marshall, 2010; Marshall et al., 2006; Mason et al., 2010). Other tests and checklists might also be able to identify low performers reliably (e.g. Anderson & Reilly, 2002 for ASL; Baker & Jansma, 2005 for Dutch-NGT).

The tests that have been developed for research purposes may not necessarily be available to language/communication professionals to use with children in their schools. Instead, schools generally develop their own in-house assessments. The manner in which this is done differs from school to school, but developmental professionals (e.g. ASL specialists, school psychologists, speech and language therapists) may create ways to assess the children in their schools, such as by using video to capture language samples and analyzing the product based on checklists of linguistic/communicative features (Quinto-Pozos et al., 2011). The efforts and gains that have been made by these professionals are noteworthy, especially since they have not been able to turn to commercially available normed instruments to serve as resources.

Availability of literature resources

Perhaps a related issue concerns the lack of writings on signed language communication disorders. There is typically not much discussion of signed language at professional gatherings of researchers and practitioners (e.g. speech and language therapists), where the focus is normally on audition and speech, and researchers who work on signed languages do not have access to a body of research on communication disorders in the visual-gesture modality. Generally speaking, there appears to be minimal discussion at scholarly meetings of communication disorders experts about the typical or atypical acquisition of a signed language by deaf children, with only some representation in the form of an occasional oral or poster presentation.[14] In addition, some school professionals who work with deaf children (e.g. speech language therapists, school psychologists, physical and occupational therapists, etc.) may not be familiar with the general milestones that deaf children should reach at different stages of their signed language development.

It is the case, however, that signed language is used by researchers and clinicians for augmentative or alternative communication with hearing patients, such as with children who are diagnosed with ASD (see Bonvillian *et al.*, 1981, Seal & Bonvillian, 1997). In some of those cases, the learning of signs by the autistic children has been reported to aid communication. However, it is likely that the children in these cases were not generally exposed to the full linguistic system of a signed language – including both lexical items and grammatical structures. Rather, the autistic children exposed to signed language may have mostly learned isolated signs, and it is questionable whether the same children use the signs regularly (i.e. outside the experimental setting) for communication (Bonviallian & Blackburn, 1991).

In addition to the dearth of published research studies on signed communication disorders, there is also a lack of documented intervention strategies in the literature for assisting deaf and hard of hearing children to improve in areas of signed language development that are noticeably delayed or atypical. It is the case that some clinicians have developed their own strategies, which are based on their experiences with interventions with children acquiring English (e.g. Quinto-Pozos *et al.*, 2011), yet the grammatical differences between English and ASL and the difference in modality between the two languages (e.g. perception, production, etc.) does not allow for a straightforward comparison. Unfortunately, a similar situation exists in the cases of deaf adults who are in need of language therapy after a neurological insult such as a stroke or brain injury; the rehabilitation that speech and language therapists have been able to engage in with this population in the past has been limited (Marshall *et al.*, 2003).

Characteristics of the target population

Characteristics of the target population also present challenges for work on communication disorders in signed languages. If a researcher would like to avoid the confound of late exposure to language, one issue concerns the estimated size of the target population of deaf signers who are exposed to a natural signed language from birth. Most deaf children have parents or caregivers who are hearing (over 90%, according to estimates; Mitchell & Karchmer, 2004); presumably, the vast majority of these adults who interact with young deaf children regularly do not sign. According to GRI data from 2010–2011, only 5.8% of Deaf and hard of hearing children (slightly over 2100 children) are exposed to ASL in the home. For a subset of the remainder of D/HH children, it may be the case that atypical aspects of signed language development are caused by delayed exposure to rich linguistic input rather than some other cognitive or neurological aspect of development. If one were conducting research on communication disorders in signed language with a focus on deaf children who are exposed to a sign language from birth, there would be a small number of children who would be potential participants in a research study. This is clearly a challenge for investigators. Among other things, this makes it difficult to design a group study in order to address individual variation within this population. This constraint also forces a researcher to work with multiple schools in order to locate various children who are appropriate for a study.

In this volume, Quinto-Pozos, Singleton, Hauser and Levine describe a multiple case-study methodology that they have employed for studies of atypical development in native signing children who are acquiring ASL. They focus on children who experience robust exposure to ASL (in the home and at school) in order to rule out effects that may be caused by delayed or impoverished input. In the chapter, the authors outline the challenges of performing research on atypical signed language development, and they also describe the ways in which they work closely with schools for the deaf in order to recruit and study focal children (i.e. atypically developing deaf children). Quinto-Pozos and colleagues also describe their approach for assessing the focal children – by using a combination of linguistic and cognitive assessments. As they point out, their approach may not be suitable for all cases of suspected deficit, but it does allow for careful examination of individual children that can potentially inform theory and provide much needed information for creating intervention strategies for such children.

Comparatively less demographic information has been reported for hearing children who are born into households with (Deaf) signing parents or siblings. These children (like those discussed in this volume in the Baker & van den Bogaerde and Chen Pichler, Lee & Lillo-Martin chapters) are exposed to signed language from a young age, and they are developing as bilingual bimodal children. Unfortunately, the development of these children is not the focus of many studies, which restricts the degree to which we understand their development as native users of signed language.

It has been reported that timely identification of atypical signed language development may also be an issue that needs to be addressed (Quinto-Pozos *et al.*, 2011). As suggested in the introduction, it is not uncommon for professionals to view atypicality as a developmental phase and something that is expected to 'go away' as they get older. This lack of early identification may be due, in part, to the lack of marketed assessment instruments – whether they be diagnostic or not – that professionals at schools can use to chart a child's developmental progress. As noted, it can also be difficult to determine if a child with late exposure to signed language has language problems in addition to being delayed with the acquisition of the signed language.

Where Do We Go From Here?

There is much to be learned about communication disorders by considering data from signed languages. As has been described in this chapter, there exist similarities and differences across language modalities with respect to perception, processing and production. The similarities allow for logical comparisons across modalities, and the differences force researchers and clinicians to carefully consider aspects of signed languages that have previously not been included in our general knowledge base about human communication.

For the future, it would be useful to continue in the quest to determine which disorders are influenced by language modality versus those that could potentially be universal for language users across both modalities. Presumably, there would be various similarities because of the ways in which language is acquired – and lost – across signers and speakers. Many notable similarities about communication have been pointed out in spite of differences in the primary channels of communication. However, as outlined in this chapter, there are important differences across modalities that should be considered (e.g. characteristics of the signal and the articulators and articulator space for signed languages) which could provide insights about those aspects of language processing and production that are not necessarily universal. Not only could this research provide evidence for what is unique to hearing or vision with respect to language perception and processing, it would inform the research community about what is generalizable for all users of language. Additionally, since there are notable differences with respect to the motor abilities needed for the production of speech versus sign, a focus on those differences and the types of impairments that occur (or may be predicted to occur) in sign would be extremely useful.

In regard to applying what is learned to the practice of intervention, one approach is for researchers and schools to form more mutually beneficial partnerships. Developmental professionals at schools could benefit from additional resources for assessing their students and providing key aspects to diagnostics. In addition, speech and language therapists could benefit from studies that explore intervention strategies that provide approaches for signed language therapy. This area of research is ripe for translational approaches. With respect to assessment instruments, regular communication between researchers who design tests and schools could support the creation of assessments that are valid reflections of the types of language knowledge and skill that are expected from typically developing children at various ages. This would allow for benchmarks from which to compare children who may be underperforming in various areas. In addition, researchers could benefit from having partnerships with schools that assist with the recruitment of potential research participants (both typically and atypically developing children) so that the body of research data on this topic could continue to grow and benefit researchers, clinical practitioners, educators and language professionals at schools, and the deaf individuals who are struggling with linguistic and/or cognitive deficits.

As mentioned in the introduction, over five decades of inquiry into signed languages have given us the opportunity to advance our linguistic knowledge of structural variation, patterns of language learning and the cognitive processing of language by children and adults. Unfortunately, comparatively little work during this same period has focused on signed language communication disorders, but the authors of the chapters in this present work would like us to believe that this will change in the near future. I optimistically agree with that sentiment.

Acknowledgements

The author wishes to thank Richard P. Meier, Jill Morford and Martha Tyrone for their comments on earlier versions of this chapter. Any errors and misinterpretations of the literature are the author's own.

Notes

(1) With respect to the United States, Gallaudet Research Institute (GRI) data from 2010 report nearly 38,000 deaf and hard of hearing school-aged students throughout the country. If SLI was represented among deaf children in rates similar to those reported for spoken language acquisition (approximately 7% of population, see Mason et al., 2010; Tomblin et al., 1997), there would be over 2600 children in the US who might exhibit SLI with respect to their ASL acquisition.

(2) In some cases, additional salient aspects of a sign's articulation may be important for the specification of a sign such as where, if at all, contact occurs between the articulators, and whether specific non-manual signals are used. Movement can also be divided into path movement and hand-internal movement.

(3) It should also be noted that a study of typically developing native signers of ASL reports that handshape is the phonological parameter with most errors for young children, whereas place of articulation exhibits the fewest errors; path movement lies between these two (Cheek et al., 2001). Interestingly, no handshape errors were reported for the atypically developing children that were discussed in Quinto-Pozos et al. (2011).

(4) Also see MacSweeney et al. (2002) for a review of comprehension studies.

(5) The term *classifier*, in the context of signed languages, is used to refer to various communicative devices that depict the motion, location and/or geometric description of objects. It most commonly refers to handshapes that are used to depict an object in its entirety, such as an ASL 3-handshape to refer to a vehicle and a bent-V handshape to refer to an animal. Other devices called classifiers are used to describe objects (i.e. provide information about the size and/or shape of an object) or how objects are handled. See Supalla (1982) for an early description of ASL classifiers, including developmental milestones for their acquisition, and Schembri (2003) for a general discussion of signed language classifiers.

(6) Of course, it is also true that light must be present in order to perceive physical changes in the environment, which makes viewing signed language in dark spaces difficult or impossible without tactile information.

(7) The next section provides details about the articulators of signed language and articulation rate. Also see Mayberry and Waters (1990) for evidence that word memory and production rate may be related for fingerspelling but not for lexical signs.

(8) Of course, signers also use kinesthetic and tactual feedback when producing signs. In fact, these types of sensory information comprise the full signal for deaf-blind signers who use tactile sign language, which provides evidence for the robust nature of those signals for communication.

(9) It may also be the case that differences in planning and coordination demands between sign and speech may lead to differences in the prevalence of stuttering across modalities.

(10) The slower articulation time in sign versus speech has also been used as an argument to account for sign errors data (i.e. slips of the hand) and the comparably faster repair of sign errors (i.e. towards the beginning of a sign's articulation) over speech errors (Hohenberger et al., 2002).

(11) See Penn et al. (2007) for data from deaf adults that support this premise.

(12) Foreign items could also appear in spoken languages and follow constraints that are different from core or native items (e.g. Brentari & Padden, 2001 cite Ito & Mester, 1995 for Japanese; also see Hancock, 1995 for a description of Vlax Romani), although spoken languages do not capitalize on iconicity of forms to the extent that signed languages do.

(13) Other proposals suggest that signs are organized in a mental lexicon according to lexical families that can be described in phonological and semantic terms (Fernald & Napoli, 2000) or with primacy to phonological onsets but not to any single phonological aspects of a sign such as handshape or place of articulation (see Emmorey, 2007 for a review).

(14) Two notable counter examples are the thematic panel sessions held at the Symposium on Research in Child Language Disorders (SRCLD) in 2002 and the Society for Research on Child Development (SRCD) in 2009 and 2013.

References

Anderson, D. and Reilly, J. (2002) The MacArthur Communicative Development Inventory: Normative data for American Sign Language. *Journal of Deaf Studies and Deaf Education* 7 (2), 83–119.

Aronoff, M., Meir, L. and Sandler, W. (2005) The paradox of sign language morphology. *Language* 81, 301–344.

Atkinson, J.A., Woll, B. and Gathercole, S. (2002) The impact of developmental visuospatial learning difficulties on British Sign Language. *Neurocase* 8, 424–441.

Atkinson, J., Campbell, R., Marshall, J., Thacker, A. and Woll, B. (2004) Understanding 'not': Neuropsychological dissociations between hand and head markers of negation in BSL. *Neuropsychologia* 42, 214–229.

Baddeley, A. (1986) *Working Memory.* Oxford: Clarendon Press.

Baker, A.E. and Jansma, S. (2005) *NGT-Observatiepakket voor Peuters.* Amsterdam: University of Amsterdam.

Baker, A. and Woll, B. (eds) (2008) *Sign Language Acquisition.* Amsterdam: John Benjamins.

Battison, R. (1978) Lexical borrowing in American Sign Language. Silver Spring, MD: Linstok Press.

Bavelier, D., Newport, E.L., Hall, M.L., Supalla, T. and Boutla, M. (2006) Persistent differences in short-term memory span between sign and speech. *Psychological Science* 17, 1090–1092.

Bedore, L. and Peña, A. (2008) Assessment of bilingual children for identification of language impairment: Current findings and implications for practice. *International Journal of Bilingual Education and Bilingualism* 11, 1–28.

Bellugi, U. and Fischer, S. (1972) A comparison of sign language and spoken language. *Cognition* 1, 173–200.

Bellugi, U., O'Grady, L., Lillo-Martin, D., O'Grady, M., van Hoek, K. and Corina, D. (1990) Enhancement of spatial cognition in deaf children. In V. Volterra and C. Erting (eds) *From Gesture to Language in Hearing and Deaf Children* (pp. 278–298). New York: Springer.

Bialystok, E. (2009) Bilingualism: The good, the bad, and the indifferent. *Bilingualism, Language and Cognition* 12, 3–11.

Bonvillian, J.D. and Blackburn, D.W. (1991) Manual communication and autism: Factors relating to sign language acquisition. In P. Siple and S. Fischer (eds) *Theoretical Issues in Sign Language Research,* Vol. 2: *Psychology* (pp. 255–277). Chicago, IL: University of Chicago Press.

Bonvillian, J.D., Nelson, K.E. and Rhyne, J.M. (1981) Sign language and autism. *Journal of Autism and Developmental Disorders* 11, 125–137.

Bonvillian, J.D., Orlansky, M.D. and Novack, L.L. (1983) Developmental milestones: Sign language acquisition and motor development. *Child Development* 54, 1435–1445.

Bosworth, R. and Emmorey, K. (2010) Effects of iconicity and semantic relatedness on lexical access in American Sign Language. *Journal of Experimental Psychology* 36, 1573–1581.

Boutla, M., Supalla, T., Newport, E.L. and Bavelier, D. (2004) Short-term memory span: Insights from sign language. *Nature Neuroscience* 7 (9), 997–1002.

Brentari, D. (2002) Modality differences in sign language phonology and morphophonemics. In R.P. Meier, K. Cormier and D. Quinto-Pozos (eds) *Modality and Structure in Signed and Spoken Languages* (pp. 35–64). Cambridge: Cambridge University Press.

Brentari, D. (2012) *Sign Languages.* Cambridge Language Surveys. Cambridge: Cambridge University Press.

Brentari, D. and Padden, C.A. (2001) Native and foreign vocabulary in American Sign Language: A lexicon with multiple origins. In D. Brentari (ed.) *Foreign Vocabulary: A Cross-linguistic Investigation of Word Formation* (pp. 87–119). Mahwah, NJ: Lawrence Erlbaum Associates.

Brentari, D., Poizner, H. and Kegl, J. (1995) Aphasic and Parkinsonian signing: Differences in phonological disruption. *Brain and Language* 48, 69–105.

Broomfield, J. and Dodd, B. (2004) Children with speech and language disability: Caseload characteristics. *International Journal of Communication Disorders* 39, 303–324.

Capek, C.M., Grossi, G., Newman, A.J., McBurney, S.L., Corina, D., Roeder, B. and Neville, H.J. (2009) Brain systems mediating semantic and syntactic processing in deaf native signers: Biological invariance and modality specificity. *Proceedings of the National Academy of Sciences* 106, 8784–8789.

Cheek, A., Cormier, K., Repp, A. and Meier, R.P. (2001) Prelinguistic gesture predicts mastery and error in the production of early signs. *Language* 77, 292–323.

Civier, O., Tasko, S.M. and Guenther, F.H. (2010) Overreliance on auditory feedback may lead to sound/syllable repetitions: Simulations of stuttering and fluency-inducing conditions with a neural model of speech production. *Journal of Fluency Disorders* 35 (3), 246–279.

Clark, M.D., Gilbert, G. and Anderson, M. (2011) Morphological knowledge and decoding skills of deaf readers. *Psychology* 2, 109–116.

Corina, D.P. (1998) The processing of sign language: Evidence from aphasia. In H. Whitaker and B. Stemmer (eds) *Handbook of Neurology.* San Diego, CA: Academic Press.

Cormier, K., Schembri, A. and Tyrone, M. (2008) One hand or two? Nativisation of fingerspelling in ASL and BANZSL. *Sign Language & Linguistics* 11 (1), 3–44.

Cormier, K., Quinto-Pozos, D., Sevcikova, Z. and Schembri, A. (2012) Lexicalisation and de-lexicalisation processes in sign languages: Comparing depicting constructions and viewpoint gestures. *Language and Communication* 32 (4), 329–348.

Denmark, T. (2011) Do children with autism spectrum disorder show deficits in the comprehension and production of emotional and linguistic facial expressions in British Sign Language? Unpublished doctoral dissertation, University College London.

Dolata, J.K., Davis, B.L. and MacNeilage, P.F. (2008) Characteristics of the rhythmic organization of vocal babbling: Implications for an amodal linguistic rhythm. *Infant Behavior & Development* 31, 422–431.

Dudis, P.G. (2004) Body partitioning and real-space blends. *Cognitive Linguistics* 15, 223–238.

Emmorey, K. (2002) *Language, Cognition, and the Brain.* Mahwah, NJ: Lawrence Erlbaum.

Emmorey, K. (2007) The psycholinguistics of signed and spoken languages: How biology affects processing. In M.G. Gaskell (ed.) *The Oxford Handbook of Psycholinguistics* (pp. 703–721). Oxford: Oxford University Press.

Emmorey, K. and Corina, D. (1990) Lexical recognition in sign language: Effects of phonetic structure and morphology. *Perceptual and Motor Skills* 71, 1227–1252.

Emmorey, K. and Kosslyn, S. (1996) Enhanced image generation abilities in deaf signers: A right hemisphere effect. *Brain and Cognition* 32, 28–44.

Emmorey, K. and Petrich, J. (2012) Processing orthographic structure: Associations between print and fingerspelling. *Journal of Deaf Studies and Deaf Education* 17 (2), 194–204.

Emmorey, K. and Reilly, N. (1998) The development of quotation and reported action: Conveying perspective in ASL. In E. Clark (ed.) *Proceedings of the Twenty-ninth Annual Child Language Research Forum* (pp. 81–90). Stanford, CA: CSLI Press.

Emmorey, K. and Wilson, M. (2004) The puzzle of working memory for sign language. *TRENDS in Cognitive Science* 8, 521–523.

Emmorey, K., Kosslyn, S. and Bellugi, U. (1993) Visual imagery and visual-spatial language: Enhanced imagery abilities in deaf and hearing ASL signers. *Cognition* 46, 139–181.

Emmorey, K., Corina, D. and Bellugi, U. (1995) Differential processing of topographic and referential functions of space. In K. Emmorey and J. Reilly (eds) *Language, Gesture, and Space* (pp. 43–62). Mahwah, NJ: Lawrence Erlbaum.

Emmorey, K., Klima, E.S. and Hickok, G. (1998) Mental rotation within linguistic and nonlinguistic domains in users of American Sign Language. *Cognition* 68, 221–246.

Emmorey, K., Gertsberg, N., Korpics, F. and Wright, C.E. (2009) The influence of visual feedback and register changes on sign language production: A kinematic study with deaf signers. *Applied Psycholinguistics* 30, 187–203.

Emmorey, K., Grabowski, T., McCullough, S., Ponto, L.L.B., Hichwa, R.D. and Damasio, H. (2005) The neural correlates of spatial language in English and American Sign Language: A PET study with hearing bilinguals. *Neuroimage* 24, 832–840.

Emmorey, K., McCullough, S., Mehta, S., Ponto, L.L.B. and Grabowski, T.J. (2013) Biology of linguistic expression impacts neural correlates for spatial language. *Journal of Cognitive Neuroscience* 25 (4), 517–533.

Enns, C. and Lafond, L.D. (2007) Reading against all odds: A pilot study of two deaf students with dyslexia. *American Annals of the Deaf* 152, 63–72.

Falchook, A.D., Mayberry, R., Poizner, H., Burtis, D.B., Doty, L. and Heilman, K.M. (2012) Sign language aphasia from a neurodegenerative disease. *Neurocase: The Neural Basis of Cognition.* doi:10.1080/13554794.2012.690427.

Fernald, T.B. and Napoli, D.J. (2000) Exploitation of morphological possibilities in signed languages. *Sign Language & Linguistics* 3, 3–58.

Freel, B.L. Clark, M.D., Anderson, M.L., Gilbert, G., Musyoka, M.M. and Hauser, P.C. (2011) Deaf individuals' bilingual abilities: American Sign Language proficiency, reading skills, and family characteristics. *Psychology* 2 (1), 18–23. doi:10.4236/psych.2011.21003.

Gallaudet Research Institute (2011) *Regional and National Summary Report of Data from the 2009–10 Annual Survey of Deaf and Hard of Hearing Children and Youth.* Washington, DC: GRI, Gallaudet University.

Grosjean, F. (1981) Sign and word recognition: A first comparison. *Sign Language Studies* 32, 195–219.

Grosjean, F. (2010) Bilingualism, biculturalism, and deafness. *International Journal of Bilingual Education and Bilingualism* 13, 133–145.

Guardino, C.A. (2008) Identification and placement for students with multiple disabilities: Choosing the path less followed. *American Annals of the Deaf* 153 (1), 55–64.

Hancock, I. (1995) *A Handbook of Vlax Romani.* Columbus, OH: Slavica Publishers.

Hermans, D., Knoors, H., Ormel, E. and Verhoeven, L. (2008) The relationship between the reading and signing skills of deaf children in bilingual education programs. *Journal of Deaf Studies and Deaf Education* 13, 519–530.

Hickok, G., Say, K., Bellugi, U. and Klima, E.S. (1996) The basis of hemispheric asymmetries for language and spatial cognition; clues from focal brain damage in two deaf native signers. *Aphasiology* 10, 577–591.

Hickok, G., Pickell, H., Klima, E. and Bellugi, U. (2009) Neural dissociation in the production of lexical versus classifier signs in ASL: Distinct patterns of hemispheric asymmetry. *Neuropsychologia* 47 (2), 382–387.

Hohenberger, A., Happ, D. and Leuninger, H. (2002) Modality-dependent aspects of sign language production: Evidence from slips of the hand and their repairs in German Sign Language. In R.P. Meier, K. Cormier and D. Quinto-Pozos (eds) *Modality and Structure in Signed and Spoken Languages* (pp. 112–142). Cambridge: Cambridge University Press.

Hwang, S. (2011) Windows into sensory integration and rates in language processing: Insights from signed and spoken languages. Unpublished doctoral dissertation. University of Maryland, College Park.

Ito, J. and Mester, A. (1995) The core-periphery structure of the lexicon and constraints on reranking. In J. Beckman *et al.* (eds) *University of Massachusetts Occasional Papers 18: Papers in Optimality Theory* (pp. 181–210). Amherst, MA: Graduate Linguistic Student Association, University of Massachusetts.

Jantunen, T. and Takkinen, R. (2010) Syllable structure in sign language phonology. In D. Brentari (ed.) *Sign Languages* (pp. 312–331). Cambridge: Cambridge University Press.

Johnston, T. and Schembri, A. (2007) *Australian Sign Language (Auslan). An Introduction to Sign Language Linguistics.* Cambridge: Cambridge University Press.

Jones, T. and Jones, J. (2003) Educating young children with multiple disabilities. In B. Bodner-Johnson and M. Sass-Leher (eds) *The Young Deaf or Hard of Hearing Child* (pp. 297–329). Baltimore, MD: Brookes Publishing.

Jones, T.W., Jones, J. and Ewing, K. (2006) Students with multiple disabilities. In D.F. Moores and D.S. Martin (eds) *Deaf Learners, Developments in Curriculum and Instruction* (pp. 127–143). Washington, DC: Gallaudet University Press.

Kanto, L., Huttunen, K. and Laakso, M-L. (2013) Relationship between the linguistic environments and early bilingual language development of hearing children in Deaf-parented families. *Journal of Deaf Studies and Deaf Education* 18, 242–260.

Kargin, T., Guldenoglu, I.B., Miller, P., Hauser, P., Rathmann, C., Kubus, O. and Superegon, E. (2012) Investigation of the differences in the word processing skills between Deaf and hearing readers: Reading in different orthographies. *Journal of Development and Physical Disabilities* 24 (1), 65–83. doi:10.1007/s10882-011-9255-z.

Kegl, J. and Poizner, H. (1998) Shifting the burden to the interlocutor: Compensation for pragmatic deficits in signers with Parkinson's disease. *Journal of Neurolinguistics* 11, 137–152.

Klima, E. and Bellugi, U. (1979) The signs of language. Cambridge, MA: Harvard University Press.

Knoors, H. and Vervloed, M. (2003) Educational programming for deaf children with multiple disabilities. Acccomodating special needs. In M. Marschark and P. E. Spencer (eds) *The Oxford Handbook of Deaf Studies, Language, and Education* (pp. 82–94). New York: Oxford University Press.

Kohnert, K. (2010) Bilingual children with primary language impairment: Issues, evidence and implications for clinical actions. *Journal of Communication Disorders* 43, 456–473.

Laing, E. and Jarrold, C. (2007) Comprehension of spatial language in Williams syndrome: Evidence for impaired spatial representation of verbal descriptions. *Clinical Linguistics & Phonetics* 21, 689–704.

Landau, B. and Zukowski, A. (2003) Objects, motions, and paths: Spatial language in children with Williams syndrome. *Developmental Neuropsychology* 23, 105–137.

Leonard, L. (1998) *Children with Specific Language Impairment.* Cambridge, MA and London: MIT Press.

Lieberman, A.M., Hatrak, M. and Mayberry, R.I. (2011) The development of eye gaze control for linguistic input in deaf children. In N. Danis, K. Mesh and H. Sung (eds) *Proceedings of the 35th Boston University Conference on Language Development* (pp.391–403). Somerville, MA: Cascadilla Press.

Lieberman, A.M., Hatrak, M. and Mayberry, R.I. (2013) Learning to look for language: Development of joint attention in young deaf children. *Language Learning and Development.* doi:10.1080/15475441.2012.760381.

Lieberth, A.K. and Bellile Gamble, M.E. (1991) The role of iconicity in sign language learning by hearing adults. *Journal of Communication Disorders* 24, 89–99.

Loew, R.C., Kegl, J.A. and Poizner, H. (1997) Fractionation of the components of role play in a right-hemisphere lesioned signer. *Aphasiology* 11 (3), 263–281.

MacNeilage, P. (1998) The frame/content theory of evolution of speech production. *Behavioral and Brain Sciences* 21, 499–546.

MacSweeney, M., Woll, B., Campbell, R., McGuire, P.K., David, A.S., Williams, S.C.R., Suckling, J., Calvert, G.A. and Brammer, M.J. (2002) Neural systems underlying British Sign Language and audio-visual English processing in native users. *Brain* 125, 1583–1593.

Mann, W. and Marshall, C.R. (2010) Building an Assessment Use Argument for sign language: The BSL Nonsense Sign Repetition Test. *International Journal of Bilingual Education and Bilingualism* 13, 243–258.

Mann, W., Marshall, C.R., Mason, K. and Morgan, G. (2010) The acquisition of sign language: The impact of phonetic complexity on phonology. *Language Learning and Development* 6, 1–27.

Marist, J.A. and Hutton, C. (1957) Effects of auditory masking upon the speech of stutterers. *Journal of Speech and Hearing Disorders* 22, 385–389.

Markham, P.T. and Justice, E.M. (2004) Sign language iconicity and its influence on the ability to describe the function of objects. *Journal of Communication Disorders* 37, 535–546.

Marshall, C.R., Denmark, T. and Morgan, G. (2006) Investigating the underlying causes of SLI: A non-sign repetition test in British Sign Language. *Advances in Speech-Language Pathology* 8 (4), 347–355. doi:10.1080/14417040600970630.

Marshall, J., Atkinson, J., Thacker, A. and Woll, B. (2003) Is speech and language therapy meeting the needs of language minorities? The case of Deaf people with neurological impairments. *International Journal of Language and Communication Disorders* 38, 85–94.

Marshall, J., Atkinson, J., Smulovitch, E., Thacker, A. and Woll, B. (2004) Aphasia in a user of British Sign Language: Dissociation between sign and gesture. *Cognitive Neuropsychology* 21, 537–554.

Marshall, C.R., Rowley, K., Mason, K., Herman, R. and Morgan, G. (2013) Lexical organization in deaf children who use British Sign Language: Evidence from a semantic fluency task. *Journal of Child Language* 40 (1), 193–220.

Masataka, N. (1995) Absence of mirror-reversal tendency in cutaneous pattern perception and acquisition of a signed language in deaf children. *Journal of Developmental Psychology* 13, 97–106.

Mason, K., Rowley, K., Marshall, C.R., Atkinson, J.R., Herman, R., Woll, B. and Morgan, G. (2010) Identifying specific language impairment in deaf children acquiring British Sign Language: Implications for theory and practice. *British Journal of Developmental Psychology* 28 (1), 33–49. doi:10.1348/026151009X484190.

Mayberry, R.I. and Waters, G.S. (1990) Children's memory for sign and fingerspelling in relation to production rate and sign language input. In P. Siple and S.D. Fischer (eds) *Theoretical Issues in Sign Language Research 2* (pp. 211–229). Chicago, IL: University of Chicago Press.

Mayberry, R.I., del Giudice, A. and Lieberman, A. (2010) Reading achievement in relation to phonological coding and awareness in deaf readers: A meta-analysis. *Journal of Deaf Studies and Deaf Education* 16 (2), 164–188. doi:10.1093/deafed/enq049.

McKee, D. (1987) An analysis of specialized cognitive functions in deaf and hearing signers. Unpublished doctoral dissertation, University of Pittsburgh.

McQuarrie, L. and Parrila, R. (2009) Phonological representations in Deaf children: Rethinking the 'Functional Equivalence' hypothesis. *Journal of Deaf Studies & Deaf Education* 14 (2), 137–154.

Meier, R.P. (1987) Elicited imitation of verb agreement in American Sign Language: Iconically or morphologically determined? *Journal of Memory and Language* 26, 362–376.

Meier, R.P. (2002) Why different, why the same? Explaining effects and non-effects of modality upon linguistic structure in sign and speech. In R.P. Meier, K. Cormier and D. Quinto-Pozos (eds) *Modality and Structure in Signed and Spoken Languages* (pp. 1–26). Cambridge: Cambridge University Press.

Meier, R.P., Mauk, C., Cheek, A. and Moreland, C. (2008) The form of children's early signs: Iconic or motoric determinants? *Language, Learning and Development* 4, 1–36.

Meronen, A. and Ahonen, T. (2008) Individual differences in sign language abilities in deaf children. *American Annals of the Deaf* 152 (5), 495–504.

Miller, M.S. (1987) Sign iconicity: Single-sign receptive vocabulary skills of nonsigning hearing preschoolers. *Journal of Communication Disorders* 20 (5), 359–365.

Miller, P. and Clark, M.D. (2012) Phonological awareness is not necessary to become a skilled deaf reader (Review). *Journal of Development and Physical Disabilities* 23, 459–476.

Miller, P., Kargin, T., Guldenoglu, B., Rathmann, C., Kubus, O., Hauser, P. and Spurgeon, E. (2012) Factors distinguishing skilled and less skilled Deaf readers: Evidence from four orthographies. *Journal of Deaf Studies & Deaf Education* 17, 439–462.

Mitchell, R. and Karchmer, M. (2004) Chasing the mythical ten percent: Parental hearing status of deaf and hard of hearing students in the United States. *Sign Language Studies* 4 (2), 138–163. doi: 10.1353/sls.2004.0005.

Mitchell, R. and Karchmer, M. (2006) Demographics in deaf education: More students in more places. *American Annals of the Deaf* 151 (2), 95–103.

Moores, D. (2001) *Educating the Deaf* (5th edn). Boston: Houghton Mifflin.

Morford, J.P. and MacFarlane, J. (2003) Frequency characteristics of American Sign Language. *Sign Language Studies* 3, 213–225.

Morford, J.P., Wilkinson, E., Villwock, A., Piñar, P. and Kroll, J.F. (2011) When deaf sign-ers read English: Do written words activate their sign translations? *Cognition* 118 (2), 286–292.

Morgan, G. (2002) The encoding of simultaneity in children's British Sign Language nar-ratives. *Sign Language and Linguistics* 5, 131–165.

Morgan, G. (2005) Biology and behaviour: Insights from the acquisition of sign language. In A. Cutler (ed.) *Twenty-first Century Psycholinguistics: Four Cornerstones* (pp. 191–208). Mahwah, NJ: Lawrence Erlbaum.

Morgan, G., Herman, R. and Woll, B. (2006) Language impairments in sign language: Breakthroughs and puzzles. *International Journal of Language and Communication Disorders* 42, 97–105.

Morgan, G., Herman, R., Barriere, I. and Woll, B. (2008) The onset and master of spatial language in children acquiring British Sign Language. *Cognitive Development* 23, 1–19.

Musselman, C. (2000) How do children who can't hear learn to read an alphabetic script? A review of the literature on reading and deafness. *Journal of Deaf Studies and Deaf Education* 5 (1), 9–31.

Myers, C., Clark, M.D., Musyoka, M.M., Anderson, M.L., Gilbert, G.L., Agyen, S. and Hauser, P.C. (2010) Black deaf individuals' reading skills: Influence of ASL, culture, family characteristics, reading experience, and education. *American Annals of the Deaf* 155 (4), 449–457.

Neilson, M.D. and Neilson, P.D. (1987) Speech motor control and stuttering: A computa-tional model for adaptive sensory-motor processing. *Speech Communication* 6 (4), 325–333.

Neville, H.J., Bavelier, D., Corina, D., Rauschecker, J., Karni, A. and Lalwani, A. (1998) Cerebral organization for language in deaf and hearing subjects: Biological constraints and effects of experience. *Proceedings of the National Academy of Science* 95, 922–929.

Newman, A.J., Bavelier, D., Corina, D., Jezzard, P. and Neville, H.J. (2002) A critical period for right hemisphere recruitment in American Sign Language processing. *Nature Neuroscience* 5, 76–80.

Newport, E.L. and Meier, R.P. (1985) The acquisition of American Sign Language. In D.I. Slobin (ed.) *The Crosslinguistic Study of Language Acquisition* (Vol. 2, pp. 881–938). Mahwah, NJ: Lawrence Erlbaum.

Nudelman, H., Herbrich, K., Hoyt, B. and Rosenfield, D. (1989) A neuro-science model of stuttering. *Journal of Fluency Disorders* 14, 399-427.

Ormel, E., Hermans, D., Knoors, H. and Verhoeven, L. (2009) The role of sign phonology and iconicity during sign processing: The case of deaf children. *Journal of Deaf Studies and Deaf Education* 14, 436–448.

Padden, C. (1998) The ASL lexicon. *Sign Language and Linguistics* 1, 39–60.

Padden, C. (2006) Learning fingerspelling twice: Young children's acquisition of finger-spelling. In M. Marschark, B. Schick and P. Spencer (eds) *Advances in Sign Language Development of Deaf Children* (pp. 189–201). New York: Oxford University Press.

Padden, C. and Gansauls, C. (2003) How the alphabet came to be used in a sign language. *Sign Language Studies* 4 (1), 10–33.

Penn, C., Commerford, A. and Ogilvy, D. (2007) Spatial and facial processing in the signed discourse of two groups of deaf signers with clinical language impairment. *Clinical Linguistics & Phonetics* 21, 369–391.

Perfetti, C. and Sandak, R. (2000) Reading optimally builds on spoken language: Implications for deaf readers. *Journal of Deaf Studies and Deaf Education* 5 (1), 32–50.

Perniss, P.M. (2012) Use of sign space. In R. Pfau, M. Steinbach, and B. Woll (eds) *Sign Language: An International Handbook* (pp. 412–431). Berlin: Mouton de Gruyter.

Perniss, P., Thompson, R. and Vigliocco, G. (2010) Iconicity as a general property of lan-guage: Evidence from spoken and signed languages. *Frontiers in Psychology* 1, 227. See http://www.frontiersin.org/Journal/Abstract.aspx?ART_DOI = 10.3389/fpsyg.2010.00227&name = language_sciences.

Petitto, L.A. (1987) On the autonomy of language and gesture: Evidence from the acquisition of personal pronouns in American Sign Language. *Cognition* 27, 1–52.

Petitto, L.A., Katerelos, M., Levy, B.G., Gauna, K., Tétreault, K. and Ferraro, V. (2001) Bilingual signed and spoken language acquisition from birth: Implications for the mechanisms underlying early bilingual language acquisition. *Journal of Child Language* 28, 453–496.

Picard, M. (2004) Children with permanent hearing loss and associated disabilities: Revisiting current epidemiological data and causes of deafness. *Volta Review* 104, 221–236.

Piñar, P., Dussias, P.E. and Morford, J.P. (2011) Deaf readers as bilinguals: An examination of deaf readers' print comprehension in light of current advances in bilingualism and second language processing. *Language and Linguistics Compass* 5 (10), 691–704.

Poizner, H., Bellugi, U. and Iragui, V. (1984) Apraxia and aphasia for a visual-gestural language. *American Journal of Physiology – Regulatory, Integrative and Comparative Physiology* 246, R868–R883.

Poizner, H., Klima, E.S. and Bellugi, U. (1987) *What the Hands Reveal About the Brain.* Cambridge, MA: MIT Press.

Pyers, J.E., Shusterman, A., Senghas, A., Spelke, E. and Emmorey, K. (2010) Evidence from an emerging sign language reveals that language supports spatial language. *Proceedings of the National Academy of Sciences* 107 (27), 12116–12120.

Quinto-Pozos, D. (2002) Deixis in the visual/gestural and tactile/gestural modalities. In R.P. Meier, K. Cormier and D. Quinto-Pozos (eds) *Modality and Structure in Signed and Spoken Languages* (pp. 442–467). Cambridge: Cambridge University Press.

Quinto-Pozos, D. and Parrill, F. (submitted) Signers and co-speech gesturers adopt similar strategies for portraying viewpoint in narratives.

Quinto-Pozos, D. (2010) Rates of fingerspelling in American Sign Language. Poster given at the *10th Theoretical Issues in Sign Language Research Conference*, Purdue University, West Lafayette, IL.

Quinto-Pozos, D., Forber-Pratt, A. and Singleton, J. (2011) Do developmental signed language disorders exist? Perspectives from professionals. *Language, Speech, and Hearing Services in Schools* 42, 1–21.

Quinto-Pozos, D., Singleton, J. and Hauser, P. (in preparation) A case for Specific Language Impairment (SLI) in American Sign Language.

Quinto-Pozos, D., Singleton, J., Hauser, P., Levine, S., Garberoglio, C.L. and Hou, L. (in press) Atypical signed language development: A case study of challenges with visual-spatial processing. *Cognitive Neuropsychology.*

Sandler, W. and Lillo-Martin, D. (2006) *Sign Language and Linguistic Universals.* Cambridge: Cambridge University Press.

Schembri, A. (2003) Rethinking 'classifiers' in signed languages. In K. Emmorey (ed.) *Perspectives on Classifier Constructions in Sign Languages.* Mahwah, NJ: Lawrence Erlbaum.

Schwartz, R.G. (2009) Specific language impairment. In R.G. Schwartz (ed.) *Handbook of Child Language Disorders* (pp. 3–43). New York: Psychological Press.

Seal, B.C. and Bonvillian, J.D. (1997) Sign language and motor functioning in students with autistic disorder. *Journal of Autism and Developmental Disorders* 27, 437–466.

Sheng, L., Peña, E., Bedore, L. and Fiestas, C.E. (2012) Semantic deficits in Spanish–English bilingual children with language impairment. *Journal of Speech, Language, and Hearing Research* 55, 1–15.

Shield, A. and Meier, R.P. (2012) Palm reversal errors in native-signing children with autism. *Journal of Communication Disorders* 45, 439–454.

Supalla, T. (1982) Structure and acquisition of verbs of motion and location in American Sign Language. Unpublished doctoral dissertation, University of California, San Diego.

Talbot, K.F. and Haude, R.H. (1993) The relationship between sign language skill and spatial visualization ability: Mental rotation of three-dimensional objects. *Perceptual and Motor Skills* 77, 1387–1391.

Tallal, P. and Benasich, A.A. (2002) Developmental language learning impairments. *Development and Psychopathology* 14, 559–579.

Taub, S. (2001) *Language from the Body: Iconicity and Metaphor in American Sign Language.* New York: Cambridge University Press.

Thompson, R., Emmorey, K. and Gollan, T. (2005) Tip-of-fingers experiences for ASL signers: Insights into the organization of a sign-based lexicon. *Psychological Science* 16, 856–860.

Thompson, R.L., Vinson, D.P., Woll, B. and Vigliocco, G. (2012) The road to language learning is iconic: Evidence from British Sign Language. *Psychological Science* 23 (12), 1443–1448.

Tomblin, B., Records, N., Buckwater, P., Zhang, X., Smith, E. and O'Brien, M. (1997) Prevalence of specific language impairment in kindergarten children. *Journal of Speech, Language and Hearing Research* 40, 1245–1260.

Tyrone, M. (2007) Simultaneity in atypical signers. In M. Vermeerbergen, L. Leeson and O. Crasborn (eds) *Simultaneity in Signed Languages, Form and Function* (pp. 317–335). Amsterdam: John Benjamins.

Tyrone, M. and Woll, B. (2008) Sign phonetics and the motor system: Implications from Parkinson's disease. In J. Quer (ed.) *Signs of the Time: Selected Papers from TISLR 2004. International Studies on Sign Language and Communication of the Deaf* 51, 43–58.

Tyrone, M.E., Atkinson, J.R., Marshall, J. and Woll, B. (2009) The effects of cerebellar ataxia on sign language production: A case study. *Neurocase* 15 (5), 419–426.

Verhoeven, J., De Pauw, G. and Kloots, H. (2004) Speech rate in a pluricentric language: A comparison between Dutch in Belgium and the Netherlands. *Language and Speech* 47, 297–308.

Visual Language and Visual Learning Science of Learning Center (2012) *Eye Gaze and Joint Attention.* Research Brief No. 5. Washington, DC: Amy M. Lieberman.

Wilbur, R.B. and Allen, G.D. (1991) Perceptual evidence against internal structure in ASL syllables. *Language and Speech* 34, 27–46.

Wilbur, R.B. and Nolen, S.B. (1986) The duration of syllables in American Sign Language. *Language and Speech* 29, 263–280.

Wilbur, R. and Petersen, L. (1997) Backwards signing and ASL syllable structure. *Language and Speech* 40, 63–90.

Wilson, M., Bettger, J., Niculae, I. and Klima, E. (1997) Modality of language shapes working memory: Evidence from digit span and spatial span in ASL signers. *Journal of Deaf Studies and Deaf Education* 2, 150–160.

Windsor, J., Kohnert, K., Loxtercamp, A.L. and Pui-Fong, K. (2008) Performance on non-linguistic visual tasks by children with language impairment. *Applied Psycholinguistics* 29 (2), 237–268.

Woll, B. (2012) Atypical signing. In R. Pfau, M. Steinbach and B. Woll (eds) *Sign Language: An International Handbook* (pp. 762–787). Berlin: Mouton de Gruyter.

Woll, B. and Morgan, G. (2012) Language impairments in the development of sign: Do they reside in a specific modality or are they modality-independent deficits? *Bilingualism, Language and Cognition* 15, 75–87.

Woll, B. and Sutton-Spence, R. (1999) *The Linguistics of British Sign Language: An Introduction.* Cambridge: Cambridge University Press.

Zakia, R.D. and Haber, R.N. (1971) Sequential letter and word recognition in deaf and hearing subjects. *Perception & Psychophysics* 9, 110–114.

Part 1

Developmental Language Disorders in the Signed Modality

2 Profiling SLI in Deaf Children who are Sign Language Users

Rosalind Herman, Katherine Rowley, Chloë Marshall, Kathryn Mason, Joanna Atkinson, Bencie Woll and Gary Morgan

Introduction

Specific language impairment (SLI) is traditionally defined as a deficit in language acquisition which occurs in the absence of any cognitive, social or neurological difficulty (Leonard, 1998). It is estimated that the disorder occurs in approximately 7% of children (Tomblin *et al.*, 1997). While there is some debate as to how specific to language development the problems are (cf. Botting, 2005), it is still the case that language is relatively more impaired than other cognitive domains in children diagnosed with SLI. Deficits have been identified in syntax, morphology, phonology, the lexicon and pragmatics, and in receptive and expressive language. However, currently there is widespread disagreement as to the underlying cause of SLI.

Cross-linguistic studies (reviewed by Leonard, 2009) have added to our knowledge of how SLI may present across different spoken languages. However, until recently there has been almost no research determining whether or not SLI occurs in deaf children acquiring signed languages. One reason for this is that hearing loss is specifically excluded when diagnosing SLI, meaning that deaf children are not identified or included in studies of SLI in spoken languages. The rationale is obvious – a hearing impairment would be expected to affect spoken language development. In contrast, there is no reason to expect a hearing impairment to impact on the acquisition of a language in the visuo-gestural modality. Furthermore, if genetic contributions to SLI hold true for all children, then the incidence of SLI should be at least the same in children who are born deaf (or who are the hearing offspring of deaf signing parents) as in the general population, if not higher due to neural predispositions caused by organic aetiologies of deafness (e.g. conditions related to premature birth). SLI should therefore be identifiable in deaf children acquiring a signed language and, if so, may provide insights moving beyond the immediate population of deaf children to theories about the nature of the deficit underlying SLI in the general population.

One problem for identification of SLI is that 90–95% of deaf children are from hearing families (Mitchell & Karchmer, 2004). Although many such children eventually become fluent users of sign language, they frequently experience delayed and impoverished sign language exposure at the crucial early stages of language development and throughout their school years, since parents and professionals are often unable to provide fluent sign language models. Thus, distinguishing the consequences of language delay from SLI is challenging.

A further complexity arises when distinguishing signs from gestures. While a linguistic description is available for British Sign Language (BSL) in its fully formed adult model (Sutton-Spence & Woll, 1999) young deaf children (especially those with hearing non-signing parents) are adept at using the visual modality creatively to communicate. For example, many iconic signs for actions resemble same-meaning gestures used by hearing children. However, lexical signs differ from gestures on many levels. Like words, signs have a phonological structure, and minimal pairs can be found which contrast in handshape, location and movement. For example, the signs AFTERNOON and NAME in BSL differ only in location (chin and forehead respectively). There are phonotactic constraints (for example, if both hands move, signs must have identical handshapes and symmetrical movements), and sign languages differ in their phonological inventories (for example, some handshapes which occur in BSL are not found in American Sign Language – ASL). Although signs may enter the language via gesture, there is no distinction between iconic and non-iconic signs in phonological structure, and there is also evidence that signs and gestures dissociate in neurological conditions, with evidence of spared gesture use in adults with sign language aphasia (Marshall et al., 2004).

At the syntactic level, some linguists have suggested that sign languages incorporate both language and gesture. Signers mark person by modifying the direction the sign moves, either towards present referents or towards abstract locations in the signing space in front of the signer. Signers also describe the location and movement of persons and objects through devices termed 'classifiers' in sign space (see Sandler & Lillo-Martin, 2006). Liddell (2003) has argued that such visual-spatial devices in sign languages have a semi-gestural status, similar to pointing and co-speech gesture.

We did consider the possibility that children with a language impairment in sign acquisition may be more reliant on gesture to communicate because they lack models of sign language. To rule out this possibility, the involvement from the beginning of the research of both sign language linguists and native signers was crucial. In addition, in our studies we focused on children exposed to good models of BSL for several years before diagnosing SLI.

As we gain greater knowledge about native and non-native sign language acquisition, differences between sign languages, gesture and artificial sign-based communication systems, and with the availability of standardized sign language assessments (Herman *et al.*, 1999, 2004), we are in a stronger position to investigate SLI among deaf children who sign. Indeed, a small number of studies in recent years have reported SLI in deaf children who are learning BSL (Mason *et al.*, 2010; Morgan *et al.*, 2007) and ASL (Quinto-Pozos *et al.*, 2011). This chapter presents a detailed overview of findings from our work documenting the sign language comprehension and production abilities of the same group of children with SLI initially identified by Mason *et al.* (2010) and, in particular, describes how new measures were developed to further investigate and characterize SLI in sign language users.

Theories of the Origins of SLI

There are a number of theories that attempt to explain the specific difficulty with phonology, syntax and morphology found in SLI. Each differs in its view as to where the underlying deficit lies. One early framework attributed the language-learning problem to a difficulty with underlying low-level auditory processing (Tallal & Piercy, 1973). Following this argument, children with SLI have difficulty processing the temporal characteristics of rapidly changing acoustic signals (at around 60 ms) for both speech and non-verbal auditory signals. This difficulty leads to the child forming unstable phonological representations of speech sounds and so interferes with the encoding and production of speech (Tallal, 2000; but see Bishop *et al.*, 1999). Since this theory is specific to the auditory modality, it excludes the possibility of language impairment in a child exposed to a non-auditory language, i.e. a signed language, which in any event has slower temporal contrasts (Klima & Bellugi, 1979). If this theory instead focused on a rapid signal, auditory or visual it could possibly account for sign SLI.

However, other processing accounts can encompass sign language impairments more readily (e.g. Kail, 1994; Leonard, 1998). One theory focuses on a reduced ability to store information in the cognitive system that deals with phonological short-term memory (Gathercole & Baddeley, 1990), with consequences for the development of speech, which depends heavily on phonological storage capacity. Given that phonological short-term memory is also involved in the processing of visuo-spatial languages (Hall & Bavelier, 2010; Marshall *et al.*, 2011), it is possible that impaired phonological short-term memory is involved in SLI in this modality too.

Leonard (1998) makes a distinction between perceptually salient and non-salient morphemes, with children with SLI predicted to have difficulties with non-salient ones. Because this approach is cross-linguistic it can be applied to both spoken and sign languages. Saliency in spoken language is defined differently in each spoken language (e.g. Dromi *et al.*, 1999). Limited processing capacity affects those morphological targets that involve several co-occurring underlying operations. According to Kail's (1994) 'Generalized Slowing Hypothesis', children with SLI process linguistic and non-linguistic input at a slower rate than typically developing children, and it is this which affects the acquisition process. There are several candidate linguistic construction types in British Sign Language (BSL) grammar, specifically complex sentences involving verb agreement and classifier constructions, non-manual scope that stretches across multiple manual signs in negations or questions, and also the coherent use of discourse markers such as role shift (akin to reported speech) across sentences.

In contrast to the previous general processing framework, some researchers claim that SLI is caused by a deficit that is specific to the computation of language rules (Rice & Wexler, 1996; Ullman & Gopnik, 1999; van der Lely & Ullman, 2001), and therefore would also predict that SLI is not unique to one modality. There are a number of models within this approach and they vary as to where in the linguistic system the deficit is purported to exist. One of the most thoroughly articulated, the Computational Grammatical Complexity (CGC) hypothesis (Marshall, 2006; van der Lely, 2005; van der Lely & Marshall, 2011), claims that the core components of grammar, that rely on the computation of rules (syntax, morphology and phonology), are most affected in SLI. The deficit in each component of grammar lies in the formation of complex structural representations. The CGC would predict SLI in signed languages, with children manifesting particular difficulties in constructions that are complex across components of grammar, such as classifiers.

In considering competing theories, most researchers acknowledge that because SLI is a heterogeneous disorder, no one account could explain all cases of language disorder. Identification of SLI in a visuomotor language presents a unique opportunity to shed further light on current theories of SLI.

Initial Identification of Deaf Children with SLI: Developing a Sample Through a Screening Questionnaire

For several years prior to the systematic studies we carried out, professionals working with deaf children reported to us that they suspected they had signing deaf children with SLI on their clinical caseloads. During our work conducting assessments of sign language development at the Compass Centre clinic at City University London, it became obvious to us that deaf children, even those with native or high-quality sign language exposure early in development, could display language impairments above and beyond typical language delays. During that time we reported on a deaf child of deaf parents who had sign language SLI despite native input (Morgan et al., 2007). Because this child had deaf parents, his delayed language development in sign language could not be explained by late or inadequate exposure. The number of both deaf and hearing children of deaf parents who we saw in our clinic began to grow and so we planned a group study to ascertain what SLI might look like in a sign language, and to estimate the incidence of SLI in the school-age deaf signing population.

Initial identification of deaf children with suspected SLI for inclusion in the study was carried out using a questionnaire sent to schools and speech and language therapists working with deaf children (Mason et al., 2010). The questionnaire contained a screening checklist of characteristics associated with SLI (see Table 2.1). As there was no precedent for sign language, a list of transferable characteristics of SLI were taken from studies of spoken languages (as reviewed by Leonard, 1988, 2009). Although SLI in spoken languages is typically characterized by grammatical deficits, it was not felt appropriate to include them in the checklist since we were concerned that teachers and speech and language therapists might not have sufficient knowledge of BSL grammar or BSL acquisition to be able to comment on this area reliably. The intention was to identify children based on teacher or clinician concern and then follow this up with assessments of performance on a range of standardized and newly developed measures, similar to approaches used with bilingual children suspected of having language impairments in spoken languages (Paradis et al., 2005; Sheng et al., 2012).

Further background information was collected as follows:

- degree of hearing loss;
- use of cochlear implant and/or hearing aids;
- age of first exposure to signing;
- means of communication – BSL, SSE, and spoken languages used at home and at school;
- exposure to fluent signers at home and/or at school;
- medical history that might exclude the child from our sample (e.g. neurological impairments or head injury).

In addition, where a child was identified as a possible SLI case, teachers and speech and language therapists were asked to report the number of deaf children attending the same school in order to gauge the proportion of children identified across the educational settings from which the SLI sample was drawn. Questionnaires were sent out to 72 mainstream schools, schools for deaf children and units for hearing impaired children around the UK; 50 completed questionnaires were returned, each identifying a potential participant. Of the 50 children referred, one child was excluded based on a prior

Table 2.1 SLI screening checklist

*When compared to their signing peers
of the same age, does the child:*

	Yes	No	Unsure	Comments
Have difficulty following instructions in sign language?				
Often misunderstand what is signed?				
Have difficulty understanding what is being signed?				
Often ask for repetition?				
Often use gesture rather than signs?				
Have poor memory for language information?				
Become easily distracted in busy or noisy environments?				
Get labelled as a daydreamer or in their own world?				
Have social difficulties with friendships, being left out, withdrawing from conversation, being bullied or bullying others?				
Benefit less from hearing aids or CI than expected for their degree of hearing loss?				
Show strengths in maths ability, which is noticeably superior to language ability?				
Show strengths in visuospatial ability (e.g. sports, puzzles, computer games, etc.), which is noticeably superior to language ability?				
Respond best to visual aids and non-language cues?				
Is the child reading at a lower level than expected, compared with their deaf peers of the same age?				
Have problems thinking of right word/sign?				
Show hesitation during signing?				
Show frustration during signing?				
Have a noticeably poor sense of rhythm?				

diagnosis of autism and five others because of failure to obtain consent. A further five children were excluded following discussion with teachers where it emerged that only reading and not language was affected; seven children could not be tested due to difficulties in arranging visits within the time frame of the study; one child refused to take part and data from one child could not be included due to corruption of video data. This left a final sample size of 30 children (16 male) ranging in age from 5 to 15 years (mean age 11 years 5 months).

Initial Identification of the Sample: Use of Standardized Measures

The next phase of the study involved the use of standardized measures to eliminate children with low non-verbal cognitive abilities or impaired motor difficulties that might contribute to their communication difficulties, thereby excluding a possible diagnosis of SLI. In addition, standardized measures of BSL development were used to confirm that the children's language development was below that expected for their age. Worldwide, very few standardized measures of sign language exist. This is due to difficulties in obtaining a sufficiently large sample, given the size and nature of the deaf population and also because of the limited research on sign language and sign language acquisition in many countries (for a discussion of this and other issues, see Mann, 2008). We were fortunate in having two available measures. For each, the standardization was based on a sample comprising native signers, deaf children in hearing families on bilingual (sign language/English) educational programmes, and deaf children in hearing families on Total Communication programmes (using a range of communication approaches including sign language and English-based sign systems). Since these assessments are based in the main on children in optimal language-learning environments, performance on these tests was used as an initial guideline. In subsequent testing, children's scores were compared with those of children from similar language-learning backgrounds.

The measures used and the corresponding cut-offs are described below. All testing was carried out in schools by a deaf native signer (second author) and a hearing researcher with a good level of fluency in BSL (fourth author).

Non-verbal cognitive abilities

Children were tested on three subtests of the British Ability Scales (BAS; Elliot *et al.*, 1996) to determine their non-verbal abilities: Matrices, Pattern Construction and Recall of Design. The BAS has been used successfully with British deaf children in recent studies (e.g. Kyle & Harris, 2006).

Our criterion for inclusion in the SLI group was a combined z score of −1.2 or below. Nine of the 30 children were excluded on the basis of low non-verbal abilities.

Motor dexterity

To establish whether language production difficulties might be related to poor fine motor skills affecting hand and eye coordination, a timed standardized bead-threading task (White *et al.*, 2006) was used. Children were timed twice as they threaded 15 large coloured beads onto a piece of string and the faster time was recorded. This was then compared to data collected for typically developing deaf and hearing children aged 3–11 years, reported in Mann *et al.* (2010). One child obtained a low score relative to age-related norms for motor dexterity, and was subsequently excluded.

BSL development

Two standardized tests of BSL development were used: the BSL Receptive Skills Test (Herman *et al.*, 1999) and the BSL Production Test (Herman *et al.*, 2004).

The BSL receptive skills test

This is a video-based test of comprehension of morphosyntax with norms derived from deaf children acquiring BSL aged 3–13 years. The child watches pre-recorded signed sentences presented individually in order of difficulty and after each has to select the picture representing the target sentence from a choice of three or four closely related alternatives. The test allows information to be derived about a child's strengths and weaknesses in different areas of BSL grammar such as negation, spatial verbs and number agreement. The cut-off for impaired performance on this task was set at a z score of −1.3 or below, based on previous research on SLI in spoken language.

The BSL production test

This test uses a story recall technique to elicit a narrative. The child watches a short story acted out by two deaf children, presented on a DVD. The child is then asked to tell the story in BSL, and is videorecorded for subsequent scoring. The assessment is scored in three parts: (1) the propositional content of the story, i.e. how much information children include in their narrative; (2) structural components of the narrative, i.e. introducing the participants and the setting, reporting the key events leading up to the climax of the story, and telling how the story ends; and (3) aspects of BSL grammar, including use of spatial location, person and object classifiers and role shift (see Sutton-Spence & Woll, 1999, for details of these aspects of BSL linguistics). The test is standardized on deaf children aged 4–11 years with early BSL exposure, and percentile scores can be calculated for each of the three parts individually.

Two raters independently scored all children and subsequently compared scores. There was over 90% agreement and for the small number of disagreements, the raters arrived at a consensus after discussion. The cut-off for impaired performance on each of the three parts of this task was set at a score at or below the 10th percentile.

Using the standardized language measures, three children were found to have language within the normal range and were therefore excluded from the sample.

Identification of a Group of Children with Sign Language SLI

A final sample of 17 children (11 male) with a mean age of 10 years (range 5;00–14;08) achieved scores within the normal range on the non-verbal and motor dexterity measures but fell outside the expected range on the two BSL development measures. Cognitive and language profiles showing relative strengths and weaknesses for these individuals are presented in Table 2.2.

At this point we were able to say that our original findings from case studies that deaf children who use sign language could present with SLI was borne out. We were able to demonstrate that this was not an anecdotal or isolated occurrence. Our recruitment process identified 17 out of 50 children initially referred who fitted the profile of SLI. We assert that SLI is a developmental disorder not restricted to spoken languages or the auditory modality. Just as language acquisition proceeds in largely the same manner across modalities (Chamberlain *et al.*, 2000; Morgan & Woll, 2002; Schick *et al.*, 2006), it would appear that developmental breakdowns specific to language comprehension and production are equally possible within the visuomotor modality. An understanding of the exact ways in which SLI in sign language manifests itself will require far more specific testing and profiling. This finding has far-reaching consequences for how we view language impairments. At a general level we can say that BSL does not offer a way for deaf children with SLI to compensate for their linguistic deficits. BSL offers just as much of a challenge for a child with a language impairment as acquiring English or any other spoken language.

Profiling Language Skills and Impairment: Developing New Tests

In the second stage of our project, the 17 children identified with SLI underwent further testing using a series of measures designed to explore

Table 2.2 Non-verbal IQ and language test scores for children with SLI

Child	BAS z-score	BSL Receptive Test z-score	BSL Production Test percentile scores		
			Narrative content	Narrative structure	BSL grammar
1	−0.6	0.3*	25*	50*	10*
2	−0.6	<−2.1	<10	<10	<10
3	−0.1	1.1*	10*	10*	25*
4	−0.9	−1.5	10*	10*	10*
5	0.6	−2.1	<10	<10	<10
6	−0.7	0.1	25	10	50
7	−1.2	<−2.1	<10	10	25
8	−1.2	0.6	<10	<10	25
9	−0.6	−2.3	10	25	10
10	0.3	−1.5	<10	<10	<10
11	−0.5	<−2.1	<10	<10	<10
12	0.7	1.1	<10	10	<10
13	−1.0	−0.7	10	50	10
14	0.2	−1.0	10	10	10
15	−0.9	−0.3	10	10	10
16	−1	−0.7	10	50	10
17	0.7	0.8	10	75	25
Range	−1.2–0.6	−2.1–1.1	<10–25	<10–50	<10–50

Notes: Cells shaded in grey represent performance below our pre-set cut-offs.

*Indicates children who are older than the standardization sample. Their performance was compared to the oldest norms available; thus the magnitude of their poor performance is in fact worse than it appears here.

their language difficulties. Our aim was to further characterize areas of sign language acquisition that were fragile or robust in the face of language impairment. There are relatively few BSL assessments in the UK; therefore, in addition to an existing measure, the Nonsense Sign Repetition Test (NSRT) (Mann *et al.*, 2010), four new tests were created for this study based on previous research into SLI in hearing children:

(1) Nonsense Sign Repetition Test (Mann *et al.*, 2010; Marshall *et al.*, 2011);
(2) Semantic Fluency Task (Marshall *et al.*, 2013);
(3) Lexical Development Test;
(4) BSL child Sentence Repetition Test (Marshall *et al.*, submitted);
(5) Narrative Details Test (Herman *et al.*, in revision).

Where existing norms were not available for the new measures, comparison data were collected from a control group of deaf children for whom there were no concerns about language acquisition or cognitive abilities, and who were matched for age, gender, parental hearing status and quality of BSL exposure. The last factor is perhaps the most crucial and to achieve this in as many cases as possible, children came from the same schools as the SLI participants. Next we describe the characteristics of the new tests, how they were developed and, as analysis is ongoing, findings for our sample where these are available.

(1) Nonsense sign repetition task (NSRT)

The ability to repeat nonsense or non-words (i.e. spoken forms that follow the phonotactics of a particular language but have no meaning) is a robust measure of SLI and of general language development in spoken languages (Gathercole & Baddeley, 1990). Children learning new words use short-term working memory to rehearse sounds they hear in order to activate meanings, as well as to lay down their first phonological representations in long-term memory. Marshall *et al.* (2006) created a test of non-sign repetition developed along similar lines to published and experimental spoken tests of non-word repetition (e.g. Gathercole & Baddeley, 1990). The task consists of 40 non-signs that are plausible BSL signs, in that they do not violate phonological rules, but they do not exist in the BSL lexicon (see Marshall *et al.*, 2006; Mann *et al.*, 2010, for more details). The nonsense signs within the test are graded for complexity linked to markedness of handshape and movement. In the test, signs are presented one by one on a computer screen and the child is required to copy them as accurately as possible. After every 10 signs, there is a brief cartoon break before the test continues (i.e. a total of three breaks). Responses are filmed and are subsequently coded according to accuracy of handshape, internal hand movement and path of movement.

Age norms are available based on 91 typically developing deaf children aged 3–11 years (Mann *et al.*, 2010), and a significant correlation has been found between the accuracy at repetition of non-signs, comprehension of BSL grammar, and motor skills based on bead-threading (Mann *et al.*, 2010).

Inter-rater reliability was established at 96.6% for overall score. The cutoff for impaired performance on this task is set at a z score of −1.3 or below. Of the 17 children identified initially as having SLI, five performed at or below this level. Thus it appears that repeating non-signs is a weak skill in only a subset of our sample of sign language users as opposed to being a defining feature as has been reported for spoken language SLI. We present some possible explanations for this somewhat unexpected finding in the general discussion section at the end of this chapter.

(2) Semantic Fluency Task

In a semantic fluency task in a spoken language, participants are asked to produce as many words as they can from a specific semantic category, such as 'animals' or 'food', within a limited time period (e.g. 1 minute). As the child produces each item, the assumption is that other semantically related items will be activated. The order of item generation is an indication of the proximity of items to each other in the lexicon. Although the time limit does not allow the child to produce an exhaustive list of the words they know, the test does reveal the items that come most readily to mind. In this way, the test gives an indication of semantic organization and the child's ability to use different language processing strategies to generate items within the specified category.

Only a few research studies have used a semantic fluency task with hearing children who have SLI. Henry *et al.* (2012) reported scores for English-speaking children with SLI below those of their chronological age-matched controls on both verbal and non-verbal fluency tasks. In a slightly different test probing lexical organization, children with SLI performed more poorly than typically developing peers matched for expressive vocabulary ability (Sheng & McGregor, 2010). However, the SLI group in Sheng and McGregor (2010) as a whole was characterized by variable performance, and some children performed age-appropriately.

We decided to use a semantic fluency task to investigate lexical organization in our SLI participants in comparison to a control group. Two semantic categories were used: 'food' and 'animals'. Children were instructed to name animal/food items in BSL as quickly as possible and timed for one minute. 'Colours' was used as a practice category. Responses were videorecorded and subsequently glossed into English for counting and coding. Inter-rater reliability was established at 90%.

Our findings indicated no differences between the SLI and control groups in terms of overall numbers or types of responses (Marshall *et al.*, 2013). However, subtle differences were observed: the SLI group produced fewer signs in the first 15 seconds than the control participants and there was also some evidence of word-finding difficulty in the SLI group, suggesting that their access to signs was poorer (Marshall *et al.*, 2013).

(3) Lexical development test

Our semantic fluency results support findings that hearing children with SLI may have slower lexical access (see Messer & Dockrell, 2006 for a review). We included a further measure of lexical knowledge in our test battery in the form of a picture-naming task.

Initially, the adaptation of existing English vocabulary tests such as the British Picture Vocabulary Scale (Dunn *et al.*, 1997) was considered. However, problems were presented by the iconicity of some signs and difficulties with the exact translation of some items. An iconic sign is one with a visual moti-vation that links the meaning of the referent to its form, e.g. WORLD in BSL, where the sign is represented by two hands outlining a large sphere. Indeed, iconic signs such as TOOTHBRUSH in BSL are readily recognized by non-signers since this sign depicts the action of brushing one's teeth (Sutton-Spence & Woll, 1999). Body part vocabulary in BSL often just requires pointing to specific parts of the body; e.g. NOSE is shown by point-ing to the nose (Sutton-Spence & Woll, 1999). These and other highly iconic signs are likely to be less challenging to acquire in a sign language than the equivalent lexical items would be in English.

As well as these issues, there are also words in English vocabulary tests that do not have an exact equivalent sign in BSL: either the same sign can be used for two different meanings or the same English word can be represented by two different signs. For these reasons it was decided to develop a measure specifically for BSL.

A key challenge in developing a lexical test in BSL is the lack of informa-tion about lexical development among children who are acquiring BSL nor-mally. Fortunately, a norming study (Vinson et al., 2008) was being conducted with adult signers at the time with the specific purpose of collecting norma-tive data about BSL for use in language processing studies. The norming study looked at age of acquisition of vocabulary by asking deaf adult partici-pants to recall when they learned particular signs. Although this appears to be relatively subjective, the data does correlate with data collected on native child signers' lexical acquisition (Thompson et al., 2012) using the BSL ver-sion of the MacArthur Communicative Development Inventory (Woolfe et al., 2009). In addition, the Vinson et al. (2008) norming study collected data about the familiarity of signs by asking adult participants to score how often the sign was seen in everyday conversation, using a Likert scale of 1–7.

Picturable items from the age of acquisition and familiarity data sets were used in the creation of the BSL vocabulary development measure. Items identified as highly iconic, easily gesturable or with high regional variation were excluded. The aim was to create a test that ranged from easy to difficult signs. The signs that were rated as being highly familiar and to have been acquired at a young age by Vinson et al. (2008) were included as easier vocab-ulary items and conversely signs that had a low familiarity rating and were acquired at a later age comprised the more difficult items on the vocabulary development measure. In addition, in order to arrive at an ecologically valid test, staff at two deaf schools were asked to suggest vocabulary that was used within the classroom environment and these items were also included.

A pilot version of the test was developed using a picture-naming proce-dure and stimuli were presented to children on a laptop. As there were some items that were not possible to depict (abstract items such as MAYBE, NEVER), an extension to the vocabulary test was developed in the form of a definitions test. For this part of the assessment, children watched a video of 22 signs presented individually by deaf adults and were asked to explain the meaning of each sign and the context in which it would be used.

Pilot versions of the vocabulary and definitions tests were trialled on six deaf adults and six deaf children who used BSL, to eliminate problematic items. Changes were made to pictures from the vocabulary test which did not effectively elicit the target response. Items from the definitions test were also removed where none of the pilot participants could give an appropriate definition or where the sign had more than one meaning.

The final version of the vocabulary test included 84 pictures to be named and 50 signs which had to be defined. A score of one point was given for an appropriate sign (vocabulary test) or description of the meaning of each sign (definitions test). An additional point was awarded for a correct example of the context in which the sign would be used (definitions test). Criteria for what constituted a correct response were compiled. For both parts of the assessments, instructions on how to do the test were pre-recorded by a deaf native signer so all children saw the same set of instructions. Responses were filmed and subsequently scored. Inter-rater reliability was established at 95.6% for this measure. The data analysis for the vocabulary test is still ongoing.

(4) BSL child sentence repetition test

Sentence repetition is a component of many different spoken language tests devised to diagnose SLI (Gardner *et al.*, 2006; Seeff-Gabriel *et al.*, 2008; Semel *et al.*, 2003). The task requires the child to repeat back a recorded or spoken sentence as accurately as they can. This type of test has been used across a range of spoken languages, such as Italian (Volterra *et al.*, 2003), German (Snow & Höfnagel-Höhle, 1978), French (Maillart & Parisse, 2008), Cantonese (Stokes & Fletcher, 2003) and Dutch (Rispens, 2004). A sign repetition test has also been developed for adult signers of ASL (Hauser *et al.*, 2008). Hauser *et al.* have shown this test to be sensitive to language proficiency with respect to language acquisition experience, with native signers performing more accurately than non-natives. However, the ASL test has not to date been used to differentiate typically developing from language-impaired signers.

The child BSL sentence repetition test required children to repeat 20 signed sentences (including three practice items). All sentences were developed and recorded by a native BSL signer. The sentences were presented in order of complexity, as defined by the number of signs and clauses in the sentence. A glossed example from the start of the test is BOY WAIT (the boy is waiting), and one of the last and most demanding sentences is GIRL WALK SUDDENLY RAIN AWFUL WET (the girl was walking, when suddenly there was a downpour and she became awfully wet).

Many standardized sentence repetition tests are scored simply as 'correct' or 'incorrect' regardless of the nature of the error. In order to make more detailed comparisons between the SLI and control groups, we devised an in-depth scoring system that allowed investigation of error patterns. Participants' repetition accuracy was scored for: (1) exact replication of the lexical items used by the model in the target sentence; (2) accurate reproduction of the overall meaning of the sentence even where different lexical items were used; (3) accurate and consistent use of spatial placement; (4) accurate reproduction of facial expression (for those sentences to which it applied); (5) order of items in the sentence; and (6) verbatim repetition, i.e. if the child reproduced the sentence exactly as it was signed, they would obtain an overall score of five or six (some items did not include facial expression or placement). If the child did not reproduce the sentence accurately, they would lose points where they made errors, e.g. wrong lexical item, altering the overall meaning, inaccurate placement, inaccurate facial expression and/or using a different sign order. Inter-rater reliability using this method of scoring was 96.4%.

The test is presented on a laptop. First, participants view instructions in BSL presented by a native signer directing them to repeat each sentence exactly immediately after the screen fades to black. Three practice sentences are shown and participants are encouraged to repeat each one as accurately as possible. If the child does not copy the practice sentence exactly, it is demonstrated by the tester. Once it is established that the child understands what is required, the 17 test sentences follow. Each sentence is viewed once. The child's responses are videorecorded for later scoring and analysis. Participant performance in comparison to our control group is reported in Marshall *et al.* (in revision).

(5) Narrative details test

Narrative skills develop over a protracted period, beginning with early word combinations and reaching peak complexity at around the ages of 10–12 years (Berman & Slobin, 1994). Development involves coordinating cohesion at the local (sentence) level, through grammatical morphology and reference and at the global (hierarchical) level with connectives, anaphora and pragmatics.

Because of the challenges posed to young children in constructing a coherent narrative, narrative tasks have been used to investigate different aspects of language development and also patterns of SLI in spoken languages (e.g. Botting, 2002; Wetherell *et al.*, 2007). English-speaking children and adolescents with SLI have been reported to produce narratives similar to those of younger typically developing children (Merritt & Liles 1987; Wetherell *et al.*, 2007) with delays reported at the local and global levels. In a study of Italian-speaking children, Marini *et al.* (2008) found that those with SLI produced narratives with less developed sentence structure and use of verb morphology and also displayed problems with anaphoric use of pronouns.

Rathmann and colleagues (2007) provide a useful review of the structure of signed narratives and the process of acquisition based on the available research. The main linguistic devices in BSL grammar important for narrative are spatial verbs, morphological markers of verb agreement, aspect, manner, classifiers, and role shift or referential shift (Sutton-Spence & Woll, 1999). Although there is some research on how these devices develop at sentence level (e.g. for basic verb agreement, see Meier *et al.*, 2002; Morgan *et al.*, 2002, 2006), information is generally lacking as to how they are used by developing children within a narrative context, other than for role shift (see Morgan & Woll, 2003 for BSL and Loew, 1984 for ASL).

There is no previous research on narrative skills in deaf signers with SLI. Because narrative provides a rich source of data on how language is used in a real life context compared with a more formal testing context, it was decided to subject the narrative samples collected for the BSL Production Test (Herman *et al.*, 2004) to a more detailed analysis in addition to the analysis that is part of the assessment protocol. Children's stories were analysed for semantic content, narrative structure, number of clauses, number of anaphoric references and the following aspects of BSL grammar: spatial verbs, e.g. PERSON-GO-TABLE; agreement verbs, e.g. SHE-GIVES-HIM; handling classifiers, e.g. TAKE-SMALL-ROUND-OBJECT; manner inflections, e.g. PUT-REPEATEDLY; role shift.

Data collected from the SLI group were compared to equivalent narrative samples collected from a control group. Findings are reported in Herman *et al.* (in revision).

General Discussion

The work reported in this chapter demonstrates that it is possible to identify children with SLI in the deaf population where language delay is often the norm. Teachers of the deaf and specialist speech and language therapists were able to identify children with suspected sign language impairments using our screening checklist (see also Quinto-Pozos *et al.*, 2011 for ASL). Following initial teacher or clinician concerns, children were followed up using standardized measures of non-verbal abilities, motor skills and sign language proficiency and a set of more detailed language tests were developed. A distinct and measurable profile of severe language difficulties on the standardized sign language tests in contrast to good non-verbal and fine motor abilities allows us to be confident about identifying SLI in deaf children. Further analysis of findings from our new measures will allow us to say more about areas of sign language that are particularly vulnerable. This approach can lead to a confirmed diagnosis and a profile of relative strengths and weaknesses, with positive implications for targeting language interventions.

Seventeen of the 30 children tested in the first phase of our research were subsequently identified as having SLI; in many of the excluded cases, other needs were apparent such as reading, motor or learning difficulties. The tendency of teachers and clinicians to over-report the number of children in their class whom they consider to have language-learning difficulties is not surprising given the high level of comorbidity and the profile of delayed sign language acquisition that so many deaf children experience. Based on our findings to date, the SLI screening questionnaire may be a useful tool for teachers of the deaf and speech and language therapists to screen deaf children in their care. Further analysis of the prevalence of the specific SLI characteristics listed in the questionnaire among our final sample and the addition of further characteristics based on findings from our new tests is needed in order to finalize this.

We estimated a prevalence rate for SLI in BSL of 6.4% (Mason et al., 2010) based on the 13 children we had identified with SLI at that stage out of a total of 203 deaf children attending the schools who responded to our initial questionnaire. Despite this finding being based on a relatively small sample compared to studies of hearing children, the prevalence is similar to that reported by Tomblin et al. (1997) for the hearing population. Although epidemiological studies are needed, at a theoretical level, this comparability allows us to speculate that similar genetic and neurobiological causes may underlie SLI in both auditory and visual-manual language modalities (although, as mentioned above, other causes can also be assumed), and this warrants further investigation.

It is important to stress that the systematic evaluation of language disorder in deaf children in our work was made possible by two main factors: (1) A team of native Deaf and hearing sign bilingual researchers, working closely with psychologists, linguists and clinicians with skills in sign language linguistics, language and cognitive assessments and knowledge of language acquisition in deaf and hearing populations; (2) a set of language assessments with norms or control group scores for age-matched children. We were fortunate that two standardized language assessments already existed for BSL when we started this project. Such instruments do not exist for many other signed languages. Even so, we are still a long way from having the range of language assessments for BSL that are employed for SLI research in spoken languages and further work is needed. Test development across a wide range of signed languages is a crucial prerequisite to cross-linguistic diagnosis and profiling of SLI in deaf sign language users around the world. Further work in this area will allow new theoretical advances in our understanding of SLI generally, and the development of therapeutic interventions in sign language.

The picture that emerges from our findings to date is that SLI in a signed language looks very similar to SLI in spoken languages, in that both comprehension and expressive language may be affected, and in some cases, both are compromised. Analysis of data collected from the new measures indicates varying difficulties with sentence and discourse level language, including morphology and co-reference (Herman *et al.*, in revision; Marshall *et al.*, in revision). Importantly, our preliminary observations suggest that most children with sign language SLI do not sign in a deviant or unusual way but, instead, features of their language performance appear to be characteristic of children at a significantly younger age. Further analysis is needed to confirm this and to describe individual cases which differ from this pattern.

Perhaps contrary to popular belief, our research suggests that there is nothing inherently 'easy' about signed language acquisition and that it is not the case that signing protects deaf signing children from developing language impairment. Language displays complexities and difficulties in whichever modality it is crafted. This has important implications for our understanding of the underlying causes of SLI. A deficit in rapid auditory processing, of the type proposed by Tallal (Tallal, 2000; Tallal & Piercy, 1973), cannot account for SLI in a signed language. Because the visual system does not process change as rapidly as the auditory system, sign languages do not make use of rapidly changing signals equivalent to the formant transitions of speech in the auditory system (the locus of the proposed impairment in spoken languages, according to Tallal's theory). A deficit in the perception of rapid temporal transitions is therefore not relevant to a visual language which has slower temporal contrasts (Klima & Bellugi, 1979). Some hearing children with SLI acquiring spoken language might plausibly have a rapid auditory processing deficit, but the fact that this cannot explain sign impairment suggests that there are other pathways to impairment in both spoken and signed languages.

At first glance, the performance of our group of SLI children on the non-sign repetition task, on which the majority performed comparably to typically developing deaf controls, might appear to challenge the hypothesis that SLI is caused by a phonological short-term memory deficit (Gathercole & Baddeley, 1990). However, as we have argued elsewhere (Marshall *et al.*, 2011), the repetition of non-signs appears to be a difficult task even for typically developing deaf children. Our current explanation is that the phonological content of a non-sign is less predictable than the phonological content of a spoken non-word, and therefore its retention in short-term memory is more costly. The basic idea here is that signs in BSL may have less limiting constraints than spoken language words in how their sublexical components can be combined. In a sense there are more degrees of freedom for how subcomponents combine in a sign than a word and this makes processing demands higher (Marshall *et al.*, 2011). Because performance of the norming sample on this task was low and had such a large standard deviation, children had to perform particularly poorly in order to fall more than −1.3 S.D. below the mean for their age group (see Mann *et al.*, 2010). However, the fact that five children did so poorly suggests that weakness in phonological short-term memory may be part of the profile for at least some deaf children with SLI. This pattern of findings supports the notion that there may be subgroups of SLI with different aetiologies in both hearing and deaf populations.

We are not yet able, on the basis of data collected, to test the other theories discussed previously, namely the generalized slowing hypothesis (Kail, 1994), and one of the linguistic hypotheses of SLI such as the computational grammatical complexity hypothesis (van der Lely & Marshall, 2011). This would make for a fruitful line of future enquiry. We can say that any universal explanations of SLI will need to account not only for cross-linguistic data, but also cross-modality data of the type we have presented here. We have not explored this in our work up to now, but there are important implications of diagnoses of sign SLI for deaf children's acquisition of spoken or written English. It is generally the case that SLI affects both languages in hearing bilingual children (e.g. Gutiérrez-Clellen et al., 2008; Paradis, 2010) and the same would be expected for a deaf child. Indeed, a hearing child who was a native signer found to have SLI in English also had difficulties with language development in BSL (Morgan, 2005). It should therefore be expected that a deaf child with SLI in sign language might experience difficulties with the acquisition of a spoken language.

Further issues following a diagnosis of SLI concern the long-term outlook and implications for intervention. Many hearing children with language impairments have difficulties that persist over time (Conti-Ramsden et al., 2001) and although there is not yet any longitudinal research to confirm this, the same is likely to be the case for deaf children with SLI.

It is often suggested that a deaf child who does not sign well would be best placed in a signing environment where they would have more opportunities to see sign language, rather than being placed in a school where only oral communication is used. However, if the child has SLI, they will also require specialist sign language therapy, since clinical experience and research based on hearing children with SLI suggests that language enrichment interventions alone are insufficient. Specific interventions for hearing children with SLI in spoken languages have been developed to target a range of areas: vocabulary (e.g. Hyde Wright, 1993; McGregor & Leonard, 1989; Parsons et al., 2005); morphology (Ebbels, 2007; Leonard, 1975); pronouns (Courtright & Courtright, 1976); various syntactic structures such as questions (e.g. Ebbels, 2007; Ebbels & van der Lely, 2001; Wilcox & Leonard, 1978); and narrative (Swanson et al., 2005), among others. The development of guidelines for specific interventions in a sign language remain to be addressed in future work.

A first step in this direction for deaf children with SLI might use existing therapies as possible templates. However, for staff working with deaf children, there is also the issue of the knowledge and skills needed to deliver language interventions in a sign language. Although interventionists such as speech and language therapists are often native speakers of the languages they are working with and have extensive knowledge and experience of spoken language development and interventions, many lack fluency in sign language or knowledge of sign linguistics and sign language acquisition. In contrast, Deaf staff working in educational contexts generally have high levels of sign language fluency but require training in developing, delivering and evaluating language interventions. One way to address this mismatch in key skills is for staff to work collaboratively in order to achieve the necessary skill mix. This is the principle behind a training course that has been established at City University London for Deaf and hearing professionals learning to use the BSL Production Test (Herman *et al.*, 2004). Professionals attend a four-day training course in pairs with colleagues from their service. Training is delivered by Deaf and hearing researchers and practitioners, often directly in BSL. The course seeks to develop an understanding of sign linguistics and sign language acquisition, alongside principles of assessment and practice in using the BSL Production Test. On the final training day, an afternoon is set aside to discuss approaches to intervention. Participants work in small groups sharing their ideas, experience, knowledge of resources, etc., based on the children with whom they have worked. Feedback from several cohorts of course participants confirms the value of working in teams and sharing working practices in this way, the relevance of the course content, and the feelings of empowerment following such training.

Finally, there is a need to develop more centres of excellence where a diagnosis of SLI can be confirmed using a set of instruments designed for this purpose. One such centre is the Sign Language Assessment Clinic at the Compass Centre, City University London (http://www.city.ac.uk/health/public-clinics/compass-centre/sign-language-assessment-clinic). This clinic has an open referral system, allowing families and professionals throughout the UK to refer deaf individuals for whom there are concerns about communication in sign language. Deaf and hearing staff carry out individualized assessments, using available standardized and experimental measures along with collection of background information and observations of the person's communication in different contexts and with different people. Based on the assessment, a report is written that profiles the individual's strengths and difficulties and recommendations are made for local services which include the optimal communication environment, suggested intervention targets and appropriate intervention strategies.

Practical Implications/Recommendations

Our preliminary work has confirmed the existence of SLI among deaf children. This has theoretical consequences and also practical implications for professionals who work with deaf children:

- Professionals should be aware that a proportion of deaf children may have SLI.

- Our screening checklist may, with further refinement, prove to be a quick and useful preliminary tool for initial identification of deaf signing children with SLI.
- Further language assessments are needed for deaf children who sign in order to confirm a diagnosis of SLI.
- There is a need for more centres of excellence to be set up which offer specialist assessments for deaf children who sign and advice for professionals working with such children.

Acknowledgements

The research was funded by the Economic and Social Research Council of Great Britain (Grant 620-28-6001-Deafness, Cognition and Language Research Centre) and a Leverhulme Trust Early Career Fellowship to Chloë Marshall.

We would like to express our thanks to the children, their families and staff in participating schools, without whom this research would not have been possible. We would also like to thank a group of specialist speech and language therapists working in bilingualism and deafness in the UK (SALTIBAD), and in particular Jane Thomas, Katie Martin and Katy Persse, for their contributions at various stages of the study.

References

Berman, R. and Slobin, D.I. (eds) (1994) *Relating Events in Narrative: A Crosslinguistic Development Study*. Mahwah, NJ: Lawrence Erlbaum.

Bishop, D.V.M., Carlyon, R.P., Deeks, J.M. and Bishop, S.J. (1999) Auditory temporal processing impairment: Neither necessary nor sufficient for causing language impairment in children. *Journal of Speech, Language and Hearing Research* 42, 1295–1310.

Botting, N. (2002) Narrative as a tool for the assessment of linguistic and pragmatic impairments. *Child Language Teaching and Therapy* 18 (1), 1–22.

Botting, N. (2005) Non-verbal cognitive development and language impairment. *Journal of Child Psychology and Psychiatry* 46, 317–326.

Chamberlain, C., Morford, J.P. and Mayberry, R.I. (2000) *Language Acquisition By Eye*. Mahwah, NJ: Lawrence Erlbaum.

Conti-Ramsden, G., Botting, N., Simkin, Z. and Knox, E. (2001) Follow-up of children attending infant language units: Outcomes at 11 years of age. *International Journal of Language & Communication Disorders* 36, 207–219.

Courtright, J.A. and Courtright, I.C. (1976) Imitative modelling as a theoretical base for instructing language-disordered children. *Journal of Speech and Hearing Research* 19, 655–663.

Dromi, E., Leonard, L.B., Adam, G. and Zadoneisky-Ehrlich, S. (1999) Verb agreement morphology in Hebrew speaking children with specific language impairment. *Journal of Speech, Language and Hearing Research* 42 (6), 1414–1431.

Dunn, L.M., Dunn, D.M., Whetton, C. and Burley, J. (1997) *The British Picture Vocabulary Scale* (2nd edn). Windsor: NFER-Nelson.

Ebbels, S.H. (2007) Teaching grammar to school-aged children with specific language impairment using Shape Coding. *Child Language Teaching and Therapy* 23 (1), 67–93.

Ebbels, S.H. and van der Lely, H. (2001) Meta-syntactic therapy using visual coding for children with severe persistent SLI. *International Journal of Language & Communication Disorders* 36 (1), 345–350.

Elliot, C.D., Smith, P. and McCulloch, K. (1996) *The British Ability Scales*. Windsor: NFER-Nelson.

Gardner, H., Froud, K., McClelland, A. and van der Lely, H.K.J. (2006) Development of the Grammar and Phonology Screening, GAPS, test to assess key markers of specific language and literacy difficulties in young children. *International Journal of Language & Communication Disorders* 41, 513–540.

Gathercole, S.E. and Baddeley, A.D. (1990) Phonological memory deficits in language disordered children: Is there a causal connection? *Journal of Memory and Language* 29, 336–360.

Gutiérrez-Clellen, V.F., Simon-Cereijido, G. and Wagner, C. (2008) Bilingual children with language impairment: A comparison with monolinguals and second language learners. *Applied Psycholinguistics* 29, 3–19.

Hall, M. and Bavelier, D. (2010) Working memory, deafness and sign language. In M. Marschark and P.E. Spencer (eds) *The Handbook of Deaf Studies, Language and Education* (Vol. 2, pp. 458–472). Oxford: Oxford University Press.

Hauser, P.C., Paludnevičiene, R., Supalla, T. and Bavelier, D. (2008) American Sign Language-Sentence Reproduction Test: Development and implications. In R.M. de Quadros (ed.) *Sign Language: Spinning and Unraveling the Past, Present and Future* (pp. 160–172). Petropolis, Brazil: Editora Arara Azul.

Henry, L.A., Messer, D.J. and Nash, G. (2012) Executive functioning in children with specific language impairment. *Journal of Child Psychology and Psychiatry* 53, 37–45.

Herman, R., Holmes, S. and Woll, B. (1999) *Assessing British Sign Language Development: Receptive Skills Test*. Gloucestershire: Forest Bookshop.

Herman, R., Grove, N., Holmes, S., Morgan, G., Sutherland, H. and Woll, B. (2004) *Assessing British Sign Language Development: Production Test (Narrative Skills)*. London: City University.

Herman, R., Rowley, K., Mason., K. and Morgan, G. (in revision). Deficits in narrative abilities in child BSL users with SLI.

Hyde Wright, S. (1993) Teaching word-finding strategies to severely language-impaired children. *International Journal of Language & Communication Disorders* 28 (2), 165–175.

Kail, R. (1994) A method for studying the generalized slowing hypothesis of children with specific language impairment. *Journal of Speech and Hearing Research* 37, 418–421.

Klima, E.S. and Bellugi, U. (1979) *The Signs of Language*. Cambridge, MA: Harvard University Press.

Kyle, F.E. and Harris, M. (2006) Concurrent correlates and predictors of reading and spelling in deaf and hearing school children. *Journal of Deaf Studies & Deaf Education* 11, 273–288.

Leonard, L.B. (1975) Developmental considerations in the management of language disabled children. *Journal of Learning Disabilities* 8, 44–49.

Leonard, L.B. (1998) *Children with Specific Language Impairment*. Cambridge, MA: MIT Press.

Leonard, L. (2009) Cross-linguistic studies of child language disorders. In R. Schwartz (ed.) *Handbook of Child Language Disorders* (pp. 308–324). New York: Psychology Press.

Liddell, S. (2003) *Grammar, Gestures, and Meaning in American Sign Language*. Cambridge: Cambridge University Press.

Loew, R. (1984) Learning American Sign Language as a first language: Roles and reference. Unpublished doctoral dissertation, University of Minnesota.

Maillart, C. and Parisse, C. (2008) Dislocations as a developmental marker in French language: A preliminary study. *Clinical Linguistics & Phonetics* 22 (4–5), 255–258.

Mann, W., Marshall, C.R., Mason, K. and Morgan, G. (2010) The acquisition of sign language: The interplay between phonology and phonetics. *Language and Learning Development* 6, 60–86.

Marini, A., Tavano, A. and Fabbro, F. (2008) Assessment of linguistic abilities in Italian children with specific language impairment. *Neuropsychologia* 46 (11), 2816–2823.

Marshall, C.R. (2006) The morpho-phonological interface in specific language impairment. *Language Acquisition* 13, 373–375 (thesis synopsis).

Marshall, C.R., Denmark, T. and Morgan, G. (2006) Investigating the underlying causes of SLI: A non-sign repetition test in British Sign Language. *Advances in Speech–Language Pathology* 8 (4), 347–355.

Marshall, C.R., Mann, W. and Morgan, G. (2011) Short term memory in signed languages: Not just a disadvantage for serial recall. *Frontiers in Psychology* 2, 102. doi: 10.3389/fpsyg.2011.00102.

Marshall, C.R., Rowley, K., Mason, K., Herman, R. and Morgan, G. (2013) Lexical organisation in deaf children who use British Sign Language: Evidence from a semantic fluency task. *Journal of Child Language* 40, 193–220.

Marshall, C., Mason, K., Rowley, K., Herman, R., Atkinson, J., Woll, B. and Morgan, G. (in revision) Sentence repetition in deaf children with SLI in BSL.

Marshall, J., Atkinson, J., Smulovitch, E., Thacker, A. and Woll, B. (2004) Aphasia in a user of British Sign Language: Dissociation between sign and gesture. *Cognitive Neuropsychology* 21 (5), 537–554.

Mason, K., Rowley, K., Marshall, C.R., Atkinson, J.R., Herman, R., Woll, B. and Morgan, G. (2010) Identifying SLI in Deaf children acquiring British Sign Language: Implications for theory and practice. *British Journal of Developmental Psychology* 28, 33–49.

McGregor, K.K. and Leonard, L.B. (1989) Facilitating word-finding skills of language-impaired children. *Journal of Speech and Hearing Disorders* 54, 141–147.

Meier, R.P., Cormier, K. and Quinto-Pozos, D. (eds) (2002) *Modality and Structure in Signed and Spoken Languages.* Cambridge: Cambridge University Press.

Merritt, D.D. and Liles, B.Z. (1987) Story grammar ability in children with and without language disorder: Story generation, story retelling, and story comprehension. *Journal of Speech and Hearing Research* 30, 539–552.

Messer, D. and Dockrell, J.E. (2006) Children's naming and word-finding difficulties: Descriptions and explanations. *Journal of Speech, Language & Hearing Research* 49, 309–324.

Mitchell, R.E. and Karchmer, M.A. (2004) When parents are deaf versus hard of hearing: Patterns of sign use and school placement of deaf and hard-of-hearing children. *Journal of Deaf Studies & Deaf Education* 9 (2), 133–152.

Morgan, G. (2005) Biology and behaviour: Insights from the acquisition of sign language. In A. Cutler (ed.) *Twenty-First Century Psycholinguistics: Four Cornerstones.* Mahwah, NJ: Lawrence Erlbaum.

Morgan, G. and Woll, B. (eds) (2002) *Directions in Sign Language Acquisition.* Amsterdam: John Benjamins.

Morgan, G. and Woll, B. (2003) The development of reference switching encoded through body classifiers in BSL. In K. Emmorey (ed.) *Perspectives on Classifier Constructions in Sign Languages* (pp. 297–310). Mahwah, NJ: Lawrence Erlbaum.

Morgan, G., Herman, R. and Woll, B. (2002) The development of complex verb constructions in BSL. *Journal of Child Language* 29 (3), 655–675.

Morgan, G., Barriere, I. and Woll, B. (2006) The influence of typology and modality in the acquisition of verb agreement in British Sign Language. *First Language* 26 (1), 19–43.

Morgan, G., Herman, R. and Woll, B. (2007) Language impairments in sign language: Breakthroughs and puzzles. *International Journal for Language and Communication Disorders* 42, 97–105.

Paradis, J. (2010) The interface between bilingual development and specific language impairment. *Applied Psycholinguistics* 31, 227–252.

Paradis, J., Crago, M. and Genesee, F. (2005) Domain-general versus domain-specific accounts of specific language impairment: Evidence from bilingual children's acquisition of object pronouns. *Language Acquisition* 13 (1), 33–62.

Parsons, S., Law, J. and Gascoigne, M. (2005) Teaching receptive vocabulary to children with specific language impairment: A curriculum-based approach. *Child Language Teaching and Therapy* 21 (1), 39–59.

Quinto-Pozos, D., Forber-Pratt, A. and Singleton, J.L. (2011) Do developmental communication disorders exist in the signed modality? Perspectives from professionals. *Language, Speech and Hearing Services in Schools* 42, 423–443.

Rathmann, C., Mann, W. and Morgan, G. (2007) Narrative structure and narrative development in deaf children. *Deafness and Education International* 9 (4), 187–196.

Rice, M. and Wexler, K. (1996) Toward tense as a clinical marker of specific language impairment in English-speaking children. *Journal of Speech and Hearing Research* 39, 1239–1257.

Rispens, J.E. (2004) *Syntactic and Phonological Processing in Developmental Dyslexia.* Groningen: Grodil.

Sandler, W. and Lillo-Martin, D. (2006) *Sign Language and Linguistic Universals.* Cambridge: Cambridge University Press.

Schick, B., Marschark, M. and Spencer, P.E. (eds) (2006) *Advances in the Sign Language Development of Deaf Children.* New York: Oxford University Press.

Seeff-Gabriel, B., Chiat, S. and Roy, P. (2008) *Early Repetition Battery.* London: Pearson Education.

Semel, E., Wiig, E.H. and Secord, W.A. (2003) *Clinical Evaluation of Language Fundamentals* (4th edn). San Antonio, TX: Psychological Corporation.

Sheng, L. and McGregor, K.K. (2010) Lexical-semantic organization in children with specific language impairment. *Journal of Speech, Language, & Hearing Research* 53, 146–159.

Sheng, L., Peña, E.D., Bedore, L.M. and Fiestas, C.E. (2012) Semantic deficits in Spanish–English bilingual children with language impairment. *Journal of Speech, Language, & Hearing Research* 55, 1–15. doi:10.1044/1092-4388(2011/10-0254).

Snow, C.E. and Hoefnagel-Hohle, M. (1978) Critical period for language acquisition: Evidence from second language learning. *Child Development* 49, 1263–1279. Reprinted in S. Krashen, R. Scarcella and M. Long (eds) (1982) *Child–Adult Differences in Second Language Acquisition* (pp. 93–111). Rowley, MA: Newbury House.

Stokes, S. and Fletcher, P. (2003) Aspectual forms in Cantonese children with specific language impairment. *Linguistics* 41 (2), 381–406.

Sutton-Spence, R. and Woll, B. (1999) *The Linguistics of British Sign Language: An Introduction.* Cambridge: Cambridge University Press.

Swanson, L.A., Fey, M.E., Mills, C.E. and Hood, L.S. (2005) Use of narrative-based language intervention with children who have specific language impairment. *American Journal of Speech-Language Pathology* 14, 131–143.

Tallal, P. (2000) Experimental studies of language learning impairments: From research to remediation. In D.V.M. Bishop and L.B. Leonard (eds) *Speech and Language Impairments in Children: Causes, Characteristics, Intervention and Outcome* (pp. 131–155). Hove: Psychology Press.

Tallal, P. and Piercy, M. (1973) Defects of non-verbal auditory perception in children with developmental aphasia. *Nature* 241, 468–469.

Thompson, R.L., Vinson, D.P., Woll, B. and Vigliocco, G. (2012) The road to language learning is iconic: Evidence from British Sign Language. *Psychological Science* 23 (12), 1443–1448.

Tomblin, J.B., Records, N.L., Bookwalter, P., Zhang, X., Smith, E. and O'Brien, M. (1997) Prevalence of specific language impairment in kindergarten children. *Journal of Speech, Language, & Hearing Research* 40, 1245–1260.

Ullman, M.T. and Gopnik, M. (1999) Inflectional morphology in a family with inherited specific language impairment. *Applied Psycholinguistics* 20, 51–117.

van der Lely, H.K.J. (2005) Domain-specific cognitive systems: Insight from Grammatical-SLI. *Trends in Cognitive Sciences* 9 (2), 53–59.

van der Lely, H.K.J. and Marshall, C.R. (2011) Grammatical-specific language impairment: A window onto domain-specificity. In J. Guendouzi, F. Loncke and M. Williams (eds) *The Handbook of Psycholinguistic and Cognitive Processes: Perspectives in Communication Disorders* (pp. 401–418). New York, Taylor & Francis.

van der Lely, H.K.J. and Ullman, M.T. (2001) Past tense morphology in specifically language impaired and normally developing children. *Language and Cognitive Processes* 16 (2–3), 177–217.

Vinson, D.V., Cormier, K.A., Denmark, T., Schembri, A. and Vigliocco, G. (2008) The British Sign Language (BSL) norms for age of acquisition, familiarity and iconicity. *Behavior Research Methods* 40 (4), 1079–1087.

Volterra, V., Caselli, M.C., Capirci, O., Tonucci, F. and Vicari, S. (2003) Early linguistic abilities of Italian children with Williams syndrome. *Developmental Neuropsychology* 23 (1–2), 33–58.

Wetherell, D., Botting, N. and Conti-Ramsden, G. (2007) Narrative in adolescent specific language impairment (SLI): A comparison with peers across two different narrative genres. *International Journal of Language & Communication Disorders* 42, 583–605.

White, S.A., Fisher, S.E., Geschwind, D.H., Scharff, C. and Holy, T.E. (2006) Singing mice and songbirds: Animal models for FOXP2 function and dysfunction in human speech. *Journal of Neuroscience* 26, 10376–10379.

Wilcox, J.M. and Leonard, L.B. (1978) Experimental acquisition of Wh-questions in language-disordered children. *Journal of Speech and Hearing Research* 21, 220–239.

Woolfe, T., Herman, R., Roy, P. and Woll, B. (2009) Early vocabulary development in deaf native signers: A British Sign Language adaptation of the communicative development inventories. *Journal of Child Psychology and Psychiatry* 51 (3), 322–331. doi:10.111 1/j.1469-7610.2009.02151.

3 A Case-study Approach to Investigating Developmental Signed Language Disorders

David Quinto-Pozos, Jenny L. Singleton, Peter C. Hauser and Susan C. Levine

Introduction

Research on developmental signed language disorders is important for theoretical and practical reasons. Unfortunately, researchers in this nascent area of enquiry are faced with multiple challenges. One example is that there exists a lack of normed language assessment instruments that can be used for diagnostic purposes with children of various ages. In addition, it might be difficult to distinguish a case of language disorder from delayed development due to late exposure to a signed language, which is not uncommon with more than 90% of deaf children being born into hearing households. Our case study approach, we believe, has enabled us to address these challenges and offers researchers and clinicians an approach that, at the very least, makes some headway into helping individuals who are suspected of a signed language disorder, and at most can perhaps contribute to general theories of language disorders.

In this chapter, we outline our methodological approach for conducting research in this important area of enquiry. The approach involves working closely with professionals at schools for the deaf. These liaisons are able to identify children suspected of possessing a sign language disorder because of their extensive experience working with deaf and hard of hearing children, and also seeing a particular child communicating on a daily basis. Once a case of atypicality is identified, we conduct an in-depth analysis of that *focal child's* communication abilities, drawing upon multiple sources of information. Throughout the process there are methodological and ethical considerations that help to guide the interactions that we have with the focal children (i.e. those who have been identified as exhibiting atypical acquisition of signed language) and the adults with whom they are in frequent contact (e.g. their parent[s], teachers, ASL specialists, etc.).

The structure of the chapter is designed to highlight the challenges that we feel are particularly notable about this type of research and outline the methods, in some detail, that our team employs. We begin by discussing what we feel are the most challenging aspects of this work, and that discussion is followed by our approach to identifying focal children and collecting data that are used for our case study analyses. Our goal is to provide a concise, yet thorough, introduction to a case-study methodology that we feel is successful for researchers and clinicians who are working with low-incidence atypicality, especially when standardized signed language assessment instruments are not available to provide a definitive diagnosis and comparison norms drawn from typical signers.

Assessing atypicality: Research design challenges

We begin by first acknowledging the potential limitation of generalizing our case methodology approach to other settings. Our work on sign language disorders has taken place entirely within the United States; thus, some of the challenges that we have encountered in this area of research may not be common to deaf children in other countries or even other regions of the US due to different political or educational influences of those regions.

Proper and timely identification of atypical signed language development as exhibited by a deaf child may be among the biggest issues with this area of research. This may be due, in part, to the lack of marketed language assessment instruments – whether they be diagnostic or not – that professionals at schools can use to chart a child's developmental progress in a signed language (also see Quinto-Pozos, this volume). Singleton and Supalla (2011) provide a description of various instruments that have been used over the years, mostly for research purposes (see also Mann & Haug, this volume). Among those instruments are checklists that can help a language professional to determine if a child is demonstrating linguistic features that would be expected based on age-related milestones (Anderson & Reilly, 2002; Mounty, 1994). However, it is often the case that there are no (or limited) published norms for the tests that can be used by assessment specialists to determine a child's performance with respect to a large sample mean. In addition, it is often difficult to determine whether a child with late exposure to signed language has language problems that are independent of being delayed with the acquisition of the signed language.

Another challenge for researchers working in this area concerns *the estimated size of the target population* (see Quinto-Pozos, this volume, for a discussion of estimated numbers). As one example, in comparison to the suggested percentage of hearing English-speaking children with Specific Language Impairment (SLI) in the US (7%), there may be relatively few deaf children who exhibit atypical acquisition characteristics, and those that do exist are likely scattered throughout the country. This makes it difficult to design a group study in order to address individual variation, although some research teams are able to overcome that challenge by using survey method-ologies and reaching out to multiple schools for the deaf (Mason *et al.*, 2010). Further, the small number of deaf children is compounded by the fact that most deaf children are not exposed to signed language from birth or early in development because their parents or caregivers do not sign (over 90%, according to some estimates; Mitchell & Karchmer, 2004). For those chil-dren, it may be the case that the atypical aspects of their signed language development are caused by delayed exposure to rich linguistic input rather than an underlying cognitive or neurological deficit that affects their lan-guage development. If all deaf children with atypical signing were excluded on the basis of delayed signed language exposure, the number of potential research participants for any given study of sign language disorders will be extremely small, and indeed poses a challenge for investigators.

Another important point about this research concerns *multilingualism*. Deaf children (and adults) have been described as being typically bilingual because their language and communication normally includes the written form of the ambient spoken language (Grosjean, 2010). Some deaf and hard of hearing individuals could be considered sign-speech-print bilinguals since they have chosen to use spoken language, too. Others could be considered sign-print bilinguals. Regardless, it is normally the case that at least two (if not more) languages are acquired or learned by deaf people, and they use those languages daily. This fact poses challenges for the researcher of devel-opmental signed language disorders because it requires them to consider *over-all* language development and not simply how one of their multiple languages is developing (De Houwer, 2009). Researchers must recognize that there may be influences from one language to the other, or that aspects of the languages could develop independently of each other, or be differentially impaired.

Communication disorders research within a close-knit community

There are ethical considerations when working with members of a small community – particularly concerning the topic of communication disorder. Even though its members are spread throughout the country, the Deaf com-munity is a tight-knit group of people who are linked together by linguistic and cultural characteristics, and information sharing is a key component of community involvement (Hoffmeister *et al.*, 1996). Furthermore, for many Deaf individuals, there might be some reluctance to acknowledge either to concerned professionals or to other community members that their deaf child is not developing their ASL 'normally' because for so long they have had to defend their language and their 'normalcy' to the 'hearing society.' For these reasons, it is of utmost importance to maintain strict confidentiality throughout the research process in order to respect the privacy of the children, families and schools that are involved. This must occur during the identification of atypicality (i.e. subject recruitment for the study), data collection by the researchers and presentation of results, regardless of the form in which the presentation occurs.

It is particularly important to exercise care in the reporting of data that are collected and analyzed because of the tight-knit aspect of Deaf networks. It could be possible that the identity of a focal child in a study would be revealed to an audience due to seemingly trivial information that is contained in the reporting. Maintaining confidentiality is particularly important because of the case-study nature of the research design that is being employed. If presentations are given at conferences and educational settings for deaf and hard of hearing children (e.g. schools for the deaf, Gallaudet University, Rochester Institute of Technology, etc.), the researcher should try to present the findings in a way to avoid identification of the children in the study by audience members or those who will later learn about the presentation. Singleton and colleagues (2012) discuss the increasing use of video-clips of signers in research presentations and the importance of securing informed consent about the range of uses of video-based data. In the case of working with individuals with suspected signed language disorders, it would be highly unusual to seek permission to display the child's or adolescent's videos to the public. 'Fuzzing out' a signer's face to obscure their identity is also problematic as this also destroys significant grammatical facial expressions. Alternative strategies for research presentations of sign language disorder data include the presenter describing or demonstrating the atypical signing, or displaying a video recording of a deaf actor 'recreating' the example of atypical signing.

Our Approach to This Research

For this project we adopted a case-study methodology that involves multiple steps and repeated visits with a focal child and adults familiar with the child (see Quinto-Pozos & Singleton, 2009, 2010). This approach involves working closely with schools for the Deaf throughout the process.

Our approach: Focus on deaf children who are native signers of ASL

For this project, thus far we have chosen to focus on the acquisition of language by children who are exposed to ASL from birth and who are exposed to ASL on a daily basis at school. These deaf children have at least one Deaf ASL-using parent and receive signed language input from their ASL-signing instructors, other professional staff at the school and their peers. The decision to focus on native signers is predicated on the concern that delayed or impoverished exposure to ASL may result in atypical acquisition. Researchers in the UK have provided a case study of a native BSL-signing child with atypical characteristics of language acquisition (Morgan *et al.*, 2006), and we follow in a similar vein by working with parallel case studies in the US.

Our approach: Work with schools for child identification

Schools for the deaf play key roles with respect to the identification of focal children for the research. They are important because experienced professionals have worked with many children over the years and they can serve as experts who can recognize atypicality in a child's development (Quinto-Pozos *et al.*, 2011). Because of the limited availability of normed ASL assessment instruments, the identification of children who exhibit atypical developmental characteristics (with respect to ASL acquisition) occurs in various ways. We have heard reports of some schools developing their own in-house assessments, and such tests and checklists have served as means for documenting unexpected linguistic behaviors. In some cases, professionals at schools simply realize that something is odd or unexpected about a deaf child's ASL development, and such observations are discussed among the team of professionals who interact with the child. Sometimes the parents of a deaf child also report to school officials that their child's signed language (comprehension and/or production) does not appear to be developing like that of peers of comparable ages or of their older children when they were at the focal child's age.

Our approach: Obtaining informed consent

When we first approach a school, we assemble and meet with a team of language specialists and/or school psychologists to explain our research objectives and enlist their help in identifying children who may meet our eligibility criteria (Quinto-Pozos *et al.*, 2011). We ask these professionals to disseminate our information packet to the parents of the deaf children they feel exhibit atypical characteristics in their ASL development. At this point, we do not know the identity of any suspected cases of signed language disorder. The packet includes a consent form (in English) and a DVD that contains an ASL translation of the consent form as well as a general description of the study (see Singleton *et al.*, 2012, in press, for a discussion of accessibility issues in consent procedures). The parent(s) are asked to review the material and endorse the consent forms if they wish to participate. If the parent(s) choose not to participate (for whatever reason), the research team does not learn the identity of those individuals. This participant recruitment process is carefully followed in order to maintain the high level of confidentiality that is particularly important for this project. If we receive from the parents signed consent forms approving their child's participation, giving authorization for their child's teachers or clinicians to discuss language and learning progress, and allowing researchers access to their child's school records, the process of collecting information about the child begins.

Our approach: Data collection

The process involves collection of information from multiple sources in order to create a comprehensive picture of a child's abilities. This methodology has been invaluable for the analysis of each case study of atypical signing. The data collection has generally included: (1) an interview with the parent(s) of the child; (2) interviews with the child's teacher(s) or other developmental experts at the school (e.g. a speech language pathologist or audiologist, a school psychologist, an ASL specialist, etc.); (3) a thorough review of the child's school records; (4) a neuropsychological assessment of the child's cognitive abilities; and (5) assessment of the child's language abilities. Such data collection normally requires repeated trips to a school to work with the child, with data collected diachronically. The longitudinal nature of the work allows for us to also determine how the child is developing and whether or not there is an improvement in the child's ability to comprehend and produce structures that were previously reported to be challenging.

Interviews with adults

An interview, usually conducted in ASL, is held with the parent(s) in order to obtain their views about specific aspects of their child's early years (e.g. information about childbirth, various developmental milestones and examples of communication difficulties). Questions that are used during these data collection sessions can be found Appendix A. The videorecorded interview produces much information that is used to corroborate reports that appear in the child's school records.

Interviews with school staff (e.g. teachers, speech and language pathologists, ASL specialists, etc.) who have worked closely with the child complement the information that is obtained from the parent(s). Those questions are found in Appendix B.

Most interviews are conducted face-to-face, but other reliable communication media (e.g. internet video conferencing with recordable features) can be used when the researcher cannot travel to the location of the interviewee. The important point is that the researcher must be able to reliably capture the contents of the interview (e.g. via recorded video) in order to create a transcript and review the content throughout the analysis, as needed.

School record review

Additionally, the child's school records are examined closely to ascertain patterns of behavior (whether or not the patterns are strictly linguistic) exhibited by the child and if any specific events had been documented that could provide important information about the child's behavior and development. Multiple types of information are carefully considered in order to support a holistic approach during the analysis of each case. A student's school records normally contain multiple reports from annual meetings that are designed to establish and evaluate learning and behavioral objectives set forth by a team of professionals from the school and the child's parents.[1] Those reports serve as invaluable information about linguistic matters, general academic performance, information about social and emotional development, results from recent assessments and information about past and future (i.e. planned) intervention techniques. The school records often also contain individual entries that reflect reports about testing or referral/intervention services. Results of standardized tests can be particularly useful because they show how the child performs with respect to his/her peers, which is particularly valuable for the research process.

Another important source of information from the school records – although there is less standardization with respect to the measures that are used – is what the student's teachers report. Sometimes this includes grade reports along with comments about the student. However, checklists of linguistic features (for either ASL or English) and whether or not a child has mastered those features are common. Scales sometimes include labels such as 'not present', 'emerging' or 'mastered'. While this provides a general sense of the student's development with respect to the specific features of language, we suggest that caution must be exercised when interpreting the reports because of the lack of standardization in the measures and the inability for such assessment processes to capture, in an objective manner, the student's true abilities.

Neuropsychological assessment

At some point in the data collection process we also conduct neuropsychological testing with the focal child in order to plot aspects of the child's cognitive development (see Hauser *et al.*, submitted, for a detailed account of the neuropsychological testing that we administer). An array of tests are used that are designed to examine the child's general cognitive functioning, memory, motor skills, behavior and emotional functioning, and visual perceptual processing. The standardized tests are administered by a deaf clinical neuropsychologist on the team (the third author of this chapter), and the tests are all administered in ASL. See Appendix C for a list of the instruments that are used. Only tests that are believed to be appropriate for deaf children or adolescents are used. Results from neuropsychological tests help the team to rule out other factors that could cause language developmental delays such as intelligence, visual processing or motor processing difficulties. The results also help the team identify potential cognitive functions that might be significantly weak, compared to the individual's other functions, and might contribute to the language difficulties. When these specific weaknesses are identified, they can be followed up with more specific neuropsychological testing.

Language assessment: Tests with preliminary norms

Without the availability of standardized ASL instruments with norms, we have chosen to design some new tests as well as to administer language assessments using instruments that have been developed for research purposes. In both cases, we rely on preliminary norms (i.e. means based on a limited group of typically developing test-takers)[2] made available to us by researchers or gathered by our research team. This strategy allows us at least to compare the individual with atypical signing to a small group of his/her age- and gender-matched peers.

The existing language tests with preliminary norms that we use include the American Sign Language Proficiency Assessment (*ASL-PA*; Maller *et al.*, 1999), the American Sign Language-Sentence Reproduction Test (*ASL-SRT*; Hauser *et al.*, 2008) and the Fingerspelling Reproduction Test (Science of Learning Center on Visual Language and Visual Learning Toolkit, 2011).

American Sign Language proficiency assessment

We utilize the ASL-PA since it is particularly suited for the collection of conversational data. Using this instrument, a trained native or near-native signer collects three 10-minute (or longer) language samples from a deaf child within three distinct discourse contexts: (a) Adult-Child Interview; (b) Structured Interaction with a Friend; and (c) Story Retelling (the Tortoise and the Hare narrative). All portions of the ASL-PA are videotaped and scored based on a system that focuses on 23 morphosyntactic features of ASL; the scoring system can categorize child signers, between the ages of 6 and 12, into low, moderate and high proficiency levels of ASL. Because the three discourse contexts are designed to elicit rich child productions, the 30-minute recording also serves as a natural language source data for observing language errors produced by the focal children.

American Sign Language sentence reproduction test

The ASL-SRT is a measure of global ASL fluency including receptive, processing and production skills. It contains 20 signed sentences that are presented via video. Test-takers are asked to repeat each sentence exactly as produced on the video. Deviations from the original sentence (omissions, commissions, phonological errors, etc.) are scored as incorrect. Correct reproductions are awarded a point and the maximum score for the test is 20. An earlier version of the ASL-SRT (a 39-item version) was determined to have a high inter-rater reliability ($R = 0.83$) and internal consistency (alpha coefficient of 0.88; Hauser *et al.*, 2008).

VL2 Fingerspelling reproduction test

The Fingerspelling Reproduction Test assesses a signer's ability to comprehend and copy fingerspelled words ($N = 45$) and pseudo-words ($N = 25$) that were taken from the Spelling and Spelling of Sounds subtests of the Woodcock Johnson III Tests of Achievement. The signer views video clips with the fingerspelled items and, after each clip, the participant is required to repeat (i.e. fingerspell) the item they have just seen. The test items range from 2 to 13 letters in length (mean length = 6.18 letters). In their study of associations between print and fingerspelling, Emmorey and Petrich (2012) reported that 36 adult signers of ASL (mean age 28) were administered the test in two different experiments. The mean items correct of the first administration equaled 84% (S.D. = 11%), and the second administration equaled 82% (S.D. = 18%). The authors also reported that the performance on this test correlated with ASL skill, as measured by the ASL-SRT (Hauser *et al.*, 2008) ($r = 0.494$; $p < 0.001$, based on data from 36 deaf adults [19 males, 17 native signers]).

Language assessment: Perspective-taking tests without preliminary norms

Certain aspects of linguistic and cognitive processing are not included in the existing research instruments and because we had interest in the use of space in ASL with two particular focal children, we needed to develop our own assessments: the ASL Perspective Taking Spatial Orientation Test (ASL-PTSO) and the ASL Perspective Taking Comprehension Test (ASL-PTCT). Both tests are designed to examine a child's visual-spatial cognition, specifically perspective-taking abilities, and how those skills are employed in conjunction with language tasks that involve classifiers and the arrangement of objects in the signing space.

Since these tests do not have norms, our approach has been to also test several age- and gender-matched native signing children in order to determine how peers would perform given the same tasks. As mentioned earlier in this chapter, the challenge of not having sufficient resources for assessment is a part of this relatively new area of research, so a combination of strategies must be used in order to develop rich data sets that can be used for analysis of a child's atypicality.

American Sign Language Perspective Taking Spatial Orientation Test

The ASL-PTSO (Quinto-Pozos & Hou, 2010a) is an adaptation of a paper-and-pencil perspective-taking test that was designed by Mary Hegarty and colleagues (the *Perspective Taking/Spatial Orientation (PTSO)* Test; Hegarty *et al.*, 2008). The PTSO (Hegarty *et al.*, 2008) was designed to assess an individual's ability to imagine himself/herself situated within an array of objects (as shown on paper) and where other objects would be situated in relation to the imagined viewpoint. Prompts are in written English, and the test-taker's task is to draw a vector on a circle to indicate where an object would be located vis-à-vis the imagined perspective (see the 12-item instrument in Appendix D). Performance is measured by accuracy (absolute deviation, in degrees, from the correct response) and error analysis (e.g. within quadrant, opposite or 'mirror' quadrant, etc.) and is compared to Hegarty and Waller's (2004) adult norms.

The Hegarty *et al.* (2008) version of the PTSO was adapted to ASL; this version, referred to as the ASL-PTSO, requires no English instructions but presents the 12 test items via ASL. This version eliminates English within the test, which may serve as a possible limiting factor for participants whose English skills are weak, although it may also add an additional challenge of processing linguistic information since the item prompts employ the use of ASL classifiers and particular locations in the signing space. Some of the objects that were chosen for the circular array differed from that of the Hegarty *et al.* (2008) version, because of our desire to use objects that could each be represented with unique classifiers. See Appendix D for examples of the PTSO, the ASL-PTSO and the quadrant error analysis technique.

American Sign Language Perspective Taking Comprehension Test

The ASL-PTCT was designed to test a signer's ability to imagine a scene from various perspectives (Quinto-Pozos *et al.*, 2010b). In the ASL-PTCT the test-taker is presented with 20 videorecorded signed phrases presented on a laptop computer, each of which contains two classifiers that denote objects (from a set of three objects: a car, a dog or a woman) in specific arrangements (which object is on the left versus right) and orientations (which direction – inward or outward – one of the objects has fallen). On each item, the task is to view each signed phrase (i.e. *item*) and then choose a picture, from four choices, that corresponds with the arrangements and orientations of the objects as indicated by the signer. Item accuracy and response time are measured. In order to test a signer's ability to imagine a scene from various perspectives, the angle of perspective shift is increased throughout the 20 items on the PTCT. Distracter choices are presented from either the opposite perspective (the common vantage point for a signer), or side-by-side perspective (which does not require the viewer to substantially shift perspective). See Appendix E for a sample item and further descriptions.

We also developed a non-linguistic version of the ASL-PTCT, the *Non-linguistic Perspective Taking Comprehension Test*, in order to assess the same skills without the use of ASL as prompts (Quinto-Pozos *et al.*, 2010). Instead, the non-linguistic version utilizes picture prompts, although most other aspects of the design of this test were maintained.

In summary, the administration of various assessments (neuropsychological, visual-spatial non-linguistic cognition, linguistic [including visual-spatial processing]) occurs over multiple visits with the focal child. It is also the case that the same instrument may be administered multiple times – normally after multiple months have elapsed. This allows our team to chart the child's development over time. This approach also allows us to identify patterns that are consistent, rather than relying on particularly poor or good performance on any one testing period. In addition, we utilize multiple tests, even though the tests may be tapping into very similar linguistic and cognitive processes. The reason for this diversity of assessment administration is to establish the reliability of the results.

Our Approach: Data Management and Analysis

Not surprisingly, because of the diversity of the large data set that is created utilizing this case-study approach (i.e. longitudinal information from multiple sources), management and analysis of the data must be done carefully. In this section we highlight key strategies that we have employed to deal with the challenge of pinpointing the characteristics of a child's developmental challenges, given a large and diverse data set.

Our focus here is not on the methods for organization, cataloging and access to the data within a research lab's system; however, we do offer some general tips that have been useful to us. It seems worthwhile to establish a robust system for cross-referencing video data (e.g. footage from interviews and language data collection sessions) with printed transcripts and coding of those data. This makes it relatively easy to return to video data for review and verification of language and behavioral features that need to be confirmed during the review and analysis of a case.

It is also useful to have print data (results from tests, scores, etc.) catalogued according to a system that takes into account the different sources of information. For example, within school records we organized our data according to what was captured in IEP case conference reports, informal assessments (e.g. teacher's grades and comments about a child), formal assessments (e.g. annual state testing with reported norms or other psychological testing conducted by an assessment expert), and external referrals (e.g. referred to a speech language therapist or occupational therapist for services along with their reports). The formal assessments could then be considered alongside other standardized testing that is administered by the research team. We also found that it is useful to have a system for cataloging the data from a chronological perspective while also categorizing the data according to various aspects of development (e.g. linguistic, cognitive, emotional, motor, etc.).

Importance of a diverse set of information

We feel that it is important to consider both qualitative and quantitative information for the analysis of a child's case. Various types of data could be considered as qualitative information: interviews with adults, conversational language data produced by the child, and various types of reports contained in school records. Quantitative information includes the results of standard-ized testing and other aspects of development where the researcher is able to consider the child's performance vis-à-vis that of his/her peers (e.g. through reported norms, group means, etc.). Whereas quantitative results (e.g. perfor-mance on standardized testing) are more straightforward to interpret, it can be a challenge to understand qualitative information in context. We provide some suggestions below.

We use the parental interview as one of the points of entry in the data collection process since it allows us to begin to learn about a child's history. The information collected from the parent(s) forms part of the foundation that we refer back to regularly. Throughout the process of reviewing and analyzing additional data, whether it is data shared with us by the school or data that we collect directly from the child through our own data collection sessions, we repeatedly refer to information gained from the parent(s) in order to confirm or question what we are learning throughout the process of data analysis. Of particular importance is what we learn about a child's infancy, especially their early developmental milestones that include linguistic features (e.g. babbling, first words, first combinations of words) and non-linguistic matters (e.g. crawling, walking and eye-hand coordination). This information helps us to consider whether a child exhibits a congenital developmental dis-order or a deficit that may have been the result of a childhood experience (e.g. accident with trauma to the head, childhood illness with a possible impact on neurological development, etc.). Even though the parental interview has limi-tations (e.g. a parent's memory of what their child did, a qualitative sense that is based on a parent's interpretation, etc.) there is much to be learned by obtaining information from a caregiver who has seen the child throughout their developmental years. Unfortunately, it may also be true that such infor-mation would be difficult, if not impossible, to obtain in some cases.

The school records are read carefully and repeatedly in order to identify themes about the child's development. Like the parental interview, this infor-mation forms a portion of the foundation because it allows the research team to carefully consider what other adults reported before we began working with the child. The informal assessments (e.g. grade reports, teacher comments, etc.) are useful, although the information contained therein should be interpreted with caution – simply because it is difficult to maintain reliable standards for these types of assessments. Some teachers are more lenient graders than others or grades may be based on individual effort and not on academic performance per se. Of particular value, however, are the comments made by teachers about a child's patterns of behavior. We consider these carefully since they provide complementary information – to that received from the parent(s) – with respect to the reports from adults who interacted with a child regularly.

Among the quantitative data are the analyses of conversational lan-guage use by a child. As reported earlier, we utilize the ASL-PA protocol for obtaining our first look at how the child interacts with others – both with adults and with a school peer. The data could be analyzed in a number of ways, including utilizing the protocol for analysis suggested by Maller *et al.* (1999). That includes viewing the conversational data and identifying the use of specific linguistic features from among a list. Once it is confirmed that a child has utilized a feature correctly three times, the researcher moves on to identifying the next feature in the list. The process continues until all the features have been investigated within conversational data.

Another strategy for analyzing conversational data is to target specific linguistic items and how a child uses them throughout that setting in comparison with his/her conversational partners. In the case of one child we have worked with in the past, we have focused on the use of fingerspelling within the interview portions of the ASL-PA because it had been repeatedly reported to us (e.g. by the child's mother and school records) that this child struggles with fingerspelling reception.

Using quantitative data to chart progress over time

As opposed to the qualitative data and analyses that we have touched on above, some of the results are in the form of scores from standardized assessments, and they are perhaps easier to interpret. It is the case that standardized assessments have drawbacks (e.g. they may not be the most representative measures of a test-taker's abilities at any one given time), but they allow for a general charting of a child's development vis-à-vis that of age-matched deaf and hard of hearing peers.

With most of the children enrolled in our study, we have administered some language assessments repeatedly – with periods of 9–12 months intervening between administrations. This allows us to chart a child's development over time and establish the reliability of the results. It may be the case that a child improves over time, but multiple administrations would mitigate a result that would have been influenced by the particular testing day (e.g. if the child was not feeling well and could not attend to the testing situation fully). This procedure can be followed with multiple assessment instruments as long as the test-taker is given enough time between administrations so that memory does not become a primary influence on performance.

Assembling the puzzle

The quantitative and qualitative analyses that are produced after data collection help to create a detailed developmental profile of each focal child in the study. It is this profile that is scrutinized by the research team, which is comprised of researchers who specialize in linguistics and linguistic theory, language acquisition, psychological and cognitive development, and the development of visual-spatial skills in children. Within this area of research it is particularly important to consider children's cognitive development in addition to linguistic development to investigate the possible contribution of non-linguistic cognitive processing deficits to signed language production and comprehension (see Hauser *et al.*, 2008, for a detailed discussion of these factors).

Conclusions

The study of developmental signed language disorders has the potential to contribute significantly to theories of communication disorder and to the practical aspects of working with deaf and hard of hearing children. There is much to be learned about this particular topic, and our team has approached the enquiry by focusing on native signing deaf children and collecting information from a myriad of sources in order to create a developmental profile that is comprehensive and representative of a child's abilities. Future work on childhood signers of ASL could include group studies, which can then build upon the knowledge that we will have gained by looking very carefully at individual cases of development.

References

Anderson, D. and Reilly, J. (2002) The MacArthur Communicative Development Inventory: Normative data for American Sign Language. *Journal of Deaf Studies and Deaf Education* 7, 83–106.

Baser, C.A. and Ruff, R.M. (1987) Construct validity of the San Diego neuropsychological test battery. *Achieves of Clinical Neuropsychology* 2, 13–32.

Beery, K.E. and Beery, N.A. (2004) The Beery–Buktenica Developmental Test of Visual-Motor Integration (5th edn). Minneapolis, MN: NCS Pearson.

Benedict, R.H., Schretlen, D., Groninger, L., Dobraski, M. and Shpritz, B. (1996) Revision of the Brief Visuospatial Memory Test: Studies of normal performance, reliability, and validity. *Psychological Assessment* 8, 145–160.

Benton, A.L., Hamsher, K., Varney, N.R. and Spreen, O. (1983) *Facial Recognition: Stimuli and Multiple Choice Pictures.* New York: Oxford University Press.

De Houwer, A. (2009) *Bilingual First Language Acquisition.* Bristol: Multilingual Matters.

Elliott, C. (2007) *Differential Abilities Scales Test –* (2nd edn). San Antonio, TX: Psychological Corporation.

Emmorey, K. and Petrich, J.A. (2012) Processing orthographic structure: Associations between print and fingerspelling. *Journal of Deaf Studies and Deaf Education* 17 (2), 194–204.

Gioia, G.A., Isquith, P.K., Guy, S.C. and Kenworth, L. (2000) *Behavior Rating Inventory of Executive Function.* Odessa, FL: Psychological Assessment Resources.

Grosjean, F. (2010) Bilingualism, biculturalism, and deafness. *International Journal of Bilingual Education and Bilingualism* 13 (2), 133–145.

Hauser, P.C., Paludnevičiene, R., Supalla, T. and Bavelier, D. (2008) American Sign Language-Sentence Reproduction Test: Development and implications. In R.M. de Quadros (ed.) *Sign Language: Spinning and Unraveling the Past, Present and Future* (pp. 160–172). Petropolis: Editora Arara Azul.

Hauser, P.C., Quinto-Pozos, D. and Singleton, J. L. (submitted) Studying sign language disorders: Considering neuropsychological data. In E. Orfanidou, B. Woll and G.

Morgan (eds) *Research Methods in Sign Language Studies: A Practical Guide*. Hoboken, NJ: Wiley-Blackwell.

Hegarty, M. and Waller, D. (2004) A dissociation between mental rotation and perspective-taking spatial abilities. *Intelligence* 32, 175–191.

Hegarty, M., Kozhevnikov, M. and Waller, D. (2008) *Perspective Taking/Spatial Orientation Test*. University of California, Santa Barbara.

Hoffmeister, R., Lane, H. and Bahan, B. (1996) *Journey into the DEAF WORLD*. San Diego, CA: Dawn Sign Press.

Maller, S.J., Singleton, J.L., Supalla, S.J. and Wix, T. (1999) The development and psychometric properties of the American Sign Language Proficiency Assessment (ASL-PA). *Journal of Deaf Studies and Deaf Education* 4, 249–269.

Martin, N.A. (2006) *Test of Visual Perceptual Skills – 3* (3rd edn). Novato, CA: American Therapy Publications.

Mason, K., Rowley, K., Marshall, C.R., Atkinson, J.R., Herman, R., Woll, B. and Morgan, G. (2010) Identifying specific language impairment in deaf children acquiring British Sign Language: Implications for theory and practice. *British Journal of Developmental Psychology* 28 (1), 33–49. doi: 10.1348/026151009X484190.

Meyers, J. and Meyers, K. (1995) *Rey Complex Figure Test and Recognition Trial*. Odessa, FL: Psychological Assessment Resources.

Mitchell, R. and Karchmer, M. (2004) Chasing the mythical ten percent: Parental hearing status of deaf and hard of hearing students in the United States. *Sign Language Studies* 4 (2), 138–163. doi: 10.1353/sls.2004.0005.

Morgan, G., Herman, R. and Woll, B. (2006) Language impairments in sign language: Breakthroughs and puzzles. *International Journal of Language and Communication Disorders* 42, 97–105.

Mounty, J. (1994) *The Signed Language Development Checklist*. Princeton, NJ: Educational Testing Service.

Peters, M., Lehmann, W., Takahira, S., Takeuchi, Y. and Jordan, K. (2006) Mental rotation performance in four cross-cultural samples: Overall sex differences and the role of academic program in performance. *Cortex* 42, 1005–1014.

Quinto-Pozos, D. and Hou, L. (2010a) American Sign Language Perspective Taking Spatial Orientation Test (ASL-PTSO). Unpublished assessment, University of Texas at Austin.

Quinto-Pozos, D. and Hou, L. (2010b) Non-linguistic Perspective Taking Comprehension Test. Unpublished assessment, University of Texas at Austin.

Quinto-Pozos, D., Hou, L. and Garberoglio, C.L. (2010) American Sign Language Perspective Taking Comprehension Test (ASL-PTCT). Unpublished assessment, University of Texas at Austin.

Quinto-Pozos, D. and Singleton, J. (2009) Developmental histories and language elicitation as complementary strategies for investigating signed language disorders. Paper presented at the Society for Research in Child Development (SRCD) Conference, April, Denver, CO.

Quinto-Pozos, D. and Singleton, J. (2010) Investigating signed language disorders: Case study methods and results. Paper presented at the Theoretical Issues in Sign Language Research (TISLR) Conference, September, West Lafayette, IN.

Quinto-Pozos, D., Forber-Pratt, A. and Singleton, J. (2011) Do developmental signed language disorders exist? Perspectives from professionals. *Language, Speech, and Hearing Services in Schools* 42, 1–21.

Reynolds, C. (2004) *Behavior Assessment System for Children-2* (2nd edn). Circle Pines, MN: American Guidance Service.

Science of Learning Center on Visual Language and Visual Learning (2011) Fingerspelling Reproduction Test [computer video] (Unpublished instrument). Washington, DC.

Singleton, J.L. and Supalla, S. (2011) Assessing children's proficiency of natural signed languages. In M. Marschark and P. Spencer (eds) *Oxford Handbook of Deaf Studies, Language, and Education* (2nd edn) (pp. 306–321). New York: Oxford University Press.

Singleton, J., Jones, G. and Hanumantha, S. (2012) Deaf friendly research? Toward ethical practice in research involving Deaf participants. *DSDJ: Deaf Studies Digital Journal* 3.

Singleton, J.L., Jones, G. and Hanumantha, S. (in press) Toward ethical research practice with Deaf participants. *Journal of Empirical Research on Human Research Ethics.*

Spreen, O. and Strauss, E. (1998) *A Compendium of Neuropsychological Tests: Administration, Norms, and Commentary.* New York: Oxford University Press.

Wechsler, D.L. (1997) *Wechsler Memory Scale* – (3rd edn). San Antonio, TX: Psychological Corporation.

Wechsler, D. (2003) *Wechsler Intelligence Scale for Children* – (4th edn). San Antonio, TX: Psychological Corporation.

Woodcock, R.W., McGrew, K.S. and Mather, N. (2001) *Woodcock–Johnson III Test of Cognitive Abilities.* Rolling Meadows, IL: Riverside Publishing.

Appendix A: Interview Questions for Parent(s)

A.   What led you to believe your child's sign language development was different?

A.   With what areas of language does your child appear to have differences?

A.   Can you give examples?

B.   Has your child ever used any amplification devices?

B.   How much exposure to sign did your child receive as an infant?

B.   What languages – signed or spoken – is your child exposed to:
At his/her school?
At home?
With extended family?
Within your community?

B.   When did you first realize your child was deaf?

B.   When did your child enter a schooling program (early intervention, day programs, etc.)?

C.   At what age did your child produce his/her first sign?
What was the sign?

C.   When did your child first show signs of trying to communicate?

C.   When did your child first start:
Combining signs?
Requesting items?
To crawl?
To walk?
      Has your child reached all the motor developmental milestones on time? Late? With any difficulty?
Using classifiers (show examples)?
Using pronouns – such as ME, YOU, SHE, HE, HIM, HER, MINE?

Using signs with motion – such as GIVE, TAKE?

D.   Does your child have any medical conditions that you think influence his/her learning?
D.   Has your child ever appeared to struggle with the use of facial expressions?
D.   Is there any family history of language problems?
D.   Is your child able to comprehend more sophisticated signing, for example between yourself and another Deaf adult?

Key:
A-Questions – discuss atypical development + examples;
B-Questions – general information;
C-Questions – timeline or milestones (use checklist for school officials);
D-Questions – specific questions about X.

Appendix B: Interview Questions for Clinicians/Educators

Now that the parents of <child's name> have signed the consent form, they give us permission to ask you some specific questions about <child's name>. In our first interview we kept our questions more general, now we'll be more specific. I'll show you a copy of the interview consent form you signed for our first interview so that you can be reminded of what you signed. The same procedures apply. Do you have any questions about this before we start?

–   Is <child's name >'s situation the first time you have encountered this particular challenge with language learning? How often have you seen this kind of pattern before?
–   What is it about <child's name >'s pattern of learning that made you think it was atypical?
–   According to the school records, the school staff has conducted the following language assessments with <child's name> [list assessments here]. What was your experience with using these instruments in the assessment situation? Do you feel these are authentic reflections of <child's name >'s language development? Did you consider using other assessments?
–   What kind of intervention strategies have you tried with <child's name >? Have any of these approaches (even if informal) been successful, even if in a limited way?
–   Do you feel <child's name> comprehends more than he/she can produce in ASL?
–   Do you feel that <child's name> struggles academically?
–   Do you feel that <child's name> struggles socially?

- Do you feel that <child's name >'s language production and comprehension patterns are similar at home vs. school contexts?
- In your opinion, is <child's name> aware that their sign language development is atypical?
- What advice do you have for us as we develop a plan for observing this child in their classroom setting? What suggestions do you have regarding potential assessments that we might use?

Appendix C: Neuropsychological Assessments

Table 3.C1 Neuropsychological assessments

Area(s)	Assessments
General cognitive functioning	• Wechsler Intelligence Scale for Children – 4th Edition (WISC-IV; Wechsler, 2003), various subtests (Block Design, Similarities, Picture Concepts, Coding, Matrix Reasoning, Comprehension, Symbol Search)
Executive functioning	• Behavior Rating Inventory of Executive Functions (BRIEF; Gioia *et al.*, 2000) • Decision Speed and Visual Matching subtests of the Woodcock Johnson-III Test of Cognitive Abilities (Woodcock *et al.*, 2001)
Visualization skills and visual working memory	• Mental Rotation Test (Peters *et al.*, 2006) • Woodcock Johnson Spatial Relations subtest (Woodcock *et al.*, 2001)
Memory skills	• Wechsler Memory Scale – 3rd Edition (WMS-III; Wechsler, 1997) • Spatial Span subtest (a.k.a. Corsi Blocks) • Differential Abilities Scale – 2nd Edition (Elliott, 2007) Recall of Objects subtest • Brief Visuospatial Memory Test – Revised (BVMT-R; Benedict *et al.*, 1996) • Rey Osterrieth Complex Figure Test (Meyers & Meyers, 1995)
Visual processing	• Beery Developmental Test of Visual Motor Integration (VMI; Beery & Beery, 2004) • Benton Facial Recognition Test (Benton *et al.*, 1983) • Test of Visual Perceptual Skills – 3rd Edition (Martin, 2006)
Motor skills	• Hand Dynamometer (Spreen & Strauss, 1998) • Fingertapping Test (Spreen & Strauss, 1998) • Grooved Pegboard Test (Baser & Ruff, 1987).
Behavior and emotional functioning	• Behavior Assessment System for Children – 2nd Edition (Reynolds, 2004)

Appendix D: Visual-Spatial Assessments

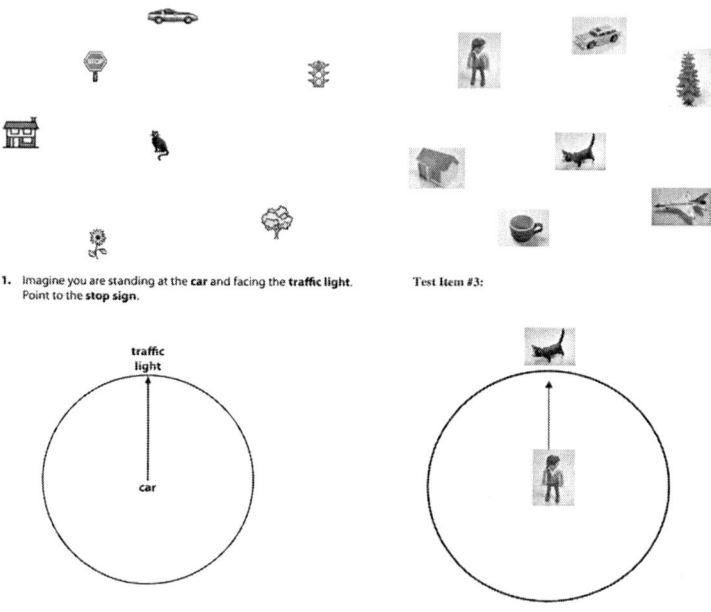

1. Imagine you are standing at the **car** and facing the **traffic light**. Point to the **stop sign**.

Test Item #3:

Imagine you are standing at the **car** and facing the **house**. Point to the **traffic light**.

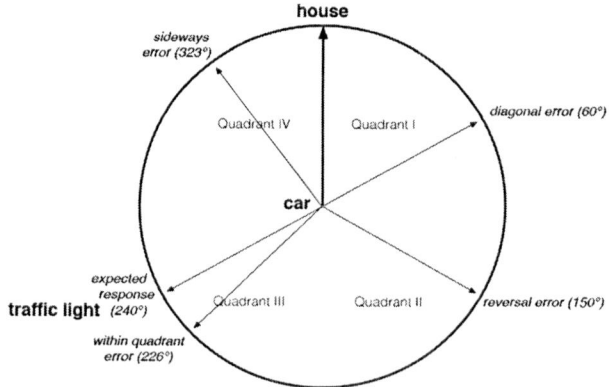

Figure 3.D1 Examples of the PTSO (upper left; Hegarty *et al.*, 2008), the ASL-PTSO (upper right, Quinto-Pozos & Hou, 2010a), and the quadrant scoring technique for each test (lower)

Appendix E: Example Item from the ASL-PTCT (Quinto-Pozos *et al.*, 2010)

Final frame of video stimuli:
Opposite perspective (180°)   Side-by-side perspective (45°)
(matches explanation below)   (for example purposes)

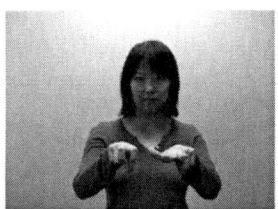
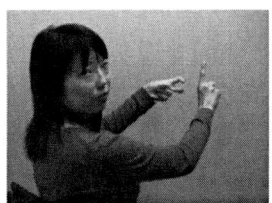

English glosses (for opposite perspective example only; this information is not viewed by test-taker):

DOG CL-animal-facing-forward (right hand), CAR CL-vehicle-facing-forward-turned-on-right-side (left hand)

English translation:

'A dog facing away from the signer is to the right of the car, which is facing in the same direction and resting on its right side (with the top of the car facing the dog).'

Participant options (they appear all at once on a screen following the stimulus video):

(a)   (b)   (c)   (d)

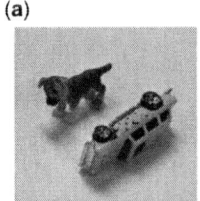
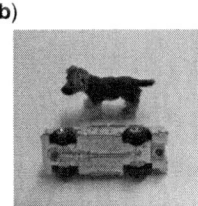
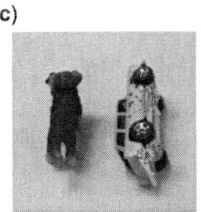
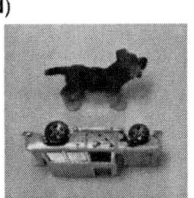

Choices (c) and (d) are incorrect because the dog is to the left of the car, and choice (a) is incorrect because the car is resting on its left side. Choice (c) is also the egocentric foil. Choice (b) is the correct answer for this item.

Notes

(1) This process is followed in order to comply with the Individualized Education Program (IEP) (see http://www.idea.gov for detailed information), a federal program that is designed to serve students with disabilities within the US educational system.

(2) In most cases, the limited norms are based on the performance of children. However, at the present time we do not have child comparison data for the Fingerspelling Reproduction Test.

4 The Acquisition of Sign Language by Deaf Children with Autism Spectrum Disorder

Aaron Shield and Richard P. Meier

Introduction

Autism spectrum disorder (ASD) consists of a set of neurobiological developmental disorders characterized by communicative and social deficits as well as repetitive, stereotyped behaviors.[1] In this chapter, we use the terms 'ASD' and 'autism' interchangeably; although 'autism' is not a clinical term, it is the term popularly used to refer to the range of disorders found in ASD.

The language deficits of hearing children with autism are well documented, and can range from the very mild in highly fluent speakers to the very severe in children with a total absence of productive spoken language. For those children who do acquire speech, the most common characteristics of autistic language include echolalia (echoing the utterances of others), pronoun reversal, idiosyncratic language use and neologisms (the creation of new words), difficulty with pragmatics (problems interpreting the use of language in context and the non-literal use of language), and abnormal intonation and vocal quality. Although relatively little research to date has focused on the sign language deficits of deaf children with autism, in this chapter we will review what is currently known about the sign language of such children. It is worth noting from the outset that virtually all work on this population has occurred since 2010, and findings are still preliminary.

Apparent dramatic increases in the rates of autism in the general population (1 in 88 children in the United States; Centers for Disease Control, 2012) have been widely publicized. Since autism is a brain disorder and occurs whether or not hearing is intact, it is likely that autism affects at least as high a percentage of the deaf population as the general population. Indeed, Szymanski *et al.* (2012) recently reported that 1 in 59 deaf or hard of hearing children in the 2009–2010 Annual Survey of Deaf and Hard of Hearing Children and Youth (Gallaudet Research Institute, 2011) carried an ASD diagnosis. Chess *et al.* (1978) reported that 7% of 243 students deafened by rubella had autistic symptoms, while Jure *et al.* (1991) found that 46 (4%) of a sample of 1150 children with hearing impairment also carried a diagnosis of autism. Conversely, there is evidence that severe hearing loss occurs at a higher rate in the autistic population (3.5%; Rosenhall *et al.*, 1999) than in the general population (0.3%; White, 2004).

In this chapter, we seek to introduce the community of sign language researchers to the theoretical and practical issues involved in autism research. Our aim is to describe what is known about the interaction of autism with sign acquisition, discuss how the social, cognitive and linguistic deficits of autism are likely to impact sign language acquisition, and suggest areas that may be particularly fruitful for future research.

Methodological problems

Sign language researchers interested in autism will immediately encounter a methodological hurdle in their research: no diagnostic instruments have yet been designed specifically for deaf children, although several instruments are – at the time of this writing – in the process of being adapted for use with deaf children. Still, current gold standard instruments such as the Autism Diagnostic Observation Schedule, Second Edition (ADOS-2; Lord *et al.*, 2012) or the Autism Diagnostic Interview – Revised (ADI-R; Lord *et al.*, 1994) have yet to be adapted for deaf children, and the ADOS explicitly warns against use with deaf children. Moreover, recent research has demonstrated that behavioral checklists widely used as ASD screening instruments lack sensitivity when used with deaf children: Szymanski (2010) found that only 50% of 52 deaf children with a reported diagnosis of an ASD scored in the clinically significant range on three common screeners for ASD, the Gilliam Autism Rating Scale – Second Edition (GARS-2; Gilliam, 2006), the Social Communication Questionnaire (SCQ; Rutter *et al.*, 2003), or the Social Responsiveness Scale (SRS; Constantino, 2002). It is thus possible that ASD could be under-identified in deaf children, given the lack of appropriate diagnostic and screening instruments. Accurately diagnosing a deaf child with ASD remains a formidable obstacle, and often requires the judgment of clinicians who are both expert in ASD and familiar with deaf children.

The translation and adaptation of such instruments for use with deaf children is likely to be complex, as some of the items are inappropriate for deaf children. For example, one item on the ADOS concerns the child's response to his/her name being called by the examiner. The purpose of this task is 'to observe the consistency of the child's response to a hierarchy of auditory stimuli' (ADOS module 1, p. 2) and to see what the examiner needs to do in order to get the child's attention. It is unclear how this item would be adapted for use with a deaf child. There is no sign language equivalent of calling a child's name, although there are conventional attention-getting behaviors in the Deaf community (hand-waving, foot-stomping, or touching a person on the shoulder). How would these various behaviors be scored, and are they all equivalent to calling the child's name? Other parts of the ADOS are problematic as well, including items scoring pointing, gesture, facial expressions and intonation of vocalizations, all of which would require significant adaptation for deaf children acquiring sign. Until appropriate test instruments are published, it will remain difficult to be certain that an autism diagnosis for a deaf child is correct. Several studies have documented that diagnosis of ASD in deaf children is often delayed, if it occurs at all: Roper et al. (2003) found that the mean age of diagnosis in their sample of nine deaf ASD British children was 15;0 (range 5;0–16;0), compared with 7;5 (4;0–11;0) in a group of hearing autistic children. Jure et al. (1991) similarly reported that autism diagnosis was delayed in their sample of 46 hearing-impaired autistic children, with some children not being diagnosed until age 17. Mandell et al. (2005) found that diagnosis of ASD in deaf children lagged behind hearing children by approximately one year.

Although we believe that it is advantageous to expose deaf children to a visual language that is more fully accessible to them than is speech, the acquisition of sign is nonetheless likely to be challenging for deaf children with ASD. This is because some of the social skills impaired in autism are particularly crucial for the acquisition of signed language, and could lead to sign-specific linguistic deficits.

Indeed, the visual-gestural modality of sign relies crucially on a set of social, perceptual and articulatory skills that are known to be impaired in autism. We will mention three obstacles that may confront children with autism. First, hearing children with autism differ both from typically developing (TD) children and from children with other kinds of developmental delay in their limited use of gesture; children with autism produce significantly fewer gestures (Buitelaar et al., 1991) and are developmentally less advanced in their use of gesture (Mundy et al., 1986). Although non-linguistic gesture should not be confused with sign, sign and gesture are both articulated with the hands, and signers gesture while they sign. Could a deficit in gesture impact how deaf children with ASD acquire sign? Secondly, the perception and comprehension of visual linguistic stimuli by autistic children could be disrupted by a variety of known deficits in the areas of eye gaze, face-scanning behavior and comprehension of facial expression. Thirdly, hearing children with autism often show impairments in the ability to imitate the body movements of others (Williams *et al.*, 2004) and exhibit a variety of motor deficits (Ming *et al.*, 2007) that could lead to articulatory problems in sign. Thus, the acquisition of sign by autistic children is likely to be affected by these social, perceptual and motoric deficits.

In the next sections, we will describe what is known about the interaction of autism with sign acquisition in both hearing and deaf children.

What is Known About the Interaction of Autism with Sign Acquisition?

Few studies have examined the signing of deaf children or adults on the autism spectrum, although there have been several case studies of deaf children with autism who do not sign. For example, Brimer and Murphy (1988) reported the case of a deaf autistic boy, but focused exclusively on his acquisition of English, and Malandraki and Okalidou (2007) described a 10-year-old deaf Greek child with autism who was trained to use the Picture Exchange Communication System (PECS; Bondy & Frost, 1994), but was not taught a sign language.

Poizner *et al.* (1990) reported a single 21-year-old deaf autistic signer who exhibited sign echolalia. Morgan and colleagues have reported extensively on the British Sign Language (BSL) acquisition of Christopher, a hearing language savant with autistic characteristics (Morgan *et al.*, 2002a, 2002b, 2007; Smith *et al.*, 2011).[2] These reports contain some of the most detailed sign language data available about a person with autism. We will discuss the findings on Christopher in a later section.

More recently, two studies in particular have investigated specific sign language structures in the signing of deaf children with autism. Denmark (Denmark, 2011; Denmark *et al.*, 2009) studied how deaf British children and adolescents on the autism spectrum produce and perceive facial grammar in BSL, while Shield (2010) and Shield and Meier (2012) analyzed formational errors in the signing of deaf American children with autism. These studies will also be described in detail in later sections.

In contrast to the few studies on the signing of deaf children with autism, there is a rich literature on the therapeutic use of signs as an alternative to speech for hearing children with severe autism. Despite the limitations of these studies, it is worth reviewing the major findings of these works, which are reported below.

Sign language and hearing children with autism

In the late 1960s, an interest developed in the ability of autistic children to learn signs – particularly children who had failed to acquire speech following intensive speech therapy. It was suggested that some non-verbal autistic children 'complied readily if gesture or demonstration were used to convey the request' (Webster *et al.*, 1973: 338). Another paper reported, 'We have found it impossible to teach some children to speak. Yet some of these same children have learned to express themselves quite rapidly once they have been shown how to use their hands' (Stull *et al.*, 1979: 144). As a result of these early studies, sign was seen as a possible alternative communication mode for autistic children who had failed to acquire speech. Numerous studies in the late 1970s and early 1980s performed interventions with non-verbal autistic hearing children (for reviews, see Bonvillian *et al.*, 1981; Carr, 1979). These children were taught manual signs either alone or in addition to speech.

Although these papers are not sufficiently detailed to enable a proper analysis of the signs that the children produced, the results showed that some autistic children were successful at learning signs, even when previous attempts to teach spoken words had failed. Bonvillian *et al.* (1981: 128), in their review of over 20 studies involving the teaching of signs to more than 100 children with autism, note that:

> results of these studies indicate that even fairly brief simultaneous communication or sign language training can be an effective means of improving communication skills in low-functioning autistic children. Despite an extensive range of individual outcomes, almost every subject acquired the ability to comprehend trained signs.

Bonvillian *et al.* reported that the children acquired vocabularies ranging from five signs to over 350 signs, although Bonvillian and Blackburn (1991: 276) suggested in a later paper that 'statements in the literature about the sign vocabulary sizes of autistic children ... may considerably over-represent their real working vocabularies' because most of the signs trained to criterion in such studies were not observed in spontaneous usage outside of training sessions. Still, researchers argued that signs could be advantageous over speech because children's hands can be guided and molded, and signs can be exaggerated, enlarged or frozen to allow for additional processing time (Jordan, 1990). As various researchers have noted (recently, Pizer *et al.*, 2011), deaf mothers of TD deaf children also sometimes enlarge their signs or mold their children's hands in the acquisition process.

Importantly, most of the signs acquired by these hearing children with autism were nouns, while there are contradictory claims in the literature about the ability of these children to master what Carr (1979: 353) called 'abstract sign language ... prepositions, pronouns, and other abstractions'. A few researchers reported success: Creedon (1973) claimed that her 21 formerly non-verbal autistic subjects between the ages of four and nine achieved great success in many areas of language acquisition after an intervention employing simultaneous communication (that is, the simultaneous use of spoken and signed English). Similarly, Bonvillian *et al.* (1981: 128) reported that 'in many cases children moved to daily production of many complex sign utterances', although it is not clear what kinds of 'complex sign utterances' were produced by these children. Indeed, any claim about the acquisition of complex structures must be looked at skeptically. As Bonvillian *et al.* (1981: 130) note:

> [the] absence of detailed records of most of the children's sign language combinations makes it impossible to determine for fairly fluent children whether there is sufficient regularity of syntax or comprehension of complex semantic aspects in the children's sign utterances to credit them with these fundamentals of language.

Thus, despite the large number of studies on the subject, the available data are insufficient to determine if sign intervention with hearing ASD children (whether using American Sign Language [ASL] or Signed English) facilitates the mastery of complex grammatical structures. For most children, the data indicate that sign learning is limited to a small number of simple signs, after which they 'make only limited progress in terms of the average length and complexity of their sign utterances' (Bonvillian *et al.*, 1981: 130).

In general, these studies provide little information about the form or use of signs produced by children with autism. Only one study (Seal & Bonvillian, 1997) looked at the form of signs produced by a sample of children with autism, all of them hearing. They analyzed the sign production of 14 low-functioning hearing autistic students (12 male, 2 female) who were enrolled at a residential school for children with developmental disorders and who ranged in age from 9;2 to 20;4 (mean age 13;8). The goal of the study was 'to determine the sign formational elements that autistic children successfully and unsuccessfully produced in making their signs' (Seal & Bonvillian, 1997: 440), with an eye towards 'uncovering associations between autistic children's signing and any underlying motor deficits' (Seal & Bonvillian, 1997: 439). Focusing on the sign parameters of handshape, location, and movement[3] (see Editor's Introduction, this volume), they analyzed 348 signs produced by the children with autism. Although there was wide variability in error rates across the participants, locations were produced more successfully (16% error rate) than either handshapes or movements (36% error rate for both). Three locations – neutral space, the chin and the torso (trunk) – accounted for nearly three-quarters of subjects' signs. The movement parameter was difficult for subjects and the source of many formational errors. Signs that exhibited a contacting action with the body were produced most accurately, while several frequently occurring movements (twisting, toward-the-body, circling and away-from-the-body) had high error rates, ranging from 43% to 53%. Also, subjects tended to add epenthetic movements – extra movements not included in the citation form

– and to reduce signs consisting of two or three sequential movements to a single movement.

The size of the students' vocabularies and their accuracy in articulating signs were highly correlated with scores on tests for fine motor age and apraxia, a neuromotor disorder that impairs the ability to perform pre-planned or voluntary motor movements. Seal and Bonvillian (1997) inter-preted this result as an indication that sign formation errors could result in part from underlying motor deficits. However, they explicitly rejected the idea that such deficits could be the sole explanation for the communicative difficulties of autistic children, allowing for the possibility that there could be cognitive and perceptual reasons for such errors as well.

A later study (Soorya, 2003) further explored the relationship between motor skills, apraxia (a motor planning disorder that results in an inability to carry out planned movements), and the acquisition of signs by hearing children with autism. In two experiments, Soorya compared 12 children with autism to TD children who were matched for either mental or chrono-logical age. She found that the children with autism performed significantly more poorly than mental-age-matched TD children on apraxia tests, but not on motor tests. However, she did not find differences between children with autism and mental-age-matched TD children on sign language production or comprehension.

Collectively, these studies on hearing children accounted for the prepon-derance of work on sign and autism until very recently. The paucity of stud-ies of deaf children – particularly studies of deaf children of deaf parents exposed to a sign language from birth – limits our ability to understand how autism affects sign language development. Two earlier studies (Bonvillian & Blackburn, 1991; Ornitz & Ritvo, 1976) reported the presence of deaf or hearing-impaired subjects within their study populations, but data from those subjects were analyzed together with the hearing subjects. Poizner *et al.* (1990) and Denmark (2011) both observed a single native deaf signer in their studies. To our knowledge, only our own study (Shield & Meier, 2012) has reported on multiple native-signing children on the autism spectrum. In studies of theoretical significance, in which the goal is to understand how autism affects cognition, it is preferable to include children exposed to sign language since birth (deaf-of-deaf children), inasmuch as deaf children of hearing parents have documented developmental and language delays (Schick *et al.*, 2007) that could obscure the effects of autism on language and cogni-tive development. Since 90–95% of deaf children are born to hearing parents (Mitchell & Karchmer, 2004), identifying and recruiting native-signing autis-tic children represents a formidable methodological challenge.

Therefore, most previous studies on the acquisition of sign by children on the autism spectrum, although useful in describing a possible alternative communication strategy for hearing children when speech training has failed, do not help us understand how the core deficits of autism interact with language acquisition in the visual-spatial modality. A question of fundamental importance is whether the linguistic characteristics of autistic signing are the same as those of autistic speech. Identifying the characteristics of autistic signing may clarify the role of modality in language acquisition, insofar as sign and speech draw upon somewhat different sets of perceptual, cognitive and social skills. Differences in the linguistic profiles of deaf and hearing autistic children would provide strong evidence for the effects of these modality differences. In the next two sections, we will examine two of the most well documented characteristics of autistic speech – echolalia and pronoun reversals – as a way to analyze the interaction of modality with the deficits of autism.

Echolalia

Echolalia[4] is the repetition of other people's vocal productions, which can occur either immediately or with a delay. It was first reported in autistic children by Kanner (1943) and is 'the most frequently cited characteristic of verbal autistic children' (Prizant & Duchan, 1981), affecting up to 85% of the autistic children in some studies (Schuler & Prizant, 1985). All children repeat other people's utterances, and indeed imitation is a necessary building block for language acquisition. It is the extreme and exact nature of autistic children's repetitions that make them noteworthy; they may reflect a 'gestalt' approach to language acquisition (Prizant, 1983) rather than the analytic mode typical of normal language acquisition (Bloom & Lahey, 1978; Peters, 1983).

Is echolalia a modality-independent function of the autistic child's approach to language, or a specific effect of the vocal-auditory modality? Several reports of echolalia in signing children with autism suggest that it is the former. Poizner et al. (1990) described the signing of a 21-year-old native-signing deaf woman with autism whom they call Judith M. Despite the rich signing environment in which she was raised – her deaf parents and two elder brothers communicated exclusively in sign – Judith M. produced her first sign at age five. Poizner et al. (1990: 68) report a simple exchange between Judith M. and her father, in which the majority of her utterances are echolalic:

Father: Do you want to see a train?[5]
Judith M.:   SEE TRAIN. [An imitation of sign just produced by her father.]
Father: First, we will...?
Judith M.:   FIRST. [Imitation.]
Father: Second, we will...?
Judith M.:   SECOND... STORE.
Father: Yes, we will go to the store. Third, we will...?
Judith M.:   THIRD. [Imitation.]

Father: Yes, we will be home soon.
Judith M.:   HOME, SOON. [Imitation.]
Father: What will we do on Wednesday?
Judith M.:   STORE... TRAIN.
Father: That again?
Judith M.:   AGAIN. [Imitation.]
Father: Father and Judith M. will go to a store.
Judith M.:   STORE... FIRST... SECOND.
Father: In the morning, we first go to the store.
Judith M.:   FIRST. [Imitation.]

The authors indicate that Judith M. exhibited no evidence of grammatical knowledge, morphology or syntax. Her signing consisted largely of imitations of signs produced immediately before by her interlocutor. She rarely initiated communication or signed spontaneously. It is worth noting that this case study demonstrates that children raised in signing households can also have severe language problems, just as some hearing children with autism do: sign is not a panacea for children with language disorders.

There are several other mentions of sign echolalia in the literature. Smith *et al.* (2011) have reported that Christopher, upon first exposure to BSL, would often repeat signs without understanding them.[6] Of 27 deaf children with autism exposed to sign language in Jure *et al.*'s (1991) study, 21 could sign words or phrases, and five of these produced echolalic utterances. Finally, follow-up analyses of the data reported in Shield (2010) revealed that one participant, a deaf girl of deaf parents age 11;9, showed markedly echolalic signing, repeating the instructions to tasks as the experimenter signed them. For example, in introducing a task in which a novel object was labeled with a nonsense sign, the experimenter signed I INVENT SIGN, YOU-COPY-ME, YOUR-TURN. The child echoed each sign produced by the experimenter, signing back I INVENT SIGN, YOU-COPY-ME, YOUR-TURN. The fact that she did not maintain pronominal or verb agreement reference strongly implies echolalic signing without comprehension. We thus feel confident, even at this early stage, in concluding that echolalia is a modality-independent phenomenon characteristic of both autistic speech and autistic signing.

In the next section, we turn to another hallmark of autistic speech, pronoun reversal. Although pronoun reversal may be related to echolalia in some instances, there is reason to suspect that the cognitive deficit underlying pronoun reversal in autistic speech may lead to quite different effects in sign.

Pronoun reversal

Pronoun reversal – especially the reversal of the first- and second-person pronouns *I/me* and *you* – is more common in children with autism than in any other group (Lee *et al.*, 1994). It was originally noted by Kanner (1943), who believed that the pronoun reversals found in his case studies were related to echolalia:

> [Don] always seemed to be parroting what he had heard said to him at one time or another. He used the personal pronouns for the persons he was quoting, even imitating the intonation. When he wanted his mother to pull his shoe off, he said: 'Pull off your shoe.' When he wanted a bath, he said: 'Do you want a bath?'

Since Kanner's seminal paper, pronoun reversals in the speech of hearing children with autism have been reported in many other studies (e.g. Bartak & Rutter, 1974; Charney, 1980). TD children also sometimes reverse pronouns early in development, between the ages of 1;7 and 2;4 (Chiat, 1982; Clark, 1978; Oshima-Takane, 1992; Schiff-Myers, 1983), but this is a transitory phase, and does not persist (Bartak & Rutter, 1974; Dale & Crain-Thoreson, 1993).

Several hypotheses have been advanced to explain the difficulty that many autistic children have in mastering first- and second-person pronouns. One theory has emphasized pragmatic factors, particularly 'in conceptualizing the notion of self and other as it is embedded in shifting discourse roles between speaker and listener' (Lee *et al.*, 1994; Tager-Flusberg, 1993, 1994, 2000). Thus, a child acquiring language must come to understand that the meaning of pronouns depends on who the speaker is: *I* is not a name for any particular person, but rather refers to the speaker of a given utterance. According to this hypothesis, not just pronouns but all deictic terms should cause problems for people with autism. Indeed, Hobson *et al.* (2010) found that a majority of children with autism in their sample (but not a single one of the children without autism) incorrectly referred to a location that was distal to themselves with the more proximal terms *this* or *here*, and scored significantly lower on a task in which they were asked to place toy animals either close to or distant from themselves after receiving instructions containing contrasting terms such as *this* and *that*, *here* and *there*, *bring* and *take*, and *come* and *go*.

A second hypothesis that is particularly interesting for the study of sign language is that the proper use of person pronouns could require a more general understanding of people's differing spatial perspectives. In one study, Loveland (1984) tested a group of 27 TD children between the ages of 2;0 and 3;3 on the comprehension and production of first- and second-person subject and possessive pronouns as well as the understanding of differing visual perspectives. She found that only children who demonstrated comprehension of other people's different spatial points of view made no errors on pronouns, suggesting that an appreciation of the spatial perspectives of others is a cognitive prerequisite for the proper acquisition of pronominal forms. In another study, Ricard *et al.* (1999) tested French- and English-speaking toddlers on visual perspective-taking skills and pronoun usage. They found that performance on perspective-taking tasks was correlated with pronoun acquisition, and that the ability to coordinate two perspectives preceded mastery of first- and second-person pronouns. Thus, there is some evidence that visual perspective-taking skills underlie the pragmatic understanding necessary for the proper use of pronouns in speech. Although results have been mixed, several studies (Hamilton *et al.*, 2009; Reed, 2002; Warreyn *et al.*, 2005) have shown that children with ASD are impaired in their ability to understand the differing visual perspectives of others.

Unlike pronouns in spoken languages, which are arbitrary combinations of sounds unrelated to their meaning, pronouns in signed languages tend to be indexical points to the intended referent. Despite this transparency, there is evidence that some TD deaf children produce pronoun reversals at a stage early in development. Petitto (1987) found reversals in first- and second-person pronominal points produced by two TD native-signing deaf children between the ages of 21 and 23 months. However, she argued that these reversals were not due to a perspective-taking failure, but rather to an over-lexicalization of indexical points, effectively turning a deictic point into a frozen lexical item. In other words, the signing child interpreted the points directed at her (the ASL pronoun YOU) as her name, and would thus produce a point outwards from herself in reference to herself. This is indeed how lexical items (but not pronouns) in signed languages typically work, as Petitto (1987: 42) observed in the same paper:

> Learning signs requires that the child be able to perform a spatial transformation, such that what she produces is the mirror image of what she sees, rather than its literal form. Failure to perform this transformation would result in perceptually-based errors. . . . Essentially, the child should sign backwards.

We will return to this important observation about the nature of sign later, in our discussion of reversal errors in autistic signing.

To date, Petitto's study is the only report of pronoun reversals in sign, although Casey (2003) has reported a similar instance of a reversed verb (GIVE-YOU to mean 'give me', produced by a two-year-old TD deaf child).[7] Hatzopoulou (2010) studied the acquisition of pronouns in Greek Sign Language by one native-signing deaf Greek child between 12 and 36 months of age, but did not find pronoun errors. While it is clear that pronoun reversals in sign are possible, it is not yet clear how pervasive this phenomenon is, and whether reversals occur in sign for the same reasons they occur in speech.

There are no documented reports of pronoun reversals in the signing of deaf children with autism, though some authors have presumed (prematurely, it would seem) that pronoun reversals will occur in autistic signing, just as in autistic speech (e.g. Collins & Carney, 2007). Some of this confusion may have stemmed from studies which have documented pronoun reversals in the *speech* of deaf children (Oshima-Takane *et al.*, 1993).

Shield (2012) analyzed the spontaneous production of pointing signs, including pronouns, by four native ASL users with autism between the ages of 4;6 and 7;5. In 20-minute samples taken from naturalistic data in his dissertation, he found that all four children produced points, and that these points included points to self (i.e. first-person pronouns), points to others (second/third person pronouns) and points to objects. Two children produced five points each, one child produced 11 points, and one child produced 25 points. He analyzed the points to self and others in discourse for intended reference but did not find evidence of reversals.

Despite the lack of documented pronoun reversals in the signing of deaf children with ASD, there may still be abnormalities in pointing behavior. In interviews reported by Shield (2010), four Deaf mothers of deaf children with autism reported abnormalities in how their children referred to themselves and to others. One mother indicated that her son would sometimes refer to himself with his name sign rather than an indexical point (pronoun), although note that she also reports correct pronominal usage:

> [My son] can point to himself as in I WANT FOOD. Before he used to sign [his sign name]. I corrected him, instructing him to not say his name and instead to point to himself. He learned that about three or four years ago [when he was between the ages of four and five]. Now he points to himself. Sometimes he alternates between pointing to himself and signing his name sign[8] ... When he refers to us, he points a little bit, but he tends to fingerspell our names. He will sign MOMMY, fingerspell his brother's name, and sign his own name sign. He seldom points to refer to us. Occasionally, if he fights with his brother, he will point to [his brother] emphatically and yell YOU WRONG (*'you're wrong!'*). He points at his brother and doesn't sign his name. But if he comes up to me, he will use his brother's name sign instead of a point.[9]

Another mother stated that her son did not use points to refer to people, but did use points to make requests:

> I don't see pointing from [my son] at all. But long ago, when he was younger, he used to point to things to express what he wanted. For example, if he wanted something like food, he would point at the refrigerator incessantly. He used to point at things to make requests, but he stopped. Since then, I don't see him pointing.

These maternal reports are consistent with studies reporting abnormal pointing behavior in the communicative gestures of hearing children with autism

(Ricks & Wing, 1975). Baron-Cohen (1989) found that protodeclarative point-ing (as in sharing or commenting on an object) is impaired in autism, though protoimperative pointing (as in requesting) is not. Other studies have con-firmed that gestures used for requesting objects, actions or social routines may be present in autism (Attwood *et al.*, 1988; Loveland & Landry, 1986), while gestures sharing an awareness of an object's existence or properties are absent (Curcio, 1978; Mundy *et al.*, 1986, 1987; Wetherby, 1986).

We cannot yet say with confidence whether pronoun reversals are char-acteristic of the signing of deaf children with autism, or indeed if they occur at all. However, converging findings in the areas of gesture imitation and sign language acquisition suggest that the same cognitive deficits that under-lie pronoun reversal in hearing children with autism will affect various levels of structure in sign, from the sub-lexical to the morphological. In the next section, we will provide evidence for this hypothesis from studies on gesture imitation in autism, and then proceed to more recent work on acquisition of sign by deaf children with autism.

Imitation of gestures in autism

Children with autism are impaired in their ability to imitate others, although the exact nature of this impairment, as well its underlying cause, has occasioned much debate. Most studies on the subject have found an imitation deficit in autistic subjects (although a few studies have not; e.g. see Morgan *et al.*, 1989). DeMyer *et al.* (1972) found that children with autism were impaired in their ability to imitate the bodily actions of others as well as motor-object actions, such as stringing beads. Curcio (1978) found that non-verbal children with autism between the ages of four and 12 performed poorly on gestural imitation, a finding that has been replicated in other stud-ies (e.g. Dawson & Adams, 1984).

These deficits have led to different accounts of what underlies the imita-tion impairment in autism. Smith and Bryson (1994: 262), in their review of 15 studies of the imitation skills of autistic children, commented that these studies 'provide some support for the existence of a specific imitative deficit in autism but are uninformative as to its nature.' In another review of 21 studies of imitation by autistic subjects, Williams *et al.* (2004) concluded that of the six major theories advanced in the literature about the nature of the imitation deficit in autism, a specific deficit in self-other mapping abil-ity (Rogers & Pennington, 1991) was most consistent with the evidence pre-sented. Self-other mapping refers to the process(es) by which children or adults are able to observe the movements of others and map those observed movements onto their own bodies, thus reproducing the movements accurately.[10]

The most compelling evidence for this theory is the striking finding of a number of studies (Brown, 1996; Hobson & Lee, 1999; Ohta, 1987; Smith &

Bryson, 1998; Whiten & Brown, 1998) that when autistic children attempt to imitate the arm and hand movements produced by others, they sometimes reverse palm orientation and the direction of these arm movements. Ohta (1987) was the first to report such errors (which he called 'partial imitations') in imitations of gestures. Children with autism showed a tendency to imitate a wave-like gesture in which the experimenter's open palm was oriented toward the child with a gesture in which the palm was oriented inward toward the child him/herself. Later, Smith and Bryson (1998) found that children with autism made significantly more 180° reversal errors in palm orientation than age-matched language-impaired and TD children in the imitation of eight ASL handshapes and eight bimanual gestures.

These errors appear to be unique to autism. They have been observed in a variety of contexts, including the imitation of object-related actions, pantomimes, and meaningful and meaningless gestures. Like the spoken language pronominal reversals discussed earlier, these errors may reflect a general ability to imitate words and gestures but a specific difficulty with the shifts in perspective needed to use spoken language pronouns correctly or to imitate manual gestures accurately. Instead, children with autism tend to replicate bodily movements as observed from their own point of view, not as they are produced by the person they are attempting to imitate. This finding has clear implications for the acquisition of sign by deaf children with autism, since palm orientation and direction of arm movements have linguistic value in sign. For example, the ASL signs PAPER and CLEAN vary only in the direction of movement of the dominant hand. If the sign-learning child reproduces a sign's direction of movement as observed from his own perspective, such an error could lead to an unintended meaning. This outcome could also arise with pairs of signs that differ primarily or solely in their palm orientation, such as the ASL signs TUESDAY (palm inward) and TOILET (palm outward); see Figure 4.1.

There is evidence that indeed, the same reversal errors found in the imitation of gesture by hearing children with autism also appear in the production of signs by deaf children with autism. These errors will be described in the next section.

Reversal errors in autistic signing

In the first linguistic studies of native-signing children with autism, Shield (2010) and Shield and Meier (2012) found palm orientation and movement reversals in the signing of such children. In a series of experiments, they observed 10 native-signing children (nine deaf children and one hearing child of deaf parents, or CODA; ages 4;7–16;3) who had been diagnosed with an ASD. Naturalistic observation revealed that three of the younger children produced numerous articulatory errors in interaction with their teachers or parents, particularly reversals in palm orientation from inward to outward,

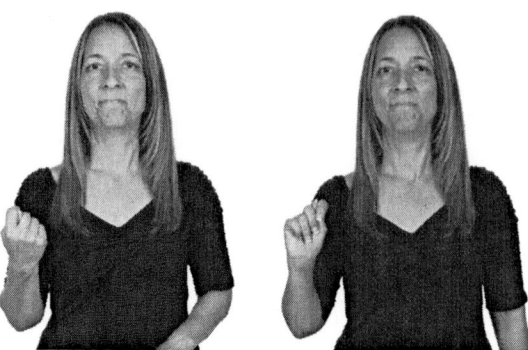

Figure 4.1 The ASL signs TUESDAY (left) and TOILET (right)

and vice versa. Shield also performed a series of experiments designed to elicit lexical signs and ASL-like nonsense signs that could lead to perspective-taking reversal errors. Although the small sample size did not yield results of great statistical power, Shield found that four of the younger children (all under the age of 10) produced inward-outward palm reversals in elicited fingerspelling, spontaneous and elicited lexical signs, and imitated nonsense signs. These types of palm orientation reversals do not appear to occur frequently in the typical acquisition of signed languages by deaf children.

Of the experimental tasks, the fingerspelling task (reported in Shield & Meier, 2012) yielded the most robust results. This task consisted of showing children a series of 10 English words (*bed, table, watch, telephone, cap, chair, door, shoes, book* and *scissors*) on cards and asking them to fingerspell those words. Three out of four young ASD subjects showed a robust tendency to finger-spell with an inward palm orientation, despite the fact that fingerspelling in ASL is in general articulated with an outward orientation. One child (age 5;8) reversed 20 of 28 fingerspelled letters (71%), another child (age 6;6) reversed 26 of 43 fingerspelled letters (61%), and the third child (age 7;5) reversed 27 of 57 fingerspelled letters (47%). A search of the literature on the acquisition of the fingerspelling system of ASL (Padden, 1991, 2006; Padden & Lemaster, 1985) found no reports of such errors. None of the 13 TD deaf children in the control group produced any fingerspellings with reversed palm orientation.

Shield and Meier considered whether the source of the palm orientation errors observed could be purely articulatory (i.e. whether the errors could be attributed to a physiological rather than a perceptual deficit). However, the subjects produced fewer errors on the handshape parameter, which is typically mastered latest in development (Cheek *et al.*, 2001; Clibbens & Harris, 1993; Karnopp, 1997; Marentette & Mayberry, 2000; Meier, 2006; Siedlecki & Bonvillian, 1993; Takkinen, 2003; von Tetzchner, 1984), than on the palm orientation and movement parameters. Moreover, in naturalistic observation and in lexical elicitation these same children also produced outward palm orientation reversals on signs specified for inward palm orientation (e.g. ASL BUTTERFLY), demonstrating that the children were capable of producing outward palm orientations. Finally, these errors are unlike those found in disorders of neuromotor control: the only palm orientation errors observed in, for example, Parkinsonian signers involved the substitution of a neutral palm orientation toward the midline for an upward/downward palm orientation (Brentari et al., 1995). Nor have inward-outward palm substitutions been found in reports of sign language paraphasias: Chiarello et al. (1982) reported two orientation errors in a signer with a left-hemisphere lesion, both involving substitution of an orientation toward the midline for an inward-facing orientation. It thus appears unlikely that motor difficulties could be the sole source of these errors.

The palm orientation errors produced by deaf signing children with autism are striking for a number of reasons: they are virtually unattested in the literature on the typical acquisition of signed languages past 18 months of age, they do not appear to be the result of articulatory difficulty, and they are suggestive of a self-other mapping error. These errors, therefore, have the potential to shed light on the cognitive processes of the autistic child in learning to represent signs mentally, although more work needs to be done in order to identify the individual cognitive processes involved. On a clinical note, these errors may serve as a marker of autism in signing children.

While the role of perspective-taking is most obvious in deictic constructions in spoken languages, it impacts the structure and acquisition of signed languages at many levels. Shield and Meier found reversal errors at the sub-lexical level, as described above, but Morgan et al. also found reversal errors in verb agreement and spatial classifier constructions in the signing of Christopher. Despite his abilities in learning other morphosyntactic constructions, Christopher had persistent problems in producing the correct direction of movement on inflecting verbs (such as HELP in British Sign Language) that change direction depending on their argument structure: in trying to copy his teacher's signing of 'you help me', Christopher produced the equivalent of 'I help you', reversing the direction of movement (Morgan et al., 2002a). It is not clear, however, whether Christopher reversed the direction of movement so as to preserve the semantics of the phrase or because of a perceptually based error (a failure to shift perspectives). Shield and Meier did not test verbs in their study, so it remains to be seen whether native-signing deaf children with autism have difficulty with verbs in which the direction of movement changes depending on their argument structure.

Returning to the earlier discussion of pronoun reversals, we now have reason to hypothesize that pronoun reversals may not occur frequently in the signing of autistic children, or at least not for the same reasons they occur in speech. Why would children who have a deficit in self-other mapping not reverse sign pronouns? Reversing pronouns in speech entails repeating pronouns exactly as they are spoken to the child: the child repeats 'you' as spoken by their conversation partner, failing to change the pronoun to 'I' or 'me'. Yet the studies on gesture imitation and lexical phonology discussed above suggest that children with autism sometimes do not reproduce signs exactly as produced by their conversational partners, but instead reproduce signs as observed from their own perspective. This could lead the signing autistic child to reproduce the pronoun YOU addressed to him as ME – in other words, the correct pronoun. Although more research is needed to test this hypothesis, the available evidence suggests that the deficit underlying pronoun reversals in autistic speech may manifest in sign language as palm orientation and movement reversals, rather than pronominal reversals per se. This may be a possible difference in the linguistic manifestations of autism in sign and speech.

We have thus demonstrated how two of the hallmarks of autistic speech – echolalia and pronoun reversal – manifest in autistic signing. Echolalia appears to be modality independent, insofar as there is already evidence from several different studies that signing children with autism produce echolalic signed utterances, much like hearing children with autism do in speech. However, at the time of this writing there is no evidence of pronoun reversals in the signing of children with autism. There is ample evidence in the literature for palm and movement reversals in gesture imitation by hearing and deaf children with autism, and for palm reversals in the spontaneous and elicited signing and fingerspelling of native-signing children with autism. These errors are suggestive of a deficit in understanding the relationship between self and other as it is embodied and reflected in language.

Joint attention, eye gaze and facial grammar

One of the most interesting aspects of sign language acquisition that is likely to be affected by ASD is facial grammar. In this section, we will discuss the linguistic consequences for signed languages of autistic deficits in eye gaze, attention and face processing. We will then proceed to a discussion of facial grammar – the encoding of linguistic information on the face in signed languages – and discuss recent work testing the abilities of autistic signers in this area.

Children with autism are impaired in the ability to engage in dyadic interactions (Leekam & Ramsden, 2006), resulting in fewer episodes of joint attention (Curcio, 1978; Loveland & Landry, 1986; Mundy et al., 1986; Sigman et al., 1999). Joint attention is positively associated with language development (Charman et al., 2003) and is thought to be a fundamental building block in the acquisition of word meanings (Tomasello & Farrar, 1986). Such an impairment could reflect a general deficit in the ability to orient to social as opposed to non-social stimuli (Dawson et al., 1998; Leekam & Ramsden, 2006; Leekam et al., 2000). Here we encounter an interesting difference between sign and speech: in sign the linguistic stimulus cannot be isolated and separated from the person producing it, while in speech the linguistic stimulus can in fact be perceived without attending to the person producing it. In other words, hearing children with autism can perceive speech without looking at the person speaking, whereas deaf children with autism cannot perceive sign without looking (at least peripherally) at the person signing.

The implications of communicating in the visual modality are broad. Deaf children with autism may face challenges in learning the meanings of signs. Bloom (e.g. Bloom, 2002) has shown that hearing children's ability to learn words is related to an ability to follow other people's gaze, and thus understand the referential intent of their interlocutor. For example, if a child is looking at an object and an adult simultaneously utters a label, a TD child will consult the adult's gaze to confirm that the adult intended to label the object in the child's gaze, and not a different object. In other words, children are more likely to make mappings between words and objects when they are able to infer that the people uttering these words intend to refer to such objects (Baldwin et al., 1996; Bloom, 2002). Yet children with autism do not appear to learn words like TD children. In one study (Baron-Cohen et al., 1997a), children with autism were tested to see if they consulted a speaker's direction of gaze in word-object mappings. They found that TD children only learned to associate a word with an object if the speaker looked at the object in question while labeling it. Children with autism, on the other hand, made significantly more mapping errors when the speaker's gaze was discrepant with the label, showing that unlike normal children, they were relatively insensitive to a speaker's gaze direction as an index of the intention to refer.

We expect that deaf children with autism will make similar mapping errors in the learning of sign labels for objects. However, to date there have been no studies testing this hypothesis. Furthermore, there could be interesting differences between deaf and hearing children with autism since sign labels are unimodal (a visual linguistic stimulus is mapped to a visual object) while spoken labels are intermodal (an acoustic linguistic stimulus is mapped to a visual object). This represents a fruitful area for future research.

The autistic impairment in joint attention and in the gauging of referential intent has implications for the learning of symbols in both sign and speech. However, a deficit in face processing has unique linguistic consequences in sign (although it may also disrupt the comprehension of pragmatic aspects of speech). Signed languages encode a variety of grammatical structures on the face, including questions (Baker, 1983), relative clauses (Liddell, 1980), conditionals (Liddell, 1986), topics (Coulter, 1979), and adverbial and lexical information (Anderson & Reilly, 1999; Liddell, 1980). A number of studies have shown that skilled deaf signers fixate on the face rather than the hands while perceiving sign language (e.g. Agrafiotis et al., 2006).

Yet children with autism have documented deficits in attending to and recognizing information from the face (Dawson *et al.*, 2005; Klin *et al.*, 1999; Schultz *et al.*, 2003), as well as deficits in the comprehension (Baron-Cohen *et al.*, 1993; Capps *et al.*, 1992; Grossman & Tager-Flusberg, 2008; Lacroix *et al.*, 2009; Rump *et al.*, 2009) and imitation (e.g. Hertzig *et al.*, 1989; Loveland *et al.*, 1994) of affective facial expressions. Several research studies have shown that the face scanning behavior of autistic individuals differs from that of non-autistic individuals (Dalton *et al.*, 2005; Klin *et al.*, 2002; Pelphrey *et al.*, 2002). Pelphrey *et al.* (2002) compared the visual scan paths of autistic adults and non-autistic controls, finding that the scan paths of the autistic group were undirected whereas the scan paths of control subjects focused on a triangle between the eyes, nose and mouth.

Several other studies of face gaze by hearing autistic subjects are suggestive of how deaf children with autism may process facial grammar. Joseph and Tanaka (2003) tested autistic and TD subjects' ability to recognize facial features that were presented in isolation or in an image of the whole face. Only the TD group showed a whole-face advantage, whereas the autism group demonstrated a mouth advantage and was impaired in recognizing the eyes. Other studies have reported similar findings: Spezio *et al.* (2007) compared nine high-functioning adults with autism to IQ-matched controls on face gaze behavior and found that the autistic adults relied on information from the mouth region while neglecting the eye region. Finally, Baron-Cohen *et al.* (1997b) analyzed autistic recognition of basic emotions and complex mental states based on whether subjects were shown pictures of whole faces, the eyes alone or the mouth alone. When compared to normal subjects, adults with Asperger's syndrome showed a significant impairment in recognizing complex mental states (such as *scheme* or *distrust*), particularly in the eyes-alone condition, indicating a difficulty in interpreting facial expressions signaled by the eyes.

These impairments pose a unique problem for the deaf child with autism acquiring sign, since the eyes and mouth sometimes encode different linguistic information (Sandler, 2009; Wilbur, 2000). For example, in ASL the mouth can encode lexical information (as in the sign NOT-YET, which is differentiated from the sign LATE by a mouth movement alone), adverbial information (e.g. a protruding tongue accompanied by exhalation 'THH' indicates carelessness when produced with a verb; Liddell, 1978), and adjectival information (e.g. puffed cheeks to indicate large size). The eye region is key for the signaling of questions (with raised or furrowed eyebrows), topicalized noun phrases, and conditionals. If deaf children with autism are impaired in their ability to gain/process information from the eye region but not the mouth, then this could differentially impact linguistic structures encoded in the eye region.

There is still relatively little work examining the eye gaze or facial processing ability of deaf people with autism. The study by Poizner *et al.* (1987) reported that Judith M. stopped making eye contact at the age of 11 months, did not vary her facial expressions and did not respond to the facial expressions of others. Smith *et al.* (2011) reported that Christopher initially avoided eye contact with his conversational partner while learning BSL, although he soon overcame his reluctance. He also did not produce appropriate question facial markers during the repetition or spontaneous production of question sentences. Based on these few reports, and given the wide variability found in the severity and symptoms of autism, it appears likely that there will be wide variability among deaf children with autism in terms of their ability to make eye contact, to infer referential intent through the following of gaze, and to comprehend and produce grammatical and affective facial expressions. It is also possible that sign language exposure could help mitigate some of the face processing deficit in autism, as deaf signing children and hearing signing adults have both been found to have a face processing advantage compared to non-signers on the Benton Facial Recognition Test (Bellugi *et al.*, 1990; Bettger, 1992).

In Shield's (2010) interviews with Deaf mothers of deaf children with autism, the mothers reported that their children were able to comprehend non-manual markers but were limited in their ability to produce grammatical facial markings. One mother remarked:

> I don't see a lot of facial expressions in [my autistic son], compared with [my non-autistic son] … [My autistic son] is more expressionless when he signs. He points to what he wants, just communication for basic needs. He doesn't elaborate his point with facial expressions … I think he can understand facial expressions, but he can't express them. Does he realize that facial expressions are an important part of communication? I don't know. [My non-autistic son] knows that, but for [my autistic son], I don't know. I'm not sure.

The mothers also reported a deficit in their children's ability to produce facial morphemes, such as the question-marking facial expression used for Wh-questions:

> On the WHY question, [my son] doesn't produce the lowering eyebrows and squinting eyes. No. Like the WHERE question, he doesn't produce the raising eyebrows and widening eyes.[11] No.

These reports, although anecdotal, are interesting because they indicate that facial grammar may be difficult for deaf children with autism, even those with native exposure from birth.

Recent studies by Denmark and colleagues (Denmark, 2011; Denmark *et al.*, 2009) provide the only systematic data available on the use of the face by deaf signers with autism. Denmark (2011) investigated deaf autistic signers' face and emotion recognition abilities as well as their comprehension and production of grammatical and affective facial markers in BSL. She compared a group of 13 deaf children and adolescents with autism (age range 8;5–18;0, M = 12;6) to a group of 12 TD deaf children (M = 11;8). The groups were matched for chronological age, BSL proficiency and non-verbal ability. Only one of the deaf subjects was a native signer with deaf parents. She found that the deaf ASD signers showed a mixed profile of abilities; however, overall they did not show characteristic impairment in their comprehension and production of linguistic and affective facial expression, as might have been expected.

The deaf ASD group showed strengths in several areas. First, deaf ASD subjects did not differ significantly from controls on the Benton Facial Recognition Test (BFRT; Benton, 1983), unlike hearing autistic subjects who demonstrate impaired performance on the BFRT. Second, on a task designed to elicit emotional facial expressions, ASD subjects were only slightly worse than controls at reproducing observed facial expressions, and there was no statistical difference in the number of expressions produced by the two groups, despite the fact that prior studies have shown that hearing children with autism produce fewer facial expressions than TD hearing children (Bieberich & Morgan, 1998; Muller & Schuler, 2006; Yirmiya et al., 1989) and their facial expressions have also been judged as more unusual or odd than those of controls (Macdonald et al., 1989; Volker et al., 2009). Third, on a task designed to elicit linguistic and affective facial expressions, ASD signers were not significantly impaired in the frequency with which they produced facial expressions, although they were impaired in terms of quality, producing fewer expressions that were judged by raters as identical to stimuli than the control group. Fourth, on tasks designed to test comprehension and production of negation and question facial expressions in BSL, the ASD group was not impaired relative to controls on the comprehension or production of either type of linguistic facial marker. As an explanation for these surprising findings, Denmark suggested that the attention to faces needed to perceive sign language forces attention to faces during development, leading to improved facial recognition ability. On a related note, other studies have found that native exposure to a sign language leads to enhanced visuospatial abilities (cf. Bosworth & Dobkins, 2002).

The ASD group did show several weaknesses, however. On an emotion recognition task, the deaf ASD group performed significantly worse than the deaf control group. Denmark concluded that this finding suggests that deaf ASD subjects glean less affective information from the face than deaf controls. Furthermore, she hypothesized a connection to an autistic deficit in prosody (Baltaxe & Guthrie, 1987; McCann & Peppé, 2003; Peppé et al., 2006; Tager-Flusberg, 1981), since affective facial expressions produced during signing could be akin to prosodic elements of speech (Dachkovsky & Sandler, 2009).

The second weakness Denmark found was on tasks designed to test the comprehension and production of adverbial facial expressions. TD deaf children were more accurate than the ASD group in comprehending adverbial facial expressions. Furthermore, the ASD group was less accurate at comprehending adverbial facial expressions when unaccompanied by a manual sign. On the production task, moreover, the ASD group produced fewer adverbial facial actions than controls. Thus, Denmark concluded that deaf people with autism may be specifically impaired in their ability to comprehend and produce adverbial facial markers. We would like to see more research that investigates this important topic.

Taken as a whole, Denmark's study represents the first attempt to understand how a known social deficit in autism – a deficit in face processing and in the comprehension and production of facial expression – impacts specific grammatical structures encoded on the face in a signed language. Surprisingly, her studies did not find evidence of a primary impairment in face processing that has linguistic effects on the use of facial expressions in BSL. Rather, she argued that the pattern of spared and impaired abilities in deaf autistic signers can be explained by deficits in emotional understanding. However, we must be cautious in generalizing from her findings. Only one of her subjects was a native BSL signer. More importantly, her participants were far beyond the typical age of acquisition for the various facial structures that were tested (4:0 for negation, 5:0 for adverbials and 6:0 for questions in ASL; Mayberry & Squires, 2006). More studies of younger subjects with autism will be needed in order to understand how grammatical facial expressions develop. Finally, her study only included children with high-functioning autism; five deaf children with severe autism who had insufficient signing skills were excluded from the study. Nevertheless, her surprising findings suggest that repeated exposure to a sign language may counteract underlying social deficits in autism and that at least some deaf children with autism are capable of acquiring facial grammar.

Conclusions and Future Directions

Research into the sign language development of children with autism is still in its infancy. We have described initial investigations into this area which, despite being suggestive of interesting interactions between autism and communication using the visual-gestural modality, need to be confirmed by future studies.

Although it is still too early to be able to make recommendations for clinicians and school psychologists with much confidence, the studies currently available do suggest a few implications for clinical practice. First, the finding of palm reversals in the signing of deaf children with ASD is a rare occurrence of a 'positive' symptom of ASD – that is, the presence of a phenomenon rather than the absence of a skill. As such, it may be particularly useful for parents and clinicians alike in signaling a possible ASD. Secondly, since perspective-taking appears to be problematic for children with ASD, parents, teachers and clinicians may find it helpful to sit beside the child, rather than opposite him or her, while signing or providing therapy to a deaf child with ASD.

As for a future research agenda, we envision several major areas where future research could be fruitful:

(1) Further research on facial grammar and eye gaze behavior, including eye-tracking studies. Studies of younger subjects in particular are needed. Such studies may depend on earlier identification of ASD in deaf children.
(2) Further research on structures in sign language grammar that require self-other mapping, including pronouns, verb agreement, classifier constructions and role shift. In particular, we currently cannot say whether the pronoun reversals that are so typical of autistic speech are also found in autistic signing.
(3) Research into the relation between non-linguistic cognitive skills, such as theory of mind, inter-subjective identification and motor imitation, and the acquisition and development of sign language structures.
(4) Longitudinal studies that document sign language development over time. Such studies could help clarify the developmental trajectory of language development in autism and the nature of developmental delay in autism.
(5) Bilingual studies of hearing children exposed to sign language and speech from birth (CODAs), which may be able to reveal important modality differences between sign and speech development. In particular, we believe that a study of pronoun use in a bilingual CODA with autism may be of special interest, since pronoun reversals are so characteristic of autistic speech but have yet to be documented in autistic signing.

The first goal of such a research agenda must be the **documentation** of the comprehension and production skills of native and non-native signing children. As we have argued in this chapter, the characteristics of autistic signing will likely differ in certain key ways from the characteristics of autistic speech. We cannot yet say with certainty whether all the hallmarks of autistic speech will also be found in the signing of deaf children with autism. Cross-linguistic studies into different signed languages will be helpful for confirming phenomena that are general to the modality, or identifying language-specific phenomena.

In the documentation process, several methodological considerations must be carefully attended to. First, utmost care must be taken in the **selection** of subjects. The diagnosis of autism must be confirmed carefully using appropriate instruments. However, as we have already pointed out, the lack of sign language translations of the current gold standard instruments poses a significant challenge to both clinicians and researchers. We thus suggest a multifaceted approach, using the available screening and diagnostic instruments with appropriate adaptations made for deaf children. It is crucial that children be evaluated by clinicians who are familiar with deaf children and are aware of the modality differences that exist between sign and speech, as well as the different social norms of Deaf culture.

A related issue is the careful **matching** of ASD subjects to subjects without ASD (both TD and with other developmental disorders). In particular, subjects should be matched for chronological age, language age, and/or nonverbal intelligence, depending on the research question.

Measures of motor skills should be taken in studies of autistic signing, so as to properly identify whether errors observed have a perceptual or motor origin. Ming *et al.* (2007) found various motor problems in a sample of 154 ASD children, including hypotonia (51%), motor apraxia (34%), toe-walking (19%) and gross motor delay (9%). Since sign language entails both gross and fine motor movements, such impairments are likely to impact how deaf children on the spectrum acquire sign.

Once there is sufficient documentation of autistic signing, these studies should be used in the **adaptation** of existing gold-standard diagnostic instruments for use with deaf children (e.g. the ADOS and ADI-R), and the **development** of appropriate sign language educational strategies and interventions. The translation of diagnostic instruments into various signed languages will in itself be a large undertaking, and will require careful consideration of differences between the visual-gestural and vocal-auditory modalities, as well as the heterogeneity of the deaf population (i.e. age of exposure to language, sign versus oral speech training, amplification and cochlear implantation, comorbidities, etc.).

Research into sign language development of deaf children on the autism spectrum has the potential to shed light on issues of interest well beyond the community of scientists who work on signed languages. In particular, in observing language acquisition in the visual-gestural modality, there is an opportunity to test hypotheses about the nature of the autistic phenotype and the core cognitive mechanisms underlying autistic impairments. Signed languages rely crucially on a set of social skills known to be impaired in autism, and careful study of deaf children on the spectrum could clarify the nature of cognitive deficits in autism, as well as the relationship between social skills and language development. Thus, despite the considerable methodological difficulties that we have highlighted, we hope that researchers will feel encouraged to pursue studies in this area. We believe that such research is feasible (albeit methodologically complex), and could benefit deaf and hearing children on the autism spectrum, as well as the Deaf community, the scientific community and society at large, by contributing insights about the nature of autism, and its complicated effects on cognition and language.

Notes

(1) Until DSM-5, subcategories of ASD included autistic disorder, Asperger's disorder, and pervasive developmental disorder-not otherwise specified (PDD-NOS).
(2) Although he lacks an official diagnosis, the authors cite Christopher's aversion to eye contact and social interaction as well as his consistent failure on false-belief tasks as evidence of his autism.
(3) Seal and Bonvillian did not examine palm orientation as a separate parameter.
(4) We use the term 'echolalia' (the automatic imitation of the vocalizations of others) here rather than 'echopraxia' (the involuntary imitation of the body movements of others) because of the linguistic nature of the signs being imitated. Both echolalia and echopraxia have been documented in hearing autistic children.
(5) Note that Poizner et al. translated the father's ASL signing into English. Thus, despite the translation, there would have been no indefinite article in this first sentence. Consequently Judith appears to have echoed the last two signs of her father's utterance verbatim.
(6) To our knowledge, there is no report of whether or not Christopher was echolalic in his production of spoken languages.
(7) It is unclear whether this example is truly an instance of verb reversal or merely an uninflected citation form of the verb give. Indeed, homonymy or near-homonymy of citation forms and 1st-to-2nd person inflected forms presents a serious methodological problem in detecting verb agreement reversals in sign.
(8) A name sign is a sign that is used to uniquely identify a person, like a name.
(9) Translated from ASL to English by Lynn Hou.
(10) Some authors have argued that the mirror neuron system of the brain, through which children match their movements to those observed in others, is impaired in ASD (cf. Dapretto et al., 2005; Iacoboni & Dapretto, 2006).
(11) Note that this mother's description of the facial marking for the ASL question word where conflicts with the standard facial marking reported in the literature (Baker, 1983; Baker-Shenk & Cokely, 1991).

References

Agrafiotis, D., Canagarajah, N., Bull, D.R., Kyle, J., Seers, H. and Dye, M. (2006) A perceptually optimised video coding system for sign language communication at low bit rates. *Signal Processing: Image Communication* 21, 531–549.
Anderson, D. and Reilly, J. (1999) PAH! The acquisition of non-manual adverbials in ASL. *Sign Language and Linguistics* 1, 115–142.
Attwood, A., Frith, U. and Hermelin, B. (1988) The understanding and use of interpersonal gestures by autistic and Down's syndrome children. *Journal of Autism and Developmental Disorders* 18, 241–257.
Baker, C.L. (1983) A microanalysis of the nonmanual components of questions in American Sign Language. *Understanding Language Through Sign Language Research* (pp. 27–57). New York: Academic Press.
Baker-Shenk, C.L. and Cokely, D. (1991) *American Sign Language: A Teacher's Resource Text on Grammar and Culture*. Washington, DC: Gallaudet University Press.
Baldwin, D.A., Markman, E.M., Bill, B., Desjardins, R.N., Irwin, J.M. and Tidball, G. (1996) Infants' reliance on a social criterion for establishing word-object relations. *Child Development* 67, 3135–3153.
Baltaxe, C.A. and Guthrie, D. (1987) The use of primary sentence stress by normal, aphasic, and autistic children. *Journal of Autism and Developmental Disorders* 17, 255–271.

Baron-Cohen, S. (1989) Perceptual role taking and protodeclarative pointing in autism. *British Journal of Developmental Psychology* 7, 113–127.

Baron-Cohen, S., Spitz, A. and Cross, P. (1993) Do children with autism recognise surprise? A research note. *Cognition & Emotion* 7, 507–516.

Baron-Cohen, S., Baldwin, D.A. and Crowson, M. (1997a) Do children with autism use the speaker's direction of gaze strategy to crack the code of language? *Child Development* 68, 48–57.

Baron-Cohen, S., Wheelwright, S. and Jolliffe, T. (1997b) Is there a 'language of the eyes'? Evidence from normal adults, and adults with autism or Asperger syndrome. *Visual Cognition* 4, 311–331.

Bartak, L. and Rutter, M. (1974) The use of personal pronouns by autistic children. *Journal of Autism and Developmental Disorders* 4, 217–222.

Bellugi, U., O'Grady, L., Lillo-Martin, D., O'Grady, M., van Hoek, K. and Corina, D. (1990) Enhancement of spatial cognition in deaf children. In V. Volterra and C. Erting (eds) *From Gesture to Language in Hearing and Deaf Children* (pp. 278–298). Washington, DC: Gallaudet University Press.

Benton, A.L., Sivan, A.B., Hamsher, K., Varney, N.R. and Spreen, O. (1983) Facial recognition: Stimulus and multiple choice pictures. In A.L. Benton, A.B. Sivan, K. Hamsher, N.R. Varney and O. Spreen (eds) *Contributions to Neuropsychological Assessment* (pp. 35–52). New York: Oxford University Press.

Bettger, J. (1992) The effects of experience on spatial cognition: Deafness and knowledge of ASL. Unpublished doctoral dissertation, University of Illinois.

Bieberich, A.A. and Morgan, S.B. (1998) Brief report: Affective expression in children with autism or Down syndrome. *Journal of Autism and Developmental Disorders* 28, 333–338.

Bloom, L. and Lahey, M. (1978) *Language Development and Language Disorders*. Somerset, NJ: John Wiley & Sons.

Bloom, P. (2002) *How Children Learn the Meanings of Words*. Cambridge, MA: MIT Press.

Bondy, A.S. and Frost, L.A. (1994) The picture exchange communication system. *Focus on Autism and Other Developmental Disabilities* 9, 1–19.

Bonvillian, J.D. and Blackburn, D.W. (1991) Manual communication and autism: Factors relating to sign language acquisition. In P. Siple and S. Fischer (eds) *Theoretical Issues in Sign Language Research, Vol. 2: Psychology* (pp. 255–277). Chicago, IL: University of Chicago Press.

Bonvillian, J.D., Nelson, K.E. and Rhyne, J.M. (1981) Sign language and autism. *Journal of Autism and Developmental Disorders* 11, 125–137.

Bosworth, R.G. and Dobkins, K.R. (2002) The effects of spatial attention on motion processing in deaf signers, hearing signers and hearing non signers. *Brain and Cognition* 49, 152–169.

Brentari, D., Poizner, H. and Kegl, J. (1995) Aphasic and Parkinsonian signing: Differences in phonological disruption. *Brain and Language* 48, 69–105.

Brimer, J. and Murphy, P. (1988) Autism and deafness: A case study of a deaf and autistic boy. In H.T. Pricket and E. Duncan (eds) *Coping with the Multi-handicapped Hearing Impaired* (pp. 37–44). Springfield, IL: Charles C. Thomas.

Brown, J.D. (1996) Imitation, play and theory of mind in autism: An observational and experimental study. Unpublished doctoral dissertation, Saint Andrew's University.

Buitelaar, J.K., van Engeland, H., de Kogel, K.H., de Vries, H. and van Hooff, J.A. (1991) Differences in the structure of social behaviour of autistic children and non-autistic retarded controls. *Journal of Child Psychology and Psychiatry, and Allied Disciplines* 32, 995–1015.

Capps, L., Yirmiya, N. and Sigman, M. (1992) Understanding of simple and complex emotions in non-retarded children with autism. *Journal of Child Psychology and Psychiatry* 33, 1169–1182.

Carr, E.G. (1979) Teaching autistic children to use sign language: Some research issues. *Journal of Autism and Developmental Disorders* 9, 345–359.

Casey, S. (2003) Relationships between gestures and signed languages: Indicating participants in action. In A. Baker, B. van den Bogaerde and O. Crasborn (eds) *Cross-linguistic Perspectives in Sign Language Research: Selected Papers from TISLR 2000* (pp. 95–117). Hamburg: Signum.

Centers for Disease Control (2012) Prevalence of autism spectrum disorders – Autism and Developmental Disabilities Monitoring Network, 14 sites, United States, 2008. *Morbidity and Mortality Weekly Report* 61, 1–19.

Charman, T., Baron-Cohen, S., Swettenham, J., Baird, G., Drew, A. and Cox, A. (2003) Predicting language outcome in infants with autism and pervasive developmental disorder. *International Journal of Language & Communication Disorders* 38, 265–285.

Charney, R. (1980) Pronoun errors in autistic children: Support for a social explanation. *International Journal of Language & Communication Disorders* 15, 39–43.

Cheek, A., Cormier, K., Repp, A. and Meier, R.P. (2001) Prelinguistic gesture predicts mastery and error in the production of early signs. *Language* 77, 292–323.

Chess, S., Fernandez, P. and Korn, S. (1978) Behavioral consequences of congenital rubella. *Journal of Pediatrics* 93, 699–703.

Chiarello, C., Knight, R. and Mandel, M. (1982) Aphasia in a prelingually deaf woman. *Brain: A Journal of Neurology* 105, 29.

Chiat, S. (1982) If I were you and you were me: The analysis of pronouns in a pronoun-reversing child. *Journal of Child Language* 9, 359–379.

Clark, E.V. (1978) From gesture to word: On the natural history of deixis in language acquisition. In J.S. Bruner and A. Garton (eds) *Human Growth and Development: Wolfson College Lectures 1976* (pp. 85–120). Oxford: Oxford University Press.

Clibbens, J. and Harris, M. (1993) Phonological processes and sign language development. In D. Messer and G. Turner (eds) *Critical Influences on Child Language Acquisition and Development* (pp. 197–208). New York: Macmillan Press.

Collins, P. and Carney, S. (2007) Autism spectrum disorder, deafness and challenging behaviour. In S. Austen and D. Jeffery (eds) *Deafness and Challenging Behaviour: The 360 Perspective* (pp. 125–143). Chichester: John Wiley & Sons.

Constantino, J.N. (2002) *The Social Responsiveness Scale*. Los Angeles, CA: Western Psychological Services.

Coulter, G.R. (1979) American Sign Language typology. Unpublished doctoral dissertation, University of California.

Creedon, M.P. (1973) Language development in nonverbal autistic children using a simultaneous communication system. Paper presented at the Society for Resarch in Child Development Meeting, Philadelphia, PA.

Curcio, F. (1978) Sensorimotor functioning and communication in mute autistic children. *Journal of Autism and Developmental Disorders* 8, 281–292.

Dachkovsky, S. and Sandler, W. (2009) Visual intonation in the prosody of a sign language. *Language and Speech* 52, 287–314.

Dale, P.S. and Crain-Thoreson, C. (1993) Pronoun reversals: Who, when, and why? *Journal of Child Language* 20, 573–589.

Dalton, K.M., Nacewicz, B.M., Johnstone, T., Schaefer, H.S., Gernsbacher, M.A., Goldsmith, H., Alexander, A.L., *et al.* (2005) Gaze fixation and the neural circuitry of face processing in autism. *Nature Neuroscience* 8, 519–526.

Dapretto, M., Davies, M.S., Pfeifer, J.H., Scott, A.A., Sigman, M., Bookheimer, S.Y. and Iacoboni, M. (2005) Understanding emotions in others: Mirror neuron dysfunction in children with autism spectrum disorders. *Nature Neuroscience* 9, 28–30.

Dawson, G. and Adams, A. (1984) Imitation and social responsiveness in autistic children. *Journal of Abnormal Child Psychology* 12, 209–226.

Dawson, G., Meltzoff, A.N., Osterling, J., Rinaldi, J. and Brown, E. (1998) Children with autism fail to orient to naturally occurring social stimuli. *Journal of Autism and Developmental Disorders* 28, 479–485.

Dawson, G., Webb, S.J. and McPartland, J. (2005) Understanding the nature of face processing impairment in autism: Insights from behavioral and electrophysiological studies. *Developmental Neuropsychology* 27, 403–424.

DeMyer, M.K., Alpern, G.D., Barton, S., DeMyer, W.E., Churchill, D.W., Hingtgen, J.N., Bryson, C.Q., *et al.* (1972) Imitation in autistic, early schizophrenic, and non-psychotic subnormal children. *Journal of Autism and Developmental Disorders* 2, 264–287.

Denmark, T. (2011) Do deaf children with Autism Spectrum Disorder show deficits in the comprehension and production of emotional and linguistic facial expressions in British Sign Language? Unpublished doctoral dissertation, University College London.

Denmark, T., Swettenham, J., Atkinson, J. and Campbell, R. (2009) What's in the face? The comprehension and production of facial expressions in sign language by deaf children with autism. Poster presented at the International Meeting for Autism Research (IMFAR), Chicago, IL.

Gallaudet Research Institute (2011) *Regional and National Summary Report of Data from the 2009–2010 Annual Survey of Deaf and Hard of Hearing Children and Youth.* Washington, DC: GRI, Gallaudet University.

Gilliam, J.E. (2006) *Gilliam Autism Rating Scale* – (2nd edn). Austin, TX: Pro-Ed.

Grossman, R.B. and Tager-Flusberg, H. (2008) Reading faces for information about words and emotions in adolescents with autism. *Research in Autism Spectrum Disorders* 2, 681–695.

Hamilton, A., Brindley, R. and Frith, U. (2009) Visual perspective taking impairment in children with autistic spectrum disorder. *Cognition* 113, 37–44.

Hatzopoulou, M. (2010) Acquisition of reference to self and others in Greek Sign Language (Stockholm University, 2008). *Sign Language & Linguistics* 13, 83–91.

Hertzig, M.E., Snow, M.E. and Sherman, M. (1989) Affect and cognition in autism. *Journal of the American Academy of Child & Adolescent Psychiatry* 28, 195.

Hobson, R.P. and Lee, A. (1999) Imitation and identification in autism. *Journal of Child Psychology and Psychiatry* 40, 649–659.

Hobson, R.P., García-Pérez, R.M. and Lee, A. (2010) Person-centred (deictic) expressions and autism. *Journal of Autism and Developmental Disorders* 40, 403–415.

Iacoboni, M. and Dapretto, M. (2006) The mirror neuron system and the consequences of its dysfunction. *Nature Reviews Neuroscience* 7, 942–951.

Jordan, R. (1990) Signing and autistic children. *Communication* 19, 9–12.

Joseph, R.M. and Tanaka, J. (2003) Holistic and part-based face recognition in children with autism. *Journal of Child Psychology and Psychiatry* 44, 529–542.

Jure, R., Rapin, I. and Tuchman, R. (1991) Hearing-impaired autistic children. *Developmental Medicine and Child Neurology* 33, 1062–1072.

Kanner, L. (1943) Autistic disturbances of affective contact. *Nervous Child* 2, 217–250.

Karnopp, L.B. (1997) Phonological acquisition in sign languages. *Letras de Hoje* 32, 147–162.

Klin, A., Sparrow, S.S., de Bildt, A., Cicchetti, D.V., Cohen, D.J. and Volkmar, F.R. (1999) A normed study of face recognition in autism and related disorders. *Journal of Autism and Developmental Disorders* 29, 499–508.

Klin, A., Jones, W., Schultz, R., Volkmar, F. and Cohen, D. (2002) Visual fixation patterns during viewing of naturalistic social situations as predictors of social competence in individuals with autism. *Archives of General Psychiatry* 59, 809–816.

Lacroix, A., Guidetti, M., Rogé, B. and Reilly, J. (2009) Recognition of emotional and nonemotional facial expressions: A comparison between Williams syndrome and autism. *Research in Developmental Disabilities* 30, 976–985.

Lee, A., Hobson, R.P. and Chiat, S. (1994) I, you, me, and autism: An experimental study. *Journal of Autism and Developmental Disorders* 24, 155–176.

Leekam, S.R. and Ramsden, C.A. (2006) Dyadic orienting and joint attention in preschool children with autism. *Journal of Autism and Developmental Disorders* 36, 185–197.

Leekam, S.R., Lopez, B. and Moore, C. (2000) Attention and joint attention in preschool children with autism. *Developmental Psychology* 36, 261–273.

Liddell, S.K. (1978) Nonmanual signals and relative clauses in American Sign Language. In P. Siple (ed.) *Understanding Language Through Sign Language Research* (pp. 59–90). San Diego, CA: Academic Press.

Liddell, S.K. (1980) *American Sign Language Syntax*. The Hague: Mouton.

Liddell, S.K. (1986) Head thrust in ASL conditional marking. *Sign Language Studies* 52, 243–62.

Lord, C., Rutter, M. and Le Couteur, A. (1994) Autism Diagnostic Interview – Revised: A revised version of a diagnostic interview for caregivers of individuals with possible pervasive developmental disorders. *Journal of Autism and Developmental Disorders* 24, 659–685.

Lord, C., Rutter, M., DiLavore, P.C., Risi, S., Gotham, K., and Bishop, S.L. (2012) *Autism Diagnostic Observation Schedule, Second Edition (ADOS-2)*. Torrance, CA: Western Psychological Services.

Loveland, K.A. (1984) Learning about points of view: Spatial perspective and the acquisition of I/you. *Journal of Child Language* 11, 535–556.

Loveland, K.A. and Landry, S.H. (1986) Joint attention and language in autism and developmental language delay. *Journal of Autism and Developmental Disorders* 16, 335–349.

Loveland, K.A., Tunali-Kotoski, B., Pearson, D.A., Brelsford, K.A., Ortegon, J. and Chen, R. (1994) Imitation and expression of facial affect in autism. *Development and Psychopathology* 6, 433–444.

Macdonald, H., Rutter, M., Howlin, P., Rios, P., Conteur, A.L., Evered, C. and Folstein, S. (1989) Recognition and expression of emotional cues by autistic and normal adults. *Journal of Child Psychology & Psychiatry* 30, 865–877.

Malandraki, G.A. and Okalidou, A. (2007) The application of PECS in a deaf child with autism: A case study. *Focus on Autism & Other Developmental Disabilities* 22, 23–32.

Mandell, D.S., Novak, M.M. and Zubritsky, C.D. (2005) Factors associated with age of diagnosis among children with autism spectrum disorders. *Pediatrics* 116, 1480–1486.

Marentette, P.F. and Mayberry, R.I. (2000) Principles for an emerging phonological system: A case study of early ASL acquisition. In C. Chamberlain, J.P. Morford and R.I. Mayberry (eds) *Language Acquisition by Eye* (pp. 71–90). Mahwah, NJ: Lawrence Erlbaum.

Mayberry, R. and Squires, B. (2006) Sign language acquisition: Language acquisition. In K. Brown (ed.) *Encyclopedia of Language and Linguistics* (2nd edn) (pp. 291–296). Oxford: Elsevier.

McCann, J. and Peppe, S. (2003) Prosody in autism spectrum disorders: A critical review. *International Journal of Language & Communication Disorders* 38, 325–350.

Meier, R.P. (2006) The form of early signs: Explaining signing children's articulatory development. In B. Schick, M. Marschark and P.E. Spencer (eds) *Advances in the Sign Language Development of Deaf Children* (pp. 202–230). New York: Oxford University Press.

Ming, X., Brimacombe, M. and Wagner, G.C. (2007) Prevalence of motor impairment in autism spectrum disorders. *Brain and Development* 29, 565–570.

Mitchell, R.E. and Karchmer, M.A. (2004) Chasing the mythical ten percent: Parental hearing status of deaf and hard of hearing students in the United States. *Sign Language Studies* 4, 138–163.

Morgan, G., Smith, N., Tsimpli, I. and Woll, B. (2002a) Language against the odds: The learning of British Sign Language by a polyglot savant. *Journal of Linguistics* 38, 1–41.

Morgan, G.D., Woll, B., Tsimpli, I. and Smith, N.V. (2002b) The effects of modality on BSL development in an exceptional learner. In R.P. Meier, D. Quinto-Pozos and K. Cormier (eds) *Modality and Structure in Signed and Spoken Language* (pp. 422–441). Cambridge: Cambridge University Press.

Morgan, G., Smith, N., Tsimpli, I. and Woll, B. (2007) Classifier learning and modality in a polyglot savant. *Lingua* 117, 1339–1353.

Morgan, S.B., Cutrer, P.S., Coplin, J.W. and Rodrigue, J.R. (1989) Do autistic children differ from retarded and normal children in Piagetian sensorimotor functioning. *Journal of Child Psychology and Psychiatry* 30, 857–864.

Muller, E. and Schuler, A. (2006) Verbal marking of affect by children with Asperger syndrome and high functioning autism during spontaneous interactions with family members. *Journal of Autism and Developmental Disorders* 36, 1089–1100.

Mundy, P., Sigman, M., Ungerer, J. and Sherman, T. (1986) Defining the social deficits of autism: The contribution on non-verbal communication measures. *Journal of Child Psychology & Psychiatry & Allied Disciplines* 27, 657–669.

Mundy, P., Sigman, M., Ungerer, J. and Sherman, T. (1987) Nonverbal communication and play correlates of language development in autistic children. *Journal of Autism and Developmental Disorders* 17, 349–364.

Ohta, M. (1987) Cognitive disorders of infantile autism: A study employing the WISC, spatial relationship conceptualization, and gesture imitations. *Journal of Autism and Developmental Disorders* 17, 45–62.

Ornitz, E.M. and Ritvo, E.R. (1976) The syndrome of autism: A critical review. *American Journal of Psychiatry* 133, 609–621.

Oshima-Takane, Y. (1992) Analysis of pronominal errors: A case-study. *Journal of Child Language* 19, 111–131.

Oshima-Takane, Y., Cole, E. and Yaremko, R.L. (1993) Semantic pronominal confusion in a hearing-impaired child: A case study. *First Language* 13, 149–168.

Padden, C.A. (1991) The acquisition of fingerspelling by deaf children. In P. Siple and S.D. Fischer (eds) *Theoretical Issues in Sign Language Research, Vol. 2: Psychology* (pp. 191–210). Chicago, IL: University of Chicago Press.

Padden, C.A. (2006) Learning to fingerspell twice: Young signing children's acquisition of fingerspelling. In B. Schick, M. Marschark and P.E. Spencer (eds) *Advances in the Sign Language Development of Deaf Children* (pp. 189–201). New York: Oxford University Press.

Padden, C. and Lemaster, B. (1985) An alphabet on hand: The acquisition of fingerspelling in deaf children. *Sign Language Studies* 14, 161–172.

Pelphrey, K.A., Sasson, N.J., Reznick, J.S., Paul, G., Goldman, B.D. and Piven, J. (2002) Visual scanning of faces in autism. *Journal of Autism and Developmental Disorders* 32, 249–261.

Peppé, S., McCann, J., Gibbon, F., O'Hare, A. and Rutherford, M. (2006) Assessing prosodic and pragmatic ability in children with high-functioning autism. *Journal of Pragmatics* 38, 1776–1791.

Peters, A.M. (1983) *The Units of Language Acquisition.* Cambridge: Cambridge University Press.

Petitto, L.A. (1987) On the autonomy of language and gesture: Evidence from the acquisition of personal pronouns in American Sign Language. *Cognition* 27, 1–52.

Pizer, G., Meier, R.P. and Shaw Points, K. (2011) Child-directed signing as a linguistic register. In R. Channon and H. van der Hulst (eds) *Formational Units in Sign Languages* (pp. 65–86). Boston, MA: Walter de Gruyter.

Poizner, H., Klima, E.S. and Bellugi, U. (1990) *What the Hands Reveal About the Brain.* Cambridge, MA: MIT Press.

Prizant, B.M. (1983) Language acquisition and communicative behavior in autism: Toward an understanding of the 'whole' of it. *Journal of Speech and Hearing Disorders* 48, 296–307.

Prizant, B.M. and Duchan, J.F. (1981) The functions of immediate echolalia in autistic children. *Journal of Speech and Hearing Disorders* 46, 241–249.

Reed, T. (2002) Visual perspective taking as a measure of working memory in participants with autism. *Journal of Developmental and Physical Disabilities* 14, 63–76.

Ricard, M., Girouard, P.C. and Gouin Décarie, T. (1999) Personal pronouns and perspective taking in toddlers. *Journal of Child Language* 26, 681–697.

Ricks, D.M. and Wing, L. (1975) Language, communication, and the use of symbols in normal and autistic children. *Journal of Autism and Developmental Disorders* 5, 191–221.

Rogers, S.J. and Pennington, B.F. (1991) A theoretical approach to the deficits in infantile autism. *Development and Psychopathology* 3, 137–162.

Roper, L., Arnold, P. and Monteiro, B. (2003) Co-occurrence of autism and deafness: Diagnostic considerations. *Autism* 7, 245–253.

Rosenhall, U., Nordin, V., Sandström, M., Ahlsén, G. and Gillberg, C. (1999) Autism and hearing loss. *Journal of Autism and Developmental Disorders* 29, 349–357.

Rump, K.M., Giovannelli, J.L., Minshew, N.J. and Strauss, M.S. (2009) The development of emotion recognition in individuals with autism. *Child Development* 80, 1434–1447.

Rutter, M., Bailey, A. and Lord, C. (2003) *Social Communication Questionnaire*. Los Angeles, CA: Western Psychological Services.

Sandler, W. (2009) Symbiotic symbolization by hand and mouth in sign language. *Semiotica* 2009, 241–275.

Schick, B., de Villiers, P., de Villiers, J. and Hoffmeister, R. (2007) Language and theory of mind: A study of deaf children. *Child Development* 78, 376–396.

Schiff-Myers, N.B. (1983) From pronoun reversals to correct pronoun usage: A case study of a normally developing child. *Journal of Speech and Hearing Disorders* 48, 394–402.

Schuler, A.L. and Prizant, B. (1985) Echolalia. In E. Schopler and G.B. Mesibov (eds) *Communication Problems in Autism* (pp. 163–184). New York: Plenum Press.

Schultz, R.T., Grelotti, D.J., Klin, A., Kleinman, J., Van der Gaag, C., Marois, R. and Skudlarski, P. (2003) The role of the fusiform face area in social cognition: Implications for the pathobiology of autism. *Philosophical Transactions of the Royal Society of London. Series B: Biological Sciences* 358, 415–427.

Seal, B.C. and Bonvillian, J.D. (1997) Sign language and motor functioning in students with autistic disorder. *Journal of Autism and Developmental Disorders* 27, 437–466.

Shield, A. (2010) The signing of deaf children with autism: Lexical phonology and perspective-taking in the visual-spatial modality. Unpublished doctoral dissertation, University of Texas at Austin.

Shield, A. (2012) Palm reversals are the pronoun reversals of sign language. Poster presented at the International Meeting for Autism Research, Toronto.

Shield, A. and Meier, R.P. (2012) Palm reversal errors in native-signing children with autism. *Journal of Communication Disorders* 45, 439–454.

Siedlecki, T. and Bonvillian, J.D. (1993) Location, handshape, and movement: Young children's acquisition of the formational aspects of American Sign Language. *Sign Language Studies* 78, 31–52.

Sigman, M., Ruskin, E., Arbelle, S., Corona, R., Dissanayake, C., Espinosa, M., Kim, N., *et al.* (1999) Continuity and change in the social competence of children with autism, Down syndrome, and developmental delays. *Monographs of the Society for Research in Child Development* 64, 1–114.

Smith, I.M. and Bryson, S.E. (1994) Imitation and action in autism: A critical review. *Psychological Bulletin* 116, 259–273.

Smith, I.M. and Bryson, S.E. (1998) Gesture imitation in autism, I: Nonsymbolic postures and sequences. *Cognitive Neuropsychology* 15, 747–770.

Smith, N., Tsimpli, I., Morgan, G. and Woll, B. (2011) *The Signs of a Savant: Language Against the Odds.* New York: Cambridge University Press.

Soorya, L.V. (2003) Evaluation of motor proficiency and apraxia in autism: Effects on sign language acquisition. Unpublished doctoral dissertation, State University of New York.

Spezio, M.L., Adolphs, R., Hurley, R.S.E. and Piven, J. (2007) Abnormal use of facial information in high-functioning autism. *Journal of Autism and Developmental Disorders* 37, 929–939.

Stull, S., Edkins, C., Krause, M., McGavin, G., Brand, L.H. and Webster, C.D. (1979) Sign language as a means of communicating with autistic and mentally handicapped children. *Child and Youth Care Forum* 8, 143–147.

Szymanski, C. (2010) Characteristics and symptomotology of autism in children who are deaf and hard of hearing. Unpublished doctoral dissertation, Gallaudet University.

Szymanski, C.A., Brice, P.J., Lam, K.H. and Hotto, S.A. (2012) Deaf children with Autism Spectrum Disorders. *Journal of Autism and Developmental Disorders* 42 (10), 2027–2037. doi:10.1007/s10803-012-1452-9.

Tager-Flusberg, H. (1981) On the nature of linguistic functioning in early infantile autism. *Journal of Autism and Developmental Disorders* 11, 45–56.

Tager-Flusberg, H. (1993) What language reveals about the understanding of minds in children with autism. In S. Baron-Cohen, H. Tager-Flusberg and D.J. Cohen (eds) *Understanding Other Minds: Perspectives From Autism* (pp. 138–157). Oxford: Oxford University Press.

Tager-Flusberg, H. (1994) Dissociations in form and function in the acquisition of language by autistic children. In H. Tager-Flusberg (ed.) *Constraints on Language Acquisition: Studies of Atypical Children* (pp. 175–194). Hillsdale, NJ: Lawrence Erlbaum.

Tager-Flusberg, H. (2000) Understanding the language and communicative impairments in autism. In L.M. Glidden (ed.) *International Review of Research on Mental Retardation: Autism* (Vol. 23). New York: Academic Press.

Takkinen, R. (2003) Variation of handshape features in the acquisition process. In A. Baker, B. van den Bogaerde and O. Crasborn (eds) *Cross-linguistic Perspectives in Sign Language Research: Selected Papers from TISLR 2000* (pp. 81–94). Hamburg: Signum.

Tomasello, M. and Farrar, M.J. (1986) Joint attention and early language. *Child Development* 57, 1454–1463.

Volker, M.A., Lopata, C., Smith, D.A. and Thomeer, M.L. (2009) Facial encoding of children with high-functioning autism spectrum disorders. *Focus on Autism and Other Developmental Disabilities* 24, 195–204.

von Tetzchner, S. (1984) First signs acquired by a Norwegian deaf child with hearing parents. *Sign Language Studies* 44, 225–257.

Warreyn, P., Roeyers, H., Oelbrandt, T. and De Groote, I. (2005) What are you looking at? Joint attention and visual perspective taking in young children with autism spectrum disorder. *Journal of Developmental and Physical Disabilities* 17, 55–73.

Webster, C.D., McPherson, H., Sloman, L., Evans, M.A. and Kuchar, E. (1973) Communicating with an autistic boy by gestures. *Journal of Autism and Developmental Disorders* 3, 337–346.

Wetherby, A.M. (1986) Ontogeny of communicative functions in autism. *Journal of Autism and Developmental Disorders* 16, 295–316.

White, K.R. (2004) Early hearing detection and intervention programs: Opportunities for genetic services. *American Journal of Medical Genetics* 103, 29–36.

Whiten, A. and Brown, J. (1998) Imitation and the reading of other minds: Perspectives from the study of autism, normal children and non-human primates. In S. Bråten (ed.) *Intersubjective Communication and Emotion in Early Ontogeny* (pp. 260–280). Cambridge: Cambridge University Press.

Wilbur, R.B. (2000) Phonological and prosodic layering of non-manuals in American Sign Language. In H. Lane and K. Emmorey (eds) *The Signs of Language Revisited: Festschrift for Ursula Bellugi and Edward Klima* (pp. 213–241). Hillsdale, NJ: Lawrence Erlbaum.

Williams, J.H., Whiten, A. and Singh, T. (2004) A systematic review of action imitation in autistic spectrum disorder. *Journal of Autism and Developmental Disorders* 34, 285–299.

Yirmiya, N., Kasari, C., Sigman, M. and Mundy, P. (1989) Facial expressions of affect in autistic, mentally retarded and normal children. *Journal of Child Psychology and Psychiatry* 30, 725–735.

5 Mapping Out Guidelines for the Development and Use of Sign Language Assessments: Some Critical Issues, Comments and Suggestions

Wolfgang Mann and Tobias Haug

Introduction

The purpose of this chapter is two-fold: to illuminate the importance of assessment in the context of language acquisition of deaf individuals, specifically children, and to provide a contextual foundation for some of the studies discussed in this book. Furthermore, with the prevailing lack of sign language assessment tests in most countries, we offer a set of guidelines for the development/adaptation of such tests for less documented sign languages.

Throughout our lifespan, we are subjected to a wide variety of assessments, ranging from developmental screening procedures or diagnostic tests during infancy to academic achievement and/or placement tests at school and in college, as well as a number of non-academic assessments, including driving exams, job interviews and/or self-assessments. Many of these procedures represent integral parts of our social life and culture (e.g. Bartram, 1990; Fulcher & Davidson, 2007; McNamara, 2000).

One of the main areas of interest to researchers, psychologists, clinicians and others in the fields of language assessment and cognitive development focuses on measuring language skills. Similar to the wide range of aforementioned assessments, which are used on a day-to-day basis, language tests can have an equally wide range of purposes. This may include tests that are part of job application procedures in English-speaking countries, such as the Test of English as a Foreign Language (*TOEFL*; e.g. Davies *et al.*, 1999) or tests to monitor children's language development (Johnston, 2007). Most of these and other comparable assessments are readily available for use in/with a variety of spoken languages. In comparison, a much smaller number of tests exists for sign languages and even fewer are: (a) suitable for use in educational settings (Mann, 2007, 2008) and/or; (b) commercially available (Haug, 2008). Aside from a few well-documented sign languages, including American Sign Language (ASL) and British Sign Language (BSL), this area of research is still considered very young, for instance, when compared to the large body of literature on the acquisition of spoken languages. The lack of standardized sign language assessments proves to be particularly challenging for practitioners in need of instruments to evaluate deaf children's sign language acquisition against normative developmental milestones. Consequently, decisions about appropriate educational placements or recommended interventions for deaf children are generally based on tests of spoken and written language skills, with only impressionistic assessments being made of sign language skills (Herman, 1998). These shortcomings are not limited to one country but exist on an international level (Germany: Haug & Hintermair, 2003; Switzerland: Audeoud & Haug, 2008; UK: Herman, 1998; US: Mann & Prinz, 2006).

One of the reasons for the international shortage of sign language assessment tools lies within the daunting process of developing such tools. For instance, only a small number of deaf children have deaf parents (less than 10%; Mitchell & Karchmer, 2004) and are considered native users of sign language. These children are critical for both test developers and researchers as they represent the normative group: children who are exposed to sign language from early on at home and who develop sign language at a pace that is comparable to hearing peers. Native signers constitute the 'ideal' population to establish developmental norms for a sign language test. In comparison, the majority of deaf children experience language very differently, partly as a result of the inconsistent input they receive from their hearing parents and/or professionals, ranging from sign language to spoken language only. For these reasons, language outcomes for deaf children with hearing parents have been widely acknowledged as notably lower than those achieved by native signers (Hermans et al., 2010; Mayer & Leigh, 2010; Spencer, 2004). Because of the limited early exposure to sign language for most of these individuals, their struggle to successfully acquire a language is understandable (Marschark, 2002).

Another, related reason for the shortage of sign language instruments is that much of the established knowledge of what constitutes 'typical' language acquisition in sign comes from studies with fairly small numbers of participants (e.g. Morgan & Woll, 2002; Schick et al., 2006). These studies tend to focus on deaf native signers and/or children of deaf adults (CODA), who are considered hearing native signers. Because of their limited numbers, the challenge of recruiting large samples of deaf native signers, specifically in smaller countries that may not have a (residential) Deaf school or program becomes apparent (see Mann et al., 2013, for a discussion of what constitutes the ideal norming sample).

The limited number of available sign language tests can be linked to a number of other, related explanations: the generalizability of findings from sign language acquisition research on deaf native signers to the (larger) deaf population, including deaf children of hearing parents, and the lack of empirical documentation on the process of language acquisition for many sign languages. Traditionally, most of the available research has focused on ASL and/or BSL (for ASL: Anderson & Reilly, 2002; Pettito, 1987; Pettito & Marentette, 1991; Reilly, 2006; for BSL: Morgan et al., 2002, 2003, 2006, 2008; Woolfe et al., 2010), although more research is becoming available on other sign languages (Australian Sign Language [Auslan]: De Beuzeville, 2006; Brazilian Sign Language: Bernardino, 2005; German Sign Language [DGS]: Hänel, 2003; Italian Sign Language [LIS]: Pizzuto, 2002; Sign Language of the Netherlands [SLN]: Slobin et al., 2003). The extensive research available on some sign languages (e.g. ASL) makes it tempting to use these results to draw conclusions about other sign languages. This approach may provide test developers with a more general understanding of the developmental aspect of a sign language. However, such 'transfer' should be done with caution and not without a critical analysis (see Haug & Mann, 2008, for a discussion).

Despite researchers' preference for using families with at least one deaf parent for studies on language development, it would be immature to consider parental deafness as the only predictor of a child's sign language proficiency. This has been demonstrated in a study by Singleton and Newport (2004), which investigated ASL development in a child with deaf, non-native, signing parents who acquired ASL after age 15. The language proficiency level of the child was based on the input from his parents. However, by the age of seven, the child outperformed both parents on an ASL morphology task, indicating that he was – despite inconsistent ASL input – able to acquire most ASL morphemes comparable to native signing deaf children (for a detailed discussion, see Singleton & Newport, 2004). This is also an important issue in sign language acquisition studies, i.e. the variability that depends, in part, on the language background of the deaf parents. Traditionally, it has been assumed that a deaf child, whose parents are deaf, will receive meaningful and consistent linguistic input from early on. At the same time, the importance of the input provided by hearing parents may have been underestimated. More than sign fluency, the frequency of adult–child interaction may provide enough meaningful input for young learners to quickly surpass their language models and to become proficient signers, similar to the reports by Singleton and Newport (2004). This raises the question whether parental hearing status alone is sufficient as matrix for language input or whether it should be broadened to 'signers at home'. For instance, Mann et al. (2013) used 'number of deaf family members' as one of their predictor variables and found that it helped to explain some of the variance in deaf children's sign production.

Because of deaf children's different language experiences, it is crucial to examine more closely the extent of variability for development of sign languages and to confirm existing findings on larger numbers of children. In this context, it may be premature to assume that deaf and hearing children in signing families are equivalent in terms of language acquisition. For instance, Herman and Roy (2006) noted that hearing children in deaf families are likely to be bilingual from an early age, whereas deaf children start off as monolingual in sign, at least until they enter school. This generates a need, at least initially, to establish monolingual norms in sign language as a basis for measuring deaf children's progress in language development.

Another issue related to sign language test development is the cultural acceptability of standardized tests. For instance, in the US, standardized tests (for educational placement, language assessment, etc.) play an important role in measuring students' academic achievement. This perception is not necessarily shared around the globe and tends to be highly culturally determined, particularly in countries where standardized testing is a less integrated part of academic assessment (e.g. in Sweden: Schönström et al., 2003; see also Haug & Mann, 2008).

Finally, when considering the development of a test for sign language (as for any other language), the purpose of the test should be clearly defined before the development begins. An assessment that is developed primarily as a research tool may look different and be devised in a different way from a test meant for carrying out large-scale norming. Similarly, a test to provide clinicians with a diagnostic tool may look very different from an assessment used by schools to monitor students' developmental progress, although some overlap of interests across targets is possible. Examples of such multi-purpose assessments include the ASL Sentence Repetition Test (ASL-SRT; Hauser et al., 2008) and the ASL/English Vocabulary Tasks (Mann, in preparation).

Types of Sign Language Assessments

Tests on sign language generally fall into one of four categories (Haug, 2008):

(a) Tests for sign language acquisition:
    Primary use: to measure deaf children's sign language skills, monitor development, and to inform intervention (where appropriate).
    Assessment instruments developed for (selected examples): BSL – *British Sign Language Receptive Skills Test* (Herman et al., 1998), *MacArthur Communicative Development Inventory for BSL* (Woolfe et al., 2010), *Web-based BSL Vocabulary Tasks* (Mann & Marshall, 2012); DGS – *German Sign Language Receptive Skills Test* (Haug, 2011); SLN – *Assessment Battery for Sign Language of the*

Netherlands (Hermans *et al.*, 2010); and ASL – *American Sign Language Proficiency Assessment* (Maller *et al.*, 1999), *MacArthur Communicative Development Inventory for ASL* (Anderson & Reilly, 2002).

(b) Tests for educational purposes:
Primary use: investigate the relationship between deaf children's sign language proficiency and their literacy skills.
Assessments instruments developed for: ASL – *American Sign Language Assessment Instrument* (Hoffmeister, 1999), *Test of American Sign Language* (Prinz *et al.*, 1994); DGS – *Computer Test for German Sign Language* (Mann, 2008); and LSF – *Test of French Sign Language* (Niederberger, 2004).

(c) Tests for linguistic research:
Primary use: to study specific grammatical features of sign language(s) and inform our understanding of how sign languages work.
Assessments developed for: ASL – *Grammatical Judgment Test for American Sign Language* (Boudreault, 1999; Boudreault & Mayberry, 2000), *American Sign Language Sentence Repetition Test* (Hauser *et al.*, 2008), *American Sign Language Morphology and Syntax* (Supalla *et al.*, 1995, unpublished); BSL – *BSL Nonsense Sign Repetition Task* (Mann *et al.*, 2008, 2010).

(d) Tests for adult second language learners:
Primary use: assessment for adults learning sign language as an additional/foreign language, and professionals who work with deaf people or have deaf colleagues.
Assessments developed for: DGS – *Aachen Test for Basic German Sign Language Competence – Adult Version* (Fehrmann *et al.*, 1995a, 1995b); ASL – *Sign Language Proficiency Interview* (Caccamise & Newell, 1995).

Approaches to the Development and/or Adaptation of Sign Language Tests

Aside from the number of different assessment tests described above, few or no sign language assessments are available, particularly in countries outside North America and Western Europe. Because of this lack, many practitioners and/or researchers looking for an appropriate tool to investigate the sign language of their countries frequently turn to existing tests that have been developed for spoken language (category 1) or to those available in other sign languages (category 2) to use as a template. Examples of the first category include the *MacArthur Communicative Inventory* (CDI; Fenson *et al.*, 1993), the *Peabody Picture Vocabulary Test* (PPVT, Dunn & Dunn, 1997), and the *Expressive/Receptive One Word Picture Vocabulary Test* (EOWPVT, Brownell, 2000; ROWPVT, Gardner, 1985). For instance, the MacArthur CDI, a parental checklist to monitor language development in young children from 8 to 36 months, has been adapted for ASL (Anderson & Reilly, 2002) and, more recently, for BSL (Woolfe *et al.*, 2010). Similar formats to the PPVT and ROWPVT/EOWPVT were used in tests to assess SLN (Hermans *et al.*, 2010) and BSL (Mann & Marshall, 2012) skills. Furthermore, the PPVT has been adapted for ASL (Schick, 2002).

An example of the second category is the BSL Receptive Skills Test (Herman *et al.*, 1998), which has been adapted to a number of different sign languages, including ASL (Enns & Herman, 2011), Auslan (Johnston, 2004), and DGS (Haug, 2011). While this approach seems plausible in light of the lack of available tests, it may give the misleading impression that sign languages are the same across countries and that linguistic structures (or features) in one sign language can easily be 'transferred' to another. However, comparative sign linguistic research (e.g. Zeshan, 2004, 2006) has shown that this is not the case. Consequently, past attempts to measure similar, or identical, features or targets across different sign languages using an adapted test have not been without complications (see Haug, 2011 for a review on adapting spoken and sign language tests). The most common factors influencing test adaptation across sign languages include differences in linguistic structures and cultural influences. Other issues that require caution comprise the adaptation of established psychometric properties, such as reliability and validity from the source test to the adapted version. This step is crucial because it means that the psychometric properties need to be established anew in an adapted test, even though strong evidence of reliability and validity may have been reported for the source test (Hambleton, 1994, 2001, 2005).

Reliability refers to whether the test is consistent in measuring what it is intended to measure (Rust & Golombok, 2000). One measure of reliability is inter-rater reliability, which refers to the level of agreement between two or more raters on a participant's performance (Davies *et al.*, 1999). This can be done, for instance, by videorecording a child's language production and then having different raters individually score the same specific grammatical structures. The core claim for the validity of a test is whether it really measures what it claims to measure (Kline, 2000). With regard to sign language, this could mean whether a test of sign language vocabulary really measures vocabulary knowledge and not, for example, the ability to guess the meaning of iconic signs (e.g. EAT, SLEEP) or gestures, which may be comparably high in non-signing, hearing children (e.g. White & Tischler, 1999). One of the several types of validity is content validity. Content validity examines whether, for example, the test items (and the test as a whole) represent the linguistic structures to be tested (Davies *et al.*, 1999). One of the prerequisites for assuring content validity in a test of sign language skills is close collaboration with deaf native signers during the developmental stage (Singleton & Supalla, 2003).

In sum, a growing number of sign language assessments have been developed over the course of the last 10–15 years, specifically for use with deaf children. Yet, only few of these assessments meet the psychometric criteria (e.g. validity and reliability) that are required for a 'good' test and are also suitable for use in educational settings. Additional tests, including linguistic/cognitive assessments, are still needed. Moreover, most of the 'available' tests focus on assessing typical sign language development, which results in a shortage of diagnostic tools. The strong need for instruments which can provide professionals with both diagnostic and acquisition information becomes evident in light of the considerable numbers of deaf individuals with additional needs (30–40%, Cone-Wesson, 2003).

Sign Language Assessments for Special Needs Groups

In addition to the limited research on sign languages and the shortage of available assessments, the characteristics of the 'typical' deaf language user (if such a person exists) keep changing. Traditionally, the distinction of deaf language users was made based on parental hearing status and type of amplification. These distinction criteria have become much more diversified due to the additional needs of certain subgroups within the deaf population. These subgroups include: (1) deaf individuals from different cultural and linguistic backgrounds; (2) children with uni/bilateral cochlear implant (CI); (3) individuals with dementia or motor disorders; and (4) individuals with additional (language) needs, which are one of the focus groups of this book. While the first three subgroups can be more easily identified, this is not always the case with children in the last subgroup, particularly those children with language and/or learning problems (e.g. Herman *et al.*, this volume). Given the delay with which many deaf children come to language, the distinction between language impairment versus language delay remains challenging. Due to the lack of any screening instruments, identification of language-impaired children usually remains with parents or teachers, who express concern for their children's sign language development (Mason *et al.*, 2010). Even then, clinicians left without the proper diagnostic tools to systematically identify particular problems struggle with establishing whether or not these children progress normally and with all the complexities of signed language development (Quinto-Pozos *et al.*, 2011)

Little is known as to what extent any of the currently available sign language tests are efficient/suitable for use with the described subgroups. The dearth of knowledge about some of these groups is mainly due to their general exclusion from empirical studies that aim to establish norms/collect average scores and to inform future assessment as part of the standardization of a test. As a result of this data shortage, we only have limited knowledge about their language skills and these subgroups continue to remain mostly underrepresented in the literature, with a exceptions (e.g. Große, 2004; Mahon *et al.*, 2011, on deaf children from migrant backgrounds; Mann, 2008;

Mann *et al.*, 2013, for a discussion of the need to include deaf children with additional needs in research; Marshall *et al.*, 2006; Mason *et al.*, 2010; Morgan, 2005; Morgan *et al.*, 2007; Quinto-Pozos *et al.*, 2011, on deaf children with language and/or communication disorders; Denmark, 2011; Shields, 2011, on deaf children with an autism spectrum disorder (ASD)).

Links to Other Chapters in the Book

The need for sign language assessments that go beyond the testing of 'typical' sign language development is highlighted by some of the other chapters in this book (e.g. Herman *et al.*, Quinto-Pozos *et al.*, Shield & Meier). For instance, Chen Pichler and colleagues (Chapter 10) argue that more sign language assessment instruments are needed in order to effectively document the bimodal development of children acquiring English and ASL. Similarly, Herman and colleagues (Chapter 2) suggest that sign language assessment tests can help identify specific language impairment (SLI) in deaf children or to test deaf children on the autism spectrum (e.g. Shield & Meier, Chapter 4). One of the overarching themes across these chapters is that standardized sign language tests should not be limited in their use to typically developing deaf children, but also be suitable for children where a different form of testing is required, such as to detect SLI.

Looking Ahead: Sign Language Assessment and Information and Communication Technologies

As mentioned before, there have been growing international efforts to address the need for appropriate assessments to use with deaf children. Many of these efforts included new technologies related to instruction, for example the use of web-based video lectures in Slovenian Sign Language for deaf students (Debevc & Peljhan, 2004), clinical assessment such as the computer-based psychiatric diagnostic interview in ASL (Montoya *et al.*, 2004), or language research (e.g. web-based vocabulary tests for BSL – Mann & Marshall, 2012, and ASL – Mann, in preparation). Other technologies include a computer-based platform for delivering content in ASL from K-12, (Hooper *et al.*, 2005; Miller *et al.*, 2005), and an interactive, web-based, multi sign language test interface (Haug, 2013).

The advantages of some of the features of information and communication technologies (ICT), such as automated score saving and/or score reporting functions, are unquestioned as they allow test developers to tailor assessments to the modality-specific needs of sign language users. For instance, a standardized testing format with a computer- or web-based interactive interface facilitates the integration of video responses (e.g. in a multiple-choice test), can be easily stored and later exported into a statistical program for analysis. In addition, set up, access and administration of tests is facilitated even further through the use of remote testing via the internet. However, this way of using ICT for language assessment is not without potential shortcomings and raises some questions related to data security (e.g. who has access to the test data? Are they stored on a secure server?). Also, the success of online testing largely depends on the availability of compatible resources/equipment at the test site and the extent to which this equipment meets the new standards, e.g. high-speed internet connection, capacity to play/store videos, on-site IT support, etc. Nevertheless, there is a clear advantage of new technologies for sign language assessment due to the highly interactive format, such as the testing of content/grammar within a narrative context, as used in the Computer Test for German Sign Language (Mann, 2005).

Taking the First Step: How to Test Sign Language Development Without Standardized Assessments

So far, we have highlighted the important role of assessment, specifically language assessment, in our lives and explained the need for (more) tests that assess sign language skills. In addition, we have presented a number of available sign language tests and discussed some of the major challenges of test development along with the possible pitfalls of adapting a test from one sign language to another. Our aim for the remaining part of this chapter is to offer some guidelines for those readers interested in assessment, who may not have access to any of the tests we mentioned. We present these guidelines in Figure 5.1, based on an adapted version of McNamara's (2000) 'testing cycle' by Haug (2011) for use with sign language (available online at http://www.signlang-assessment.info/tl_files/signlanguage/adaptation_sl_tests.pdf).

Step 1
Identifying a rationale. Test development should be approached/viewed as a cyclic rather than a linear process. There can be different reasons why language tests are developed, such as changes in the school curriculum (e.g. McNamara, 2000) or practitioners' need for a sign language test instrument (e.g. Audeoud & Haug, 2008; Haug & Hintermair, 2003; Herman, 1998; Mann & Prinz, 2006).

Step 2
Acknowledging possible constraints. Before test developers can start thinking about test content, they need to consider existing or potential limitations, including available budget and timeline, e.g. is the test part of a research project with limited funding options?

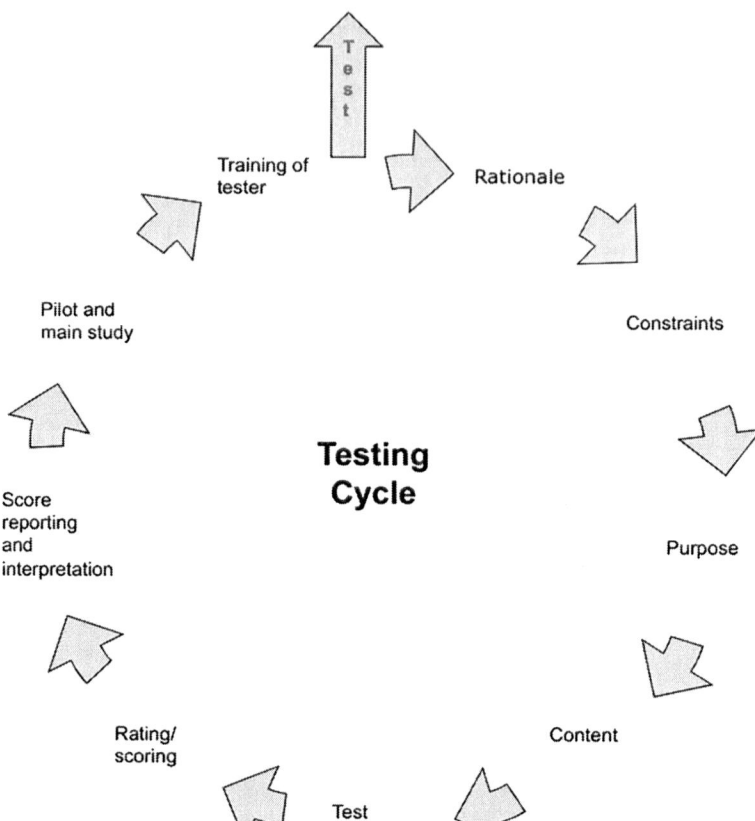

Figure 5.1 Testing cycle

Step 3

Defining the purpose of a test. This includes a clearly defined purpose of the test and an appropriate testing method. The purpose always has an influence on the testing method. The method can be viewed as two-dimensional: (1) the nature of the reference, i.e. norm- versus criterion-referenced; and (2) the nature of the sample, i.e. spontaneous versus elicited language samples. When thinking about the test method, it is most important to consider the interaction of the test participant with the test materials, most obvious with the response format, i.e. how the test participant needs to respond to the test materials (e.g. videos).

Step 4

Content of the test. Once the purpose of the test has been identified, the next step is to define the content of the test, namely which aspects of a language should be tested, e.g. the acquisition of lexical development. Other variables to take into consideration include the age of the target group and the type of language skills, e.g. comprehension and/or production to be tested.

Step 5

Test specification. These specifications represent the 'blueprint' of what needs to be done in which order, e.g. the development of the items; they are a result of the design, of the purpose, the content and the (test) method, and serve as the basis for constructing the test. Developing a new test also involves designing appropriate testing procedures and test items. Other issues that are important to consider include environmental factors of the testing situation, e.g. is the tester familiar to the test participant, familiarity/unfamiliarity of the test location (room), management and secure storage of large amounts of data (e.g. language production), and the need to report psychometric properties, i.e. validity and reliability for a new test.

Step 6

Rating/scoring. Depending on the content and the testing method it is important to have appropriate rating procedures (e.g. rating sheets) in place. These procedures may be very different for production skills, e.g. checking for correct use of classifier constructions versus comprehension skills, e.g. use of a multiple-choice format.

Step 7

Score report and interpretation of results. It is important to think about how scores will be reported and how they should be interpreted. With score reporting we mean, how does a test participant learn about the test results? For example, will s/he receive a printout of the score report along with some comments? It is also important to consider how the results will be interpreted and perhaps used to inform decisions related to placement (e.g. foreign language class), intervention (e.g. individual support sessions) and/or admittance (e.g. university).

Step 8

Pilot and main study. Before a test can be used, for example in schools for the deaf, it is important to conduct a pilot study and a main study. The pilot study can result in some revisions of the test items, the testing procedure, and/or the rating/scoring procedures. This approach also allows establishing the psychometric properties of the new test, which then need to be reported.

Step 9

Training of the tester. One of the key aspects for successful test development and administration is the training of the testers, i.e. making the tester aware of issues related to use with children, psychometrics (e.g. to administer the test to every child in the same way), and with regard to sign language acquisition.

It might appear to some readers that our guidelines make the task of developing/adapting a sign language test even more daunting. Therefore, we close this chapter with the following general recommendations, as an encouragement to those interested in exploring the field of sign language assessment.

(1)   In order to provide quality assessments for sign language(s), be it a standardized receptive skills test or a set of standardized checklists, one needs to start somewhere, no matter how simplistic a first test version might be.

(2)   At the same time, it is important for the test developer not to forget about the original purpose of the test. This is not always an easy task, given the heterogeneous nature of the deaf target population, including various subgroups (deaf children with hearing parents, deaf children from minority backgrounds, deaf children with/without CI, etc.). One way of accounting for the heterogeneity may be to collect data over a longer period of time and create language profiles for different subgroups.

(3)   Finally and above all, for any test adaptation/development to be successful, a close collaboration from early on with deaf native signers, researchers and/or practitioners/clinicians working in an educational setting is (one of) the most crucial precondition(s).

Helpful Resources

See http://www.signlang-assessment.info/.

References

Anderson, D. and Reilly, J. (2002) The MacArthur Communicative Development Inventory: Normative data for American Sign Language. *Journal of Deaf Studies and Deaf Education* 7 (2), 83–119.

Audeoud, M. and Haug, T. (2008) 'Grundsätzlich wollen wir Tests, die alle sprachlichen Ebenen überprüfen!' Eine Pilot-Studie zum Bedarf an Gebärdensprachtests für hörgeschädigte Kinder an Deutschschweizer Hörgeschädigtenschulen. *Hörgeschädigtenpädagogik* 61 (1), 15–20.

Bartram, D. (1990) Introduction. In J.R. Beech and L. Harding (eds) *Testing People: A Practical Guide to Psychometrics* (pp. 1–10). Windsor: NFER Nelson.

Bernardino, E. (2005) The acquisition of classifiers in verbs of motion and verbs of location in Brazilian Sign Language. Unpublished doctoral dissertation, Graduate School of Arts and Sciences, Boston University (ProQuest UMI number: 3186488).

Boudreault, P. (1999) Grammatical processing in American Sign Language: Effects of age of acquisition and syntactic complexity. Unpublished masters thesis, School of Communication Sciences and Disorders, McGill University.

Boudreault, P. and Mayberry, R.I. (2000) Grammatical processing in American Sign Language: Effects of age of acquisition and syntactic complexity. Poster presented at the 7th International Conference on Theoretical Issues in Sign Language Research, Amsterdam, The Netherlands, 23–27 July.

Brownell, R. (2000) *Expressive One-word Picture Vocabulary Test*. Novato, CA: Academic Therapy Publications.

Caccamise, F. and Newell, W. (1995) Evaluating sign language communication skills: The Sign Communication Proficiency Interview (SCPI). In R. Myers (ed.) *Standards of Care for the Delivery of Mental Health Services to Deaf and Hard of Hearing Persons* (pp. 33–35). Silver Spring, MD: National Association of the Deaf.

Cone-Wesson, B. (2003) Screening and assessment of hearing loss in infants. In M. Marschark and P.E. Spencer (eds) *Oxford Handbook of Deaf Studies, Language, and Education* (pp. 420–433). New York: Oxford University Press.

Davies, A., Brown, A., Elder, C., Hill, K., Lumley, T. and McNamara, T. (1999) *Dictionary of Language Testing – Studies in Language Testing 7*. Cambridge: Cambridge University Press.

De Beuzeville, L. (2006) Visual and linguistic representation in the acquisition of depicting verbs: A study of native signing deaf children of Auslan (Australian Sign Language). Unpublished doctoral dissertation, Renwick College, University of Newcastle, Australia.

Debevc, M. and Peljhan, Z. (2004) The role of video technology in on-line lectures for the deaf. *Disability and Rehabilitation* 26 (17), 1048–1059.

Denmark, T.A. (2011) Do deaf children with Autism Spectrum Disorder show deficits in the comprehension and production of emotional and linguistic facial expressions in British Sign Language? Doctoral thesis, UCL (University College London).

Dunn, L.M. and Dunn, L.M. (1997) *Peabody Picture Vocabulary Test* (3rd edn). Circle Pines, MN: American Guidance Services

Enns, C. and Herman, R. (2011) Adapting the Assessing British Sign Language Development: Receptive Skills Test into American Sign Language. *Journal of Deaf Studies and Deaf Education* 16 (3), 362–374. doi:10.1093/deafed/enr004.

Fehrmann, G., Huber, W., Jäger, L., Sieprath, H. and Werth, I. (1995a) Linguistische Konzeption des Aachener Tests zur Basiskompetenz in Deutscher Gebärdensprache (ATG). Unpublished manuscript, RWTH-Aachen, Germanistisches Institut & Neurologische Klinik, Projekt DESIRE.

Fehrmann, G., Huber, W., Jäger, L., Sieprath, H. and Werth, I. (1995b) Aufbau des Aachener Tests zur Basiskompetenz in Deutscher Gebärdensprache (ATG). Unpublished manuscript, RWTH-Aachen, Germanitisches Institut & Neurologische Klinik, Projekt DESIRE.

Fenson, L., Dale, P.S., Reznick, J.S., Thal, D., Bates, E., Hartung, J.P., Pethick, S. and Reilly, J.S. (1993) *The MacArthur Communicative Development Inventories: User's Guide and Technical Manual*. San Diego, CA: Singular Publishing Group.

Fulcher, G. and Davidson, F. (2007) *Language Testing and Assessment – An Advanced Resource Book*. London: Routledge Applied Linguistics.

Gardner, M. (1985) *Receptive One Word Picture Vocabulary Test*. Novato, CA: Academic Therapy Publishing.

Große, K-D. (ed.) (2004) *Hörbehinderte Schülerinnen und Schüler unterschiedlicher nationaler Herkunft – Eine internationale Herausforderung an die Hörgeschädigtenpädagogik*. Heidelberg: Universitätsverlag Winter.

Hänel, B. (2003) Der Erwerb der Deutschen Gebärdensprache als Erstsprache – Die frühkindliche Sprachentwicklung von Subjekt- und Objektverbkongruenz in DGS. Unpublished doctoral dissertation, Department of Linguistics, Hamburg University.

Hambleton, R.K. (1994) Guidelines for adapting educational and psychological tests: A progress report. *European Journal of Psychological Assessment* 10 (3), 229–244.

Hambleton, R.K. (2001) The next generation of the ITC test translation and adaptation guidelines. *European Journal of Psychological Assessment* 17 (3), 164–172.

Hambleton, R.K. (2005) Issues, design, and technical guidelines for adapting tests into multiple languages and cultures. In R.K. Hambleton, P.F. Merenda and C.D. Spielberger (eds) *Adapting Educational and Psychological Tests for Cross-cultural Assessment* (pp. 3–38). Mahwah, NJ: Lawrence Erlbaum.

Haug, T. (2008) Review of sign language assessment instruments. In A. Baker and B. Woll (eds) *Sign Language Acquisition* (pp. 51–85). Amsterdam: John Benjamins.

Haug, T. (2011) *Adaptation and Evaluation of a German Sign Language Test – A Computer-based Receptive Skills Test for Deaf Children 4–8 Years Old.* Hamburg: Hamburg University Press. See http://hup.sub.uni-hamburg.de/purl/HamburgUP_Haug_Adaptation.

Haug, T. (2013) *Constructing an online test framework, using the example of a sign language receptive skills test.* Manuscript submitted for publication. See http://www.signlanguagetest.com.

Haug, T. and Hintermair, M. (2003) Ermittlung des Bedarfs von Gebärdensprachtests für gehörlose Kinder – Ergebnisse einer Pilotstudie. *Das Zeichen* 64, 220–229.

Haug, T. and Mann, W. (2008) Adapting tests of sign language assessment to other sign languages – a review of linguistic, cultural, and psychometric problems. *Journal of Deaf Studies and Deaf Education* 13 (1), 138–147.

Hauser, P.C., Paludnevičienė, R., Supalla, T. and Bavelier, D. (2008) American Sign Language-Sentence Reproduction Test. In R.M. de Quadros (ed.) *Sign Languages: Spinning and Unraveling the Past, Present and Future. TISLR 9, Forty-five Papers and Three Posters from the 9.* Theoretical Issues in Sign Language Research Conference, Florianopolis, Brazil, December 2006 (pp. 160–172). Petrópolis/RJ: Editora Arara Azul.

Herman, R. (1998) The need for an assessment of deaf children's signing skills. *Deafness and Education: Journal of the British Association of the Teachers of the Deaf* 22 (3), 3–8.

Herman, R. and Roy, P. (2006) Evidence from the wider use of the BSL Receptive Skills Test. *Deafness and Education International* 8 (1), 33–47.

Herman, R., Holmes, S. and Woll, B. (1998) Design and standardization of an assessment of British Sign Language development for use with young deaf children: Final report, 1998. Unpublished manuscript, City University London.

Hermans, D., Knoors, H. and Verhoeven, L. (2010) Assessment of sign language development: The case of deaf children in the Netherlands. *Journal of Deaf Studies and Deaf Education* 15 (2), 107–119.

Hoffmeister, R. (1999) American Sign Language Assessment Instrument (ASLAI). Unpublished manuscript, Center for the Study of Communication & the Deaf, Boston University.

Hooper, S., Rose, S. and Miller, C. (2005) Assessing American Sign Language performance: Developing an environment for capturing, evaluating, and monitoring student progress. In V. Uskov (ed.) *Proceedings of the IASTED International Conference on Web-Based Education* (pp. 452–457). Calgary: ACTA Press.

Johnston, J. (2007) *Assessment of Language Learning in English Speaking Children. Encyclopedia of Language and Literacy Development* (pp. 1–9). London and Ontario: Canadian Language and Literacy Research Network. See http://www.literacyencyclopedia.ca/pdfs/topic.php?topId = 39.

Johnston, T. (2004) The assessment and achievement of proficiency in a native sign language within a sign bilingual program: The pilot Auslan receptive skills test. *Deafness and Education International* 6 (2), 57–81.

Kline, P. (2000) *Handbook of Psychological Testing* (2nd edn). London and New York: Routledge.

Mahon, M., Vickers, D., McCarthy, K., Barker, R., Merritt, R., Szagun, G., Mann, W. and Rajput, K. (2011) Cochlear-implanted children from homes where English is an additional language: Findings from a recent audit in one London centre. *Cochlear Implants International* 12 (2), 105–113. doi:10.1179/146701010X486552.

Maller, S.J., Singleton, J.L., Supalla, S.J. and Wix, T. (1999) The development and psycho-metric properties of the American Sign Language Proficiency Assessment (ASL-PA). *Journal of Deaf Studies and Deaf Education* 4 (4), 249–269.

Mann, W. (2005) Computer Test for German Sign Language (CTDGS). Unpublished Test. San Francisco State University and UC, Berkeley.

Mann, W. (2007) Examining German deaf children's understanding of referential distinc-tion in written German and German sign language (DGS). *Educational and Child Psychology* 24 (4), 59–76.

Mann, W. (2008) *Facing the Challenge of Appropriately Assessing Deaf Children's Language Skills: An Investigation into German Deaf Children's Understanding of Reference in German Sign Language and in Written German*. Saarbrücken: VDM.

Mann, W. (in preparation) Assessing different levels of deaf children's vocabulary knowl-edge in American Sign Language.

Mann, W. and Marshall, C. (2012) Investigating deaf children's vocabulary knowledge in British Sign Language. *Language Learning* 62 (4), 1024–1051. doi:10.1111/j.1467-9922.2011.00670.x.

Mann, W. and Prinz, P. (2006) The perception of sign language assessment by profession-als in deaf education. *American Annals of the Deaf* 151 (3), 356–370.

Mann, W., Marshall, C. and Morgan, G. (2008) BSL Nonsense Sign Repetition Test. Unpublished test, City University London.

Mann, W., Marshall, C., Mason, K. and Morgan, G. (2010) The acquisition of sign lan-guage: The interplay between phonology and phonetics. *Language and Learning Development* 8, 60–86. doi: 10.1080/15475440903245951.

Mann, W., Roy, P. and Marshall, C. (2013) A look at the other 90% – investigating British Sign Language knowledge in deaf children from different language learn-ing backgrounds. *Deafness & Education International* 15 (2), 91–116. doi: 10.1179/1557069X12Y.0000000017.

Marschark, M. (2002) Foundations of communication and the emergence of language in deaf children. In G. Morgan and B. Woll (eds) *Directions in Sign Language Acquisition – Trends in Language Acquisition Research* (pp. 1–28). Amsterdam: John Benjamins.

Marshall, C.R., Denmark, T. and Morgan, G. (2006) Investigating the underlying causes of SLI: A non-sign repetition test in British Sign Language. *Advances in Speech-Language Pathology* 8 (4), 347–355. doi:10.1080/14417040600970630.

Mason, K., Rowley, K., Marshall, C.R., Atkinson, J.R., Herman, R., Woll, B. and Morgan, G. (2010) Identifying specific language impairment in deaf children acquiring British Sign Language: Implications for theory and practice. *British Journal of Developmental Psychology* 28 (1), 33–49. doi:10.1348/026151009X484190.

Mayer, C. and Leigh, G. (2010) The changing context for sign bilingual education pro-grams: Issues in language and the development of literacy. *International Journal of Bilingual Education and Bilingualism* 13, 175–186. doi:10.1080/13670050903474085.

McNamara, T. (2000) *Oxford Introductions to Language Study – Language Testing*. Oxford: Oxford University Press.

Miller, C., Hooper, S. and Rose, S. (2005) Avenue ASL: Developing an environment for assessing American Sign Language performance. *Advanced Technology for Learning* 2 (3), 140–147.

Mitchell, R. and Karchmer, M. (2004) Chasing the mythical ten percent: Parental hearing status of deaf and hard of hearing students in the United States. *Sign Language Studies* 4 (2), 138–163.

Montoya, L.A., Egnatovitch, R., Eckhardt, E., Goldstein, M., Goldstein, R.A. and Steinberg, A.G. (2004) Translation challenges and strategies: The ASL translation of a computer-based, psychiatric diagnostic interview. *Sign Language Studies* 4 (4), 314–344.

Morgan, G. (2005) Biology and behavior: Insights from the acquisition of sign language. In A. Cutler (ed.) *Twenty-first Century Psycholinguistics: Four Cornerstones* (pp. 191–208). Mahwah, NJ: Lawrence Erlbaum.

Morgan, G. and Woll, B. (eds) (2002) *Directions in Sign Language Acquisition – Trends in Language Acquisition Research.* Amsterdam: John Benjamins.

Morgan, G., Herman, R. and Woll, B. (2002) The development of complex verb constructions in British Sign Language. *Journal of Child Language* 29, 655–675.

Morgan, G., Barrière, I. and Woll, B. (2003) First verbs in British Sign Language development. *Working Papers in Language and Communication Science* 2, 56–65. City University London.

Morgan, G., Barrière, I. and Woll, B. (2006) The influence of typology and modality on the acquisition of verb agreement morphology in British Sign Language. *First Language* 26, 19–43.

Morgan, G., Herman, R. and Woll, B. (2007) Language impairment in sign language: Breakthroughs and puzzles. *International Journal of Communication Disorders* 35, 95–116. doi:10.1080/13682820600783178.

Morgan, G., Herman, R., Barrière, I. and Woll, B. (2008) The onset and mastery of spatial language in children acquiring British Sign Language. *Cognitive Development* 23, 1–19.

Niederberger, N. (2004) Capacités langagières en Langue des Signes Française et en français écrit chez l'enfant sourd bilingue: quelles relations? Unpublished doctoral dissertation, University of Geneva.

Petitto, L-A. (1987) On the autonomy of language and gesture: Evidence from the acquisition of personal pronouns in American Sign Language. *Cognition* 27, 1–52.

Petitto, L-A. and Marentette, P. (1991) Babbling in the manual mode: Evidence for the ontogeny of language. *Science* 251, 1493–1496.

Pizzuto, E. (2002) The development of Italian Sign Language (LIS) in deaf preschoolers. In G. Morgan and B. Woll (eds) *Directions in Sign Language Acquisition* (pp. 77–114). Amsterdam: John Benjamins.

Prinz, P., Strong, M. and Kuntze, M. (1994) The Test of ASL. Unpublished test, California Research Institute, San Francisco State University.

Quinto-Pozos, D., Forber-Pratt, A. and Singleton, J. (2011) Do developmental communication disorders exist in the signed modality? Reporting on the experiences of language professionals and educators from schools for the deaf. *Language, Speech, and Hearing Services in Schools* 42 (4), 423–443. doi:10.1044/0161-1461(2011/10-0071).

Reilly, J. (2006) How faces come to serve grammar: The development of nonmanual morphology in American Sign Language. In B. Schick, M. Marschark and P. Spencer (eds) *Advances in the Sign Language Development of Deaf Children* (pp. 262–290). Oxford: Oxford University Press.

Rust, J. and Golombok, S. (2000) *Modern Psychometrics – The Science of Psychological Assessment* (2nd edn). London and New York: Routledge.

Schick, B. (2002) Assessing ASL skills in children: Formal tests for elementary school-aged children. Unpublished manuscript.

Schick, B., Marschark, M. and Spencer, P. (2006) *Advances in the Sign Language Development of Deaf Children.* New York: Oxford University Press.

Schönström, K., Simper-Allen, P. and Svartholm, K. (2003) Assessment of signing skills in school-aged deaf students in Sweden. In *European Days of Deaf Education* (pp. 88–95). Oerebro: EDDE.

Shields, A. (2011) The signing of Deaf children with autism: Lexical phonology and perspective-taking in the visual-spatial modality. *Sign Language & Linguistics* 14 (1), 207–212.

Singleton, J.L. and Newport, E.L. (2004) When learners surpass their models: The acquisition of American Sign Language from inconsistent input. *Cognitive Psychology* 49, 370–407.

Singleton, J.L. and Supalla, S. (2003) Assessing children's proficiency in natural signed languages. In M. Marschark and P. Spencer (eds) *Oxford Handbook of Deaf Studies, Language, and Education* (pp. 289–302). Oxford and New York: Oxford University Press.

Slobin, D.I., Hoiting, N., Kuntze, M., *et al.* (2003) A cognitive/functional perspective on the acquisition of 'classifiers'. In K. Emmorey (ed.) *Perspectives on Classifier Constructions in Sign Languages* (pp. 271–296). Mahwah, NJ: Lawrence Erlbaum.

Spencer, P.E. (2004) Individual differences in language performance after cochlear implantation at one to three years of age: Child, family, and linguistic factors. *Journal of Deaf Studies and Deaf Education* 9, 395–412.

Supalla, T., Newport, E., Singleton, J., Supalla, S., Coulter, G. and Metlay, D. (1995) *An overview of the Test Battery for American Sign Language Morphology and Syntax*. Paper presented at the Annual Meeting of the American Educational Research Association (AERA), 20 April 1995, San Francisco, CA.

Supalla, T., Newport, E., Singleton, J., Supalla, S., Coulter, G. and Metlay, D. (unpublished). Test Battery for American Sign Language Morphology and Syntax. Unpublished document.

White, A. and Tischler, S. (1999) Receptive sign vocabulary tests: Tests of single-word vocabulary or iconicity. *American Annals of the Deaf* 144 (4), 334–338.

Woolfe, T., Herman, R., Roy, P. and Woll, B. (2010) Early lexical development in native signers: A BSL adaptation of the MacArthur–Bates CDI. *Child Psychology and Psychiatry* 51 (3), 322–331.

Zeshan, U. (2004) Hand, head, and face – negative constructions in sign languages. *Linguistic Typology* 8, 1–58.

Zeshan, U. (ed.) (2006) *Interrogative and Negative Constructions in Sign Languages.* Sign Language Typology series. Nijmegen: Ishara Press.

Part 2

Fluency Disorders, Neurogenics and Acquired Communication Disorders

6 A Review of Stuttering in Signed Languages

Geoffrey Whitebread

Introduction

Developmental stuttering is defined by the World Health Organization (WHO) as 'speech that is characterized by frequent repetition or prolongation of sounds or syllables or words, or by frequent hesitations or pauses that disrupt the rhythmic flow of speech' (WHO, 2010: 227). While the WHO's definition assumes a focus on speech and spoken language, evidence on the nature of stuttering has grown markedly since the publication of that definition and several writings have described possible stuttering-like behaviors in signed languages (Cosyns et al., 2009; Montgomery & Fitch, 1988; Quinto-Pozos et al., 2011; Silverman & Silverman, 1971; Whitebread, 2004). By referencing some of these studies and his own experience, Snyder (2006) suggests that a 'paradigm shift' in stuttering research may be in order that would not only consider stuttering as a speech disorder (WHO, 2010; Yairi & Ambrose, 2005) but also as a disorder that could explain the observations of stuttering-like behavior that have been documented in other modes of expressive communication, such as signed language, music and handwriting (Meltzer, 1992; Roman, 1959; Scripture, 1909; Silverman & Bohlman, 1988). Snyder's suggestion touches on one of the central themes of current research on stuttering: whether stuttering is a motor disorder, a language disorder, or a mixture of both (for a discussion of the theories of stuttering, see Guitar, 2006).

When thinking about stuttering in signed languages, there are three characteristics of deaf people and signed languages that merit attention. First, bilingualism is a common feature in the signing Deaf community[1] and people who sign may use different modes of communication depending on the situation. For the purposes of this discussion, bilingualism refers to a person who is fluent in a signed language and is also fluent in a written language and/or a spoken language. In any given situation a Deaf person may choose to sign, speak or use both sign and speech simultaneously. A person may also be bilingual if they are fluent in multiple signed languages, but this type of bilingualism has not yet been discussed in the literature on signed stuttering.

The second characteristic is that communication can occur within a single modality (i.e. unimodally – such as only in spoken language or only in signed language) or across modalities (i.e. bimodally – such as in spoken language produced simultaneously with signed language). With respect to deaf and hard of hearing people (hereafter D/HH) who stutter, it may be particularly useful to distinguish whether they stutter in one modality or both (i.e. if they happen to use spoken language, too). If a person does stutter in both modalities, it may also be useful to consider whether a person stutters in both modalities simultaneously or if they stutter in both modalities independent of the other. Furthermore, it may also be useful to consider whether a person's level of linguistic proficiency in both modalities affects fluency.

The third characteristic that it is useful to consider is that D/HH people are not homogenous with respect to the degree to which they possess residual hearing. For this factor, there is significant variation among people who identify themselves as deaf or hard of hearing. Technological advances in hearing assistive devices mean that more deaf people have access to spoken language and sounds than in previous generations. This fact is useful to consider in stuttering in signed languages since various studies have suggested that audition, which is not used in signing, may play a key role in the manifestation of spoken stuttering (see Civier et al., 2010; Marist & Hutton, 1957; Neilson & Neilson 1987; Nudelman et al., 1989).

Keeping in mind these characteristics, there are several questions that may be useful to consider with respect to stuttering in signed languages, and some of those questions can be grouped as follows:

(1) What is the reported prevalence of stuttering within the D/HH community (in either signed or spoken language production)?
(2) What are the reported characteristics of stuttering-like disfluency in signed language production?
(3) How might language modality affect fluency for a person who stutters? For a user of signed language who also uses speech, does stuttering occur equally in both modalities? How, if at all, does stuttering in signed language interact with stuttering in spoken language?

These questions have been touched upon to varying degrees in the literature on signed language stuttering. Further consideration of these questions may yield more insight into the disfluencies observed by researchers and professional educators of the deaf.

Research on Stuttering in Signed Language

The research on signed stuttering has been growing but is still in its early stages. The literature has not yet presented a detailed picture of the nature of stuttering-like disfluencies observed in signed languages. As a result, researchers interested in the prevalence of stuttering in signed languages have been compelled to work from descriptions of stuttering-like disfluency that have been generated, in part, by the nature of stuttering in spoken language rather than from detailed descriptions of disruptions to fluency in signed languages. Researchers have typically surveyed educators and special service providers (e.g. speech and language pathologists) who work with D/HH children and relied on these professionals to recall behaviors that they believed to be stuttering in signed language and to describe what they observed.

This reliance on intuition is not unique to the literature on signed stuttering. The accuracy of observers' recognition of stuttering has been studied in spoken languages, and listeners of spoken language are shown to be relatively accurate in their identification of stuttering-like disfluencies, with errors occurring most frequently in borderline cases (Bloodstein & Bernstein Ratner, 2008; Yairi et al., 1996). It is even the case that experienced speech language pathologists are accurate, in most cases, in recognizing stuttering in foreign languages where the evaluator has a high level of proficiency (Einarsdottir & Ingham, 2009; Van Borsel & Pereira, 2005). Researchers of stuttering in American Sign Language (ASL) have relied on this same intuition in documenting stuttering in ASL by using experts with a high degree of familiarity with the language. This reliance on intuition made it possible to initially document the existence and prevalence of stuttering-like disfluencies in signed language.

Prevalence and communication modality

Bloodstein (1995) reports that the prevalence rate of developmental stuttering in English speakers in the United States is approximately 1%. Bloodstein and Bernstein Ratner (2008) aggregate 18 studies of prevalence and find that prevalence among school-aged children in the US ranges from 0.3% to 2.1%. Prevalence rates vary in monolingual speakers across cultures. Van Riper (1982) reports eight studies of prevalence in different cultures ranging between 0.8% and 1.9%, with one study reporting a prevalence rate of 0.02% in a Native American tribe. Bloodstein and Bernstein Ratner (2008) reports the results of 26 studies of prevalence in other countries and finds that prevalence rates varied between 0.5% and 1.8%, with one town in Denmark reporting a 5.2% prevalence rate. Numerous studies of prevalence have also documented the different ratios of male and female persons who stutter, with stuttering more prevalent in males than females. In the US, the gender ratio gap ranges from 2:1 to 5:1 (Andrews & Harris, 1964; Bloodstein & Bernstein Ratner, 2008; Van Riper, 1982). While there is variability in the numbers, there appears to be widespread documentation of the differences between the sexes in many cultures using spoken language.

The first studies conducted on stuttering in D/HH populations were prevalence studies focusing on school-aged children. In comparison to hearing populations, prevalence rates of stuttering in deaf populations appear to be markedly lower. Backus (1938) found stuttering to be present in 0.4% of the sampled population in 206 schools for the deaf, with 13,691 students enrolled. Harms and Malone (1939) found stuttering present in 0.3% of their sampled population in 209 deaf schools, with 14,458 students enrolled.[2] Both of these studies employed survey methods asking staff at schools for the deaf to identify students who stuttered during an era when spoken English was used as the language of instruction. As a result, the authors' findings did not differentiate between stuttering in sign and stuttering in spoken English. Reflecting what may have been an interest in the role of audition in stuttering, Backus (1938) sorted reports of stuttering by whether students were profoundly deaf or hard of hearing. Backus identified six deaf students who stuttered and an additional 55 hard of hearing students who stuttered. Harms and Malone (1939) identified eight deaf students who stuttered and 42 hard of hearing students who stuttered. Voelker and Voelker (1937) reported rare instances where stuttering exists in persons with congenital hearing loss. Table 6.1 presents the prevalence rates from various studies of children who use spoken or signed language.

Table 6.1 Prevalence of stuttering in various populations

Study	Population sampled	Prevalence rate
Van Riper (1982)*	Various populations of speakers (speech only)	0.8–1.9%
Bloodstein and Bernstein Ratner (2008)*	US schoolchildren	0.3–2.1%
Bloodstein and Bernstein Ratner (2008)*	Schoolchildren in other countries	0.5–5.2%
Backus (1938)	US deaf and hard of hearing children ($N = 13,691$)	0.4%
Harmes and Malone (1939)	US deaf and hard of hearing children ($N = 14,458$)	0.3%
Montgomery and Fitch** (1988)	US deaf and hard of hearing children ($N = 77$)	0.1%

Notes: *Rates are aggregated from multiple studies.
**Authors estimate prevalence through a survey of teachers at schools for the deaf.

An important question is whether the early studies were capturing observers' reports of disfluencies in speech, in sign, or in both modalities. As noted, Backus (1938) and Harms and Malone (1939) are not explicit about whether they are studying prevalence rates of spoken or signed language stuttering, but it appears that they are interested in the role of audition and spoken language disfluency in the deaf populations that they study. Snyder (2006) suggests that the authors may have been discussing stuttering in both spoken and manual modalities. I suggest that the early studies were focused on spoken language disfluencies because sign languages were not yet recognized as fully fledged languages, and signed language was generally not used by educators in the classroom (Baynton, 2009). In addition, the early researchers explicitly surveyed professionals at oral schools for the deaf who would interact with their students using oral communication as the method of communication. Harms and Malone (1939) also use pure-tone audiometry tests to measure the degree of hearing loss in their subjects. Follow-up studies challenging the severity of the hearing loss reported from the pure-tone audiometry tests also suggest an interest in spoken stuttering for the early studies (Bullen, 1945; Sternberg, 1946).

The prevalence of stuttering in signed language has also been explicitly examined. Montgomery and Fitch (1988) suggested that stuttering-like behaviors are more common in signed language than in spoken language in the deaf, with a prevalence of 0.12%, as reported in Bloodstein and Bernstein Ratner (2008). Silverman and Silverman (1971) find that approximately half of the teachers who used signed language and responded to their survey had observed students stuttering in signed language. It is possible that the number of teachers who report observing stuttering-like disfluency is higher in this report because the authors asked teachers to describe disfluency in sign language that they believed appropriately paralleled stuttering in spoken languages. In contrast to later studies, Silverman and Silverman do not appear to have provided respondents with guidance on what constitutes stuttering. Cosyns *et al.* (2009) asked survey respondents to identify the characteristics of stuttering-like disfluency in Flemish Sign Language. Respondents identified 13 persons who stutter aged 10–45 years, with a variety of stuttering-like behaviors. Cosyns and colleagues report that their sample size was too small to draw conclusions about wider prevalence rates.

Some of the prevalence studies also reported isolated cases of stuttering in D/HH individuals with unique profiles. Van Riper (1982) reports one incident where a person who started stuttering as a child with full hearing suddenly lost his hearing in an accident and ceased to stutter even though he continued to use speech. Unfortunately, details about this case are limited. Montgomery and Fitch (1988) mention that a female student with a severe-to-profound hearing loss and a near-hearing speaking ability was reported to stutter.

Stuttering and the role of audition

Some of the studies on signed language stuttering appear to indicate that stuttering is less prevalent in the D/HH persons (Backus, 1938; Harms & Malone, 1939). This could support a hypothesis that audition is an important part of spoken language stuttering. It was believed that audition played a central role in stuttering in the early to mid-20th century. At the time, evidence for the role of audition included the low prevalence of stuttering in the deaf (Backus, 1938; Harmes & Malone, 1939), and new discoveries of the effects of auditory masking in improving speech fluency in persons who stutter. Marist and Hutton (1957) found that the mean number of errors and length of time required for a reading decreased as auditory masking increased. In reviewing the literature, Marist and Hutton stated, 'these data seem to indicate that normal hearing acuity is a prerequisite to the onset of stuttering' (Marist & Hutton, 1957: 385). More recent studies appear to confirm the role of audition in stuttering. These studies have found marked differences in auditory functioning between persons who stutter and fluent speakers, with the former requiring more processing time and exhibiting less accuracy with auditory tasks (Neilson & Neilson, 1987; Nudelman *et al.*, 1987, 1989, 1992; Sussman & Macneilage, 1975). More recently, evidence has been presented that people who stutter may compensate for impaired speech control by over-relying on auditory feedback when producing speech (Civier *et al.*, 2010). These data, while indicating a role for audition in spoken stuttering, may not necessarily exclude the possibility for stuttering to exist in a visual modality. As Bloodstein and Bernstein Ratner (2008) note, it is possible that the role of audition is not critical to stuttering, and that stuttering and deafness may be two relatively rare conditions with a genetic influence that seldom co-occur.

Symptoms reported for stuttering-like disfluency in deaf users of signed language

It may be useful to first briefly summarize some of the common descriptions of stuttering-like behaviors given for spoken languages before discussing other considerations with respect to stuttering-like disfluencies in signed language. There are numerous ways to categorize the types of disfluency that have been reported (Bloodstein & Bernstein Ratner, 2008; Van Riper, 1982; Wingate, 1970). A recent taxonomy is known as the Illinois Disfluency Classification System, which identifies stuttering-like disfluencies and other disfluencies (Yairi & Ambrose, 2005). Stuttering-like disfluencies consist of part-word repetitions, single-syllable word repetition and disrhythmic phonation. Other disfluencies are interjection, multi-syllable word repetition, phrase repetition and revision/abandoned utterance. In an older taxonomy of stuttering-like behaviors, Van Riper (1971, 1982) classified symptoms as repetitions, prolongation and blocks. Repetitions are when a person who stutters gets 'stuck' on a sound, repeating the same syllable multiple times. Disrhythmic phonation of the Illinois Disfluency Classification system envelops two of Van Riper's core symptoms (1971, 1982) – prolongation and blocks. Prolongation is when sound or airflow continues, but one or more articulators fail to move. Blocks occur on consonant syllables when there is a stoppage of airflow and sound. In other words, it is almost as if the respiratory process essential to speaking has temporarily ceased. Inappropriate muscular tension around the larynx is also characteristic of a block, along with a squeezing of the muscles of the lips and jaw (Conture et al., 1977; Freeman & Ushijima, 1978).

Researchers studying signed language have either developed their own list of symptoms or modified lists offered up by previous researchers of speech. One challenge facing researchers who categorize the symptoms of stuttering-like disfluencies in signed language is an absence of an accepted taxonomy of stuttering-like disfluencies for sign. As previously mentioned, studies investigating stuttering in signed languages are mostly studies of incidence or prevalence instead of descriptive studies of actual cases. As might be expected in such studies, written descriptions of the nature of stuttering-like disfluency by respondents are often brief. However, other writings for stuttering in signed language have attempted to be more detailed and descriptive in nature, although the detail of these descriptions is also limited by the second-hand nature of the reports of stuttering-like disfluency in signed language. Taken together, however, these works give a picture of the characteristics of stuttering in signed languages.

In a brief report of stuttering in signed language, Silverman and Silverman (1971) mailed surveys to 78 teachers at 13 schools for the deaf and received 33 responses. Twelve respondents responded to the survey indicating that they had not observed stuttering in ASL. Of these 12, eight worked as teachers for the deaf using only spoken language for their communication with their students. Thirteen teachers, however, responded to the survey and reported observing stuttering-like disfluencies. Teachers were asked to briefly describe the symptoms they had observed. The authors briefly report the nature of the disfluencies observed by respondents and articulate the first suggested categories of signed disfluencies. These categories were: repetitions of signs, repetition of the first letter of a fingerspelled word, involuntary extra movements in fingerspelling and hesitations in fingerspelling.

Montgomery and Fitch (1988) documented stuttering-like disfluency in signed language in slightly greater detail. The authors mailed a survey to schools for the deaf around the country, and identified 12 students who exhibited stuttering-like behaviors. They found that six students stuttered in signed language only, three stuttered in speech and sign, and three stuttered only when speaking. All but one child were reported as having severe hearing loss or greater. In a qualitative section of their paper, the authors categorized, but did not describe, the nature of the stuttering-like disfluencies respondents reported having observed in children. Montgomery and Fitch reported stuttering-like disfluencies as being repetitions of the first syllable, part-word repetitions, blocks, prolongations and choppy manipulations. These disfluencies were most frequently located at the beginning of a sign.

Whitebread (2004) conducted interviews with 10 professionals in the Deaf community in an attempt to draft a more detailed description of stuttering-like disfluency in ASL than that which had previously been captured by the survey-based studies. The stuttering-like categories in ASL that Whitebread identified included: involuntary repetitions of signs that could be considered monosyllabic or polysyllabic in structure[3]; disrhythmic phonation including unnaturally gated or timed signs, with errors in the prolongation of a sign movement; disruptions in the fluidity of the sign; hesitation before or during the sign; and inappropriate muscular tension during part or the whole of a sign.

Whitebread also reported additional characteristics of disfluency that may be modality specific. These included unusual body movements unrelated to linguistic communication, such as the insertion of extra, non-linguistic movements during signing or fingerspelling (i.e. throwing an elbow upwards in the middle of the sign). Finally, Whitebread reported that interviewees noted that disfluencies were most frequent for signing deaf people who stutter at the beginning of a sign or fingerspelled word, although disfluencies could also appear later in an utterance.

Cosyns et al. (2009) surveyed sign language interpreters and employees at special needs schools to document the occurrence of stuttering-like disfluency. Cosyns and colleagues modified the list of core symptoms of stuttering in sign and descriptive research by Whitebread (2004). For example, they excluded the symptoms which concerned the timing of disfluencies and more closely aligned the descriptions of signed disfluencies with symptoms described in the literature on stuttering in speech. They achieved this by replacing some categories identified by Whitebread (i.e. replacing inappropriate muscular tension with increased muscular tension). The categories used in their survey were: repetitions, blocks, hesitations, exaggerated/prolonged signs, involuntary interjections, unusual body movements, poor fluidity or increased muscular tension. Cosyns et al. found that involuntary signed interjections were the most common disfluency. They also reported a large number of observations of poor fluidity, repetitions and unusual body movements. The categorizations of signed disfluency by Cosyns et al. are the most recent in the literature. Table 6.2 presents the categorizations of stuttering-like disfluencies for signed languages of Cosyns and colleagues alongside the categorization system by Yairi and Ambrose for spoken languages.

Quinto-Pozos et al. (2011) conducted interviews with professional staff at schools for the Deaf and inquired about their experiences with communication disorders among the students; they received a few reports of stuttering in

Table 6.2 Categorization of disfluency in sign and speech

General categorization	Signed languages	Spoken languages (Yairi & Ambrose, 2005)
Repetition	Fingerspelled repetitions[a,b,c,d] Signed repetitions[a,b,c,d,e]	Part-word repetitions Single-syllable word repetition
Disrhythmic articulation	Hesitations[a,c,d] Prolongations[b,c,d] Blocks[b,d]	Disrhythmic phonation
Interjections	Involuntary interjections[a,c,d] Unusual body movements[c,d]	Interjection
	Poor fluidity[b,c,d] Increased muscular tension[c,d]	
Other types of disfluency		Multi-syllable word repetition Phrase repetition Revision/abandoned utterance

Notes: [a]Reported in Silverman and Silverman (1971); [b]Reported in Montgomery and Fitch (1988); [c]Reported in Whitebread (2004); [d]Reported in Cosyns et al. (2009); [e]Reported in Quinto-Pozos et al. (2011).

signed language during their interviews. In particular, they provide two examples of respondents describing moments of stuttering-like disfluency that had been observed. These descriptions of disfluency could be analyzed as providing evidence for single-syllable, whole-word repetition. Their data may also suggest that the inclusion of a wave or a signed greeting may be a possible manifestation of stuttering-like disfluency, something that was not considered in previous studies.

A major limitation of the data reported regarding stuttering in ASL is that these reports come strictly from reported observations of people involved with the signing deaf community rather than from direct expert analysis of behavior. Direct observation of stuttering-like disfluencies by researchers may yield greater insight through a more detailed description of these disfluencies.

A second challenge is that studies of signed stuttering have not explicitly considered the effects of concomitant disorders. Concomitance may be important in studying stuttering in deaf people when some studies suggest that audiological deafness may be frequently accompanied by other neurological disorders or disabilities (Gallaudet Research Institute, 2008; van Naarden et al., 1999). Accurate documentation of possible concomitant disorders would increase the certainty that the symptoms described in the literature result from stuttering and not from one or more types of disorders that may compromise communication. The findings by Cosyns and colleagues illustrate the importance of this second challenge.

Yairi and Ambrose (2005) state that multiple kinds of disfluency are required for stuttering-like disfluency to be considered stuttering in speech. Cosyns and colleagues find that roughly half of those reported to exhibit stuttering-like disfluency *exhibit only one type of disfluency*. Following the criteria of Yairi and Ambrose, it may be possible that persons exhibiting only one type of stuttering-like disfluency in signed language are experiencing disfluency because of a condition *other than stuttering*. Is this an appropriate standard to use in studies in signed language? Is it possible that we are capturing disfluencies in signed language resulting from disorders other than stuttering? Exploring these questions will allow researchers to better disaggregate disfluencies resulting from concomitant disorders and disfluencies resulting from stuttering.

Bilingual persons who stutter across linguistic modalities

In addition to considering the nature of stuttering-like disfluency in signed language, another important question is whether the stuttering-like disfluencies occur when D/HH people are speaking and signing at the same time. If so, what are the characteristics of the disfluencies? Is language production in each modality equally interrupted or are the disfluencies more common in only one of the modalities? Does one modality serve as a way to counter disfluencies that occur in the other? If a bilingual signer is more proficient in one language than the other, is fluency a factor? These questions may be particularly interesting to researchers, in part because the articulatory systems for each language are different.

There have been several instances documented in the literature concerning deaf persons who stutter in both modalities. Silverman and Silverman (1971), in their survey of professionals at schools for the deaf, noted that stuttering-like behaviors may occur when signing and speaking simultaneously. Montgomery and Fitch (1988) also surveyed professionals at schools for the deaf, and they identified a total of 12 deaf children who exhibited stuttering-like disfluency. Of the 12, three of these children exhibited stuttering-like behaviors when signing and when speaking. One child exhibited disfluency when signing which is uncharacteristic of spoken language stuttering behaviors. Another participant was reported to have involuntary repetitions at the onset of spoken and signed words. A third participant is characterized as having his speech interrupted by blocks and repetitions. Montgomery and Fitch note that blocks were noted in oral communication and appear to indicate that these blocks were also present when simultaneously using signed language for all bilingual participants.

The literature on bilingual persons who stutter across modalities has not yet examined in detail the nature of the disfluencies in both languages.

However, there is one written report by a person who stutters in both modalities. Snyder (2006) provides details of his own experience as a hearing person who stutters when using simultaneous communication and he notes that disfluency, for him, is generally involuntary in speech and voluntary in sign. While an observer might conclude that he is stuttering in both modalities, Snyder maintains that he is actually only 'stuttering' in the spoken modality. It appears that because Snyder continues communicating in two modalities at once despite the disruption in the spoken modality, his signing may also become disfluent. This suggests a primacy of the spoken stutter. Disfluency in sign follows a stutter in speech. But it also appears that signing does not necessarily become disfluent when there is a spoken stutter. Snyder reports that he is also able to continue communicating in the visual modality while stuttering in the spoken modality until the asynchrony between the spoken and manual modalities becomes too great. Other studies provide evidence that seems to support Snyder's suggestion that some bilingual persons who stutter across modalities may be stuttering in speech and moving their hands to keep the 'flow' going until the involuntary spoken stutter is over (Cosyns *et al.*, 2009; Montgomery & Fitch, 1988).

My own experience as a hard of hearing person who stutters in speech mirrors the report given by Snyder (2006). I have been hard of hearing since birth and I have stuttered in speech since the first grade. I learned ASL as a second language at age 16, although I was exposed to fingerspelling at age six. I have been signing for more than 14 years, and I consider myself fully fluent in ASL. When I am only signing ASL, I experience no behaviors of disfluency associated with stuttering. If there are errors and difficulties with articulation, I do not notice them. However, when I am signing and speaking at the same time, *disruptions in my spoken language generally determine the speed and fluency of my sign production.* When a disruption occurs in speech, I tend to choose between several voluntary behaviors for my hands during this extra time. These behaviors may include whole- or part-word repetitions, prolongation of the sign, holding my hands in place, or placing my hands in a resting position. Generally, once the spoken stutter is finished, my signing and my speech then proceed in synchrony. I do not notice any significant difference in spoken fluency when speaking alone or using simultaneous communication. This suggests that I stutter in spoken language, but not in signed language.

Occasionally I may switch between spoken language and signed language within a conversation when conversing with another person fluent in both languages, rather than using both languages simultaneously. In these cases, I am generally fully fluent when signing but experience stuttering disruptions when speaking. As with simultaneous communication, disruptions in fluency in spoken language appear similar to when the entire conversation is in a spoken language. At times, I catch myself switching from English to ASL or from ASL back to English based on expected fluency. I may occasionally anticipate that I will stutter on a word using speech. When I do expect to stutter on a spoken word, I may switch to using only ASL until I get past the word I expect to stutter on, and then switch back to English. I avoid the anticipated stutter by switching to sign language, where I have a high degree of confidence in my ability to communicate fluently.

These accounts of stuttering in both sign and speech may represent an intersection of language, audition and articulatory systems which, if explored, may yield additional insight into the mechanisms behind stuttering. The experiences reported by Snyder (2006) and me appear to show that, at least for some individuals, there may be differences in fluency between spoken and signed linguistic communication. For others who use both modalities regularly for communication, disfluencies may exist in both sign and speech. It may be of interest to explore the differences between linguistic production across these two modalities.

Stuttering in Spoken Languages

The literature on spoken language stuttering has covered numerous areas that have not been covered in research on stuttering-like behaviors in sign. Each of these topics could provide interesting questions for future research for people who stutter in signed language.

It could be useful to learn if the onset and recovery patterns of spoken language disfluencies occur similarly in signed language stuttering. The onset of developmental stuttering generally occurs between 28 months and four years of age (Andrews & Harris, 1964; Mansson, 2000; Yairi, 1983; Yairi & Ambrose, 2005), although 90% of the risk of stuttering onset is over by age four (Mansson, 2000; Yairi & Ambrose, 2005). Between 65% and 80% of persons who stutter recover by the age of 15 (Andrews & Harris, 1964; Mansson, 2000; Yairi & Ambrose, 2005). Factors that have been determined to affect recovery are being female, having a family history of recovery, and having good phonological skills (Ambrose et al., 1997; Yairi & Ambrose, 1999).

Van Riper's (1971, 1982) core symptoms could also be considered with respect to the onset of stuttering. How does stuttering develop in children using signed language? For children using spoken language, single-syllable word and part-word repetitions are most common at onset. Children will repeat a word or syllable more than twice in rapid succession (Yairi, 1983; Yairi & Lewis, 1984). Prolongations tend to appear after repetitions, but may also be present at onset. Finally, blocks are commonly the last core behavior to appear but may also be present at onset (Van Riper, 1982; Yairi, 1997). Over time, blocks grow longer and more tense, leading to rapid oscillation of the muscles (Conture et al., 1977; Freeman & Ushijima, 1978).

There is considerable evidence from the spoken language literature that there may be a genetic connection to stuttering. Families with a history of stuttering are more likely to have children who stutter (Ambrose *et al.*, 1997; Kidd, 1984). Between 23% and 68% of persons who stutter have familial relatives with stuttering-like disfluency (Conture, 2001; Ooki, 2005; Yairi *et al.*, 1996). Studies have also shown higher levels of stuttering between monozygotic twins than between dizygotic twins (Andrews *et al.*, 1983; Felsenfeld *et al.*, 2000; Ooki, 2005; van Beijsterveldt *et al.*, 2010). Studies of genetics have led to research indicating that several chromosomes may be involved with stuttering, including chromosomes 1, 13, 12, 16, 18 (Riaz *et al.*, 2005; Shugart *et al.*, 2004). A major question is whether these types of genetic markers also exist for people who purportedly stutter in signed language.

Many studies have attempted to understand the differences in the brain of persons who stutter and fluent speakers. Fox (2003) proposes that stuttering may be a disorder that involves a complex interaction between speech-motor and auditory neural systems within the brain. More recently, researchers have hypothesized that stuttering results from faulty timing mechanisms between language and motor production regions of the brain (Guenther, 2006; Howell, 2011). These conclusions are based in part on the neuroimaging research which has identified structural and functional differences in the brain between persons who stutter and fluent speakers. Both the structural and functional differences in individuals who stutter affect temporal auditory cortex, frontal speech and language regions, and regions representing the articulation organs (Beal *et al.*, 2007; Chang *et al.*, 2008; Foundas *et al.*, 2001). While studies have demonstrated that structural and functional differences exist, there are persistent questions about which of these differences are pathological and which are adaptive (May & Gaser, 2006). Since some of the studies identified here have looked at speech-motor areas and the auditory cortex, it would be useful to determine if the same networks can be implicated for people who stutter in signed language.

There have also been various linguistic deficits that have been documented for persons who stutter. Children who stutter are less efficient at planning and/or retrieving units of a sentence (Anderson & Conture, 2004) and may have difficulties with semantic encoding due to lexical organization (Hartfield & Conture, 2006; Pellowski & Conture, 2005). Phonological factors on content words also affect stuttering (Dworzynski & Howell, 2004), particularly syllable onsets (Howell *et al.*, 2000). Phonological effects on stuttering become more pronounced when the speaker is experiencing a greater cognitive load (Byrd *et al.*, 2012; Weber-Fox *et al.*, 2004). Persons who stutter also have been reported to be slower in identifying linguistic sounds (Sasisekaran & Byrd, 2013; Sasisekaran *et al.*, 2006). Yet other studies have reported that persons stutter more on lexical units that are used less frequently (Hubbard & Prins, 1994) and that persons who stutter are slower in processing lexical information than fluent speakers (Bosshardt & Fransen, 1996; Byrd *et al.*, 2007). Would signers show similar deficits when their signed language abilities are measured?

Future Research on Stuttering in Signed Language

Research on signed language stuttering could provide insights into the nature of stuttering in general, and allow for the testing of modality-specific questions that arise from signed disfluencies. In addition to discussing the questions discussed in the previous section, future research should include detailing direct observations by researchers of individual cases of signed language stutterers, including the evolution and recovery of stuttering-like behaviors over time, language proficiency and the presence of any concomitant disorders. Other topics that could be addressed are reporting more details of possible secondary effects of stuttering in ASL, tracing the heritability of stuttering-like behaviors in signed language, engaging in imaging studies that could shed light on neurological questions, and comparing signed language abilities across signers who stutter and those who do not exhibit such disfluencies.

For the study of stuttering in signed language, the most pressing need is the identification and detailed description of persons who stutter in sign. This will require the use of methodologies that allow for the capture and subsequent analysis of the signed stuttering events, such as the use of video for data capture and various methods for eliciting language data. Since our understanding of signed stuttering is limited to survey methodologies, inherent weaknesses of this general approach – such as retrospective reporting of signed stuttering events by the observer and the possible presence of concomitant communication disorders for the signer(s) – have limited the strength of the results obtained.

The survey methods of previous studies have been subject to respondents' knowledge and skill and present real concerns about accuracy and representation. For example, Montgomery and Fitch (1988) received responses that included symptoms of disorders of language and what may have been concomitant neurological disorders also affecting broader non-linguistic motor functions. Silverman and Silverman (1971) did not attempt to exclude concomitant neurological disorders. Whitebread (2004) noted that participants were not able to definitively exclude the possibility of concurrent neurological conditions. Finally, Cosyns et al. (2009) also reported that the ambiguous stuttering-like criteria from previous writings increased their reliance on subjective interpretation of the symptoms by respondents.

Future studies should also carefully determine if a signer demonstrates stuttering-like disfluencies in two modalities as opposed to one (e.g. in both sign and speech versus in sign or speech alone) and whether signers stutter when (and if) they sign and speak at the same time. For example, if a person stutters in spoken language only, what are the important differences in the linguistic and articulatory systems between the two languages? By honing in on bimodal bilinguals who stutter, researchers can add important data to theoretical questions about the role of audition in stuttering. Further, questions about language perception, processing and production could allow for cross-modal comparisons – especially when the comparisons allow for insight into the nature of stuttering.

Conclusions

The evidence for stuttering in signed languages is building, but there are many questions that need to be addressed in future research. Signed language stuttering could help to shed light on theoretical questions about the nature of stuttering – including the respective roles of auditory, motor and linguistic processes. Signed language users who stutter could be the source of valuable information, but researchers must carefully tease apart whether and how stuttering occurs in signed language, in speech, and when both are used in unison. These studies could help to answer important theoretical questions about stuttering, such as the role of audition and whether language modality plays a primary role in the communication disfluencies that occur for the person who stutters.

Notes

(1) The capitalization of the d in Deaf is significant and refers to the signing Deaf community. When referring to persons who are audiologically deaf, but not signers, a lowercase d is used.
(2) Older publications refer to the percentage of the sampled populations who stutter, from Backus' (1938) and Harms and Malone's (1939) numbers as incidence rates. This terminology is inconsistent with the current definition of incidence rate. Because the percentages for these articles are calculated by dividing the number of students with stuttering by the total number of students, I refer to these as prevalence rates for Table 6.1.
(3) I use the term monosyllable sign here to refer to signs with a single movement or a single movement with morphological repetition. Reduplication is a common linguistic mechanism in ASL (Fischer, 1973; Supalla & Newport, 1978). I use the term polysyllabic signs to include signs with multiple movements. See Brentari (1998) and Wilbur (2011) for discussions of syllables in signed language.

References

Ambrose, N.G., Cox, N.C. and Yairi, E. (1997) The genetic basis of persistence and recovery in stuttering. *Journal of Speech, Language, and Hearing Research* 36, 701–706.
Anderson, J. D. and Conture, E. G. (2004) Sentence-structure priming in young children who do and do not stutter. *Journal of Speech, Language and Hearing Research* 47 (3), 552.
Andrews, G. and Harris, M. (1964) *The Syndrome of Stuttering. Clinics in Developmental Medicine*. London: William Heinemann Medical.
Andrews, G., Craig, A., Feyer, A.M., Hoddinott, S., Howie, P. and Neilson, M. (1983) Stuttering: A review of research findings and theories circa 1982. *Journal of Speech and Hearing Disorders* 48, 226–246.

Backus, O. (1938) Incidence of stuttering among the deaf. *Annals of Otology, Rhinology and Laryngology* 47, 632–635.

Baynton, D. (2009) *Forbidden Signs: American Culture and the Campaign Against Sign Language.* New York: Oxford University Press.

Beal, D., Gracco, B., Lafaille, S. and De Nil, L. (2007) Voxel-based morphometry of auditory and speech-related cortex in stutterers. *Neuro-Report* 18, 1257–1260.

Bloodstein, O. (1995) *A Handbook on Stuttering* (5th edn). London: Singular.

Bloodstein, O. and Bernstein Ratner, N.D. (2008) *A Handbook on Stuttering* (6th edn). Clifton Park, NY: Thomson-Delmar.

Bosshardt, H. and Fransen, H. (1996) Online sentence processing in adults who stutter and adults who do not stutter. *Journal of Speech and Hearing Research* 39, 785–797.

Brentari, D. (1998) *A Prosodic Model of Sign Language Phonology.* Cambridge: MIT Press.

Bullen, A. (1945) A cross-cultural approach to the problem of stuttering. *Child Development* 16, 1–88.

Byrd, C.T., Conture, E.G. and Ohde, R.N. (2007) Phonological priming in young children's picture naming: Holistic versus incremental processing. *American Journal of Speech-Language, Pathology* 16 (1), 43–53.

Byrd, C.T., Vallely, M., Anderson, J.D. and Sussman, H. (2012) Nonword repetition and phoneme elision in adults who do and do not stutter. *Journal of Fluency Disorders* 37, 188–201.

Chang, S., Erickson, K.I, Ambrose, N.G., Hasegawa-Johnson, M.A. and Ludlow, C.L. (2008) Brain anatomy differences in childhood stuttering. *Neuroimage* 39 (3), 1333–1344.

Civier, O., Tasko, S.M. and Guenther, F.H. (2010) Overreliance on auditory feedback may lead to sound/syllable repetitions: Simulations of stuttering and fluency-inducing conditions with a neural model of speech production. *Journal of Fluency Disorders* 35 (3), 246–279.

Conture, E. G. (2001) *Stuttering: Its Nature, Diagnosis, and Treatment.* Boston: Allyn and Bacon.

Conture, E., McCall, G. and Brewer, D.W. (1977) Laryngeal behavior during stuttering. *Journal of Speech and Hearing Research* 20, 661–668.

Cosyns, M., Van Herreweghe, A., Christiaens, G. and Van Borsel, J. (2009) Stutter-like disfluencies in Flemish Sign Language users. *Clinical Linguistics & Phonetics* 23 (10), 742–750.

Dworzynski, K. and Howell, P. (2004) Predicting stuttering from phonological complexity in German. *Journal of Fluency Disorders* 29 (2), 151–176.

Einarsdottir, J. and Ingham, R.J. (2009) Does language influence the accuracy of judgments in children? *Journal of Speech, Language, and Hearing Research* 52, 766–779.

Felsenfeld, S., Kirk, K.M., Zhu, G., Statham, D.J., Neale, M.C. and Martin, N.G. (2000) A study of the genetic and environmental etiology of stuttering in a selected twin sample. *Behavior Genetics* 30 (5), 359–366.

Fischer, S. (1973) Two processes of reduplication in the American Sign Language. *Foundations of Language* 9, 469–480.

Foundas, A.L, Bollich, A.M, Corey, D.M, Hurley, M. and Heilman, K.M. (2001) Anomalous anatomy of speech-language areas in adults with persistent developmental stuttering. *Neurology* 57 (2), 207–215.

Fox, P.T. (2003) Brain imaging in stuttering: Where next? *Journal of Fluency Disorders* 26, 265–272.

Freeman, F. and Ushijima, T. (1978) Laryngeal muscle activity during stuttering. *Journal of Speech and Hearing Research* 21, 538–562.

Gallaudet Research Institute (2008) Regional and national summary report of data from the 2009–08 annual survey of deaf and hard of hearing children and youth. Washington, DC: Gallaudet University.

Guenther, F.H. (2006) Cortical interactions underlying the production of speech sounds. *Journal of Communication Disorders* 39 (5), 350–365.

Guitar, B. (2006) *Stuttering: An Integrated Approach to its Nature and Treatment* (3rd edn). Baltimore, MD: Lippincott Williams Wilkins.

Harms, M.A. and Malone, J.Y. (1939) The relationship of hearing acuity to stammering. *Journal of Speech Disorders* 4, 363–370.

Hartfield, K. N. and Conture, E. G. (2006) Effects of perceptual and conceptual similarity in lexical priming of young children who stutter: Preliminary findings. *Journal of fluency disorders* 31 (4), 303–324.

Howell, P. (2011) *Recovery from Stuttering.* New York: Psychology Press.

Howell, P., Au-Yeung, J. and Sackin, S. (2000) Internal structure of content words leading to lifespan differences in phonological difficulty in stuttering. *Journal of Fluency Disorders*, 25 (1), 1–20.

Hubbard, C. and Prins, D. (1994) Word familiarity, syllabic stress pattern, and stuttering. *Journal of Communication Disorders* 37, 564–571.

Kidd, K. (1984) Stuttering as a genetic disorder. In R. Curlee and W. Perkins (eds) *Nature and Treatment of Stuttering: New Directions*. London: Taylor & Francis.

Mansson, H. (2000) Childhood stuttering: Incidence and development. *Journal of Fluency Disorders* 25 (1), 45–57.

Marist, J.A. and Hutton, C. (1957) Effects of auditory masking upon the speech of stutterers. *Journal of Speech and Hearing Disorders* 22, 385–389.

May A. and Gaser, C. (2006) Magnetic resonance-based morphometry: A window into structural plasticity of the brain. *Current Opinion in Neurology* 19 (4), 407–411.

Meltzer, A. (1992) Horn stuttering. *Journal of Fluency Disorders* 17 (4), 257–264.

Montgomery, B.M. and Fitch, J.L. (1988) The prevalence of stuttering in the hearing-impaired school age population. *Journal of Speech & Hearing Disorders* 53, 131–135.

Neilson, M.D. and Neilson, P.D. (1987) Speech motor control and stuttering: A computational model for adaptive sensory-motor processing. *Speech Communication* 6 (4), 325–333.

Nudelman, H., Herbrich, K, Hoyt, B. and Rosenfeld, D. (1987) Dynamic characteristics of vocal frequency tracking in stutterers and non-stutterers. In H.F.M. Peters and W. Hulstin (eds) *Speech Motor Dynamics in Stuttering*. Wien: Springer-Verlag.

Nudelman, H., Herbrich, K., Hoyt, B. and Rosenfield, D. (1989) A neuro-science model of stuttering. *Journal of Fluency Disorders* 14, 399–427.

Nudelman, H., Herbrich, K., Hess, K., Hoyt, B. and Rosenfield, D. (1992) A model of the phonation response time of stutterers and fluent speakers to frequently-modulated tones. *Journal of the Acoustical Society of America* 92, 1882–1888.

Ooki, S. (2005) Genetic and environmental influences on stuttering and ties in Japanese twin children. *Twin Research and Human Genetics* 8, 69–75.

Pellowski, M. W. and Conture, E. G. (2005) Lexical priming in picture naming of young children who do and do not stutter. *Journal of Speech, Language and Hearing Research* 48 (2), 278.

Quinto-Pozos, D., Forber-Pratt, A. and Singleton, J. (2011) Do developmental communication disorders exist in the signed modality? Reporting on the experiences of language professionals and educators from schools for the deaf. *Language, Speech, and Hearing Services in Schools* 42, 423–443.

Riaz, N., Steinberg, S., Ahmad, J., Pluzhnikov, A., Riazuddin, S., Cox, N.J., *et al.* (2005) Genomewide significant linkage to stuttering on chromosome 12. *American Journal of Human Genetics* 76, 647–651.

Roman, K.G. (1959) Handwriting and speech. *Logos* 2, 29–39.

Sasisekaran, J. and Byrd, C.T. (2013) A preliminary investigation of segmentation and rhyme abilities of children who stutter. *Journal of Fluency Disorders* 38 (2), 222–234.

Sasisekaran, J., De Nil, L., Smyth, R. and Johnson, C. (2006) Phonological encoding in the silent speech of persons who stutter. *Journal of Fluency Disorders* 31 (1), 1–21.

Scripture, E.W. (1909) Penmanship stuttering. *Journal of the American Medical Association* 19, 1480–1481.

Shugart, Y.Y., Mundorff, J., Kilshaw, J., Doheny, K., Doan, B., Wanyee, J., Green, E.D. and Drayna, D. (2004) Results of a genome-wide linkage scan for stuttering. *American Journal of Medical Genetics A* 124 (15), 133–135.

Silverman, F.H. and Bohlman, P. (1988) Flute stuttering. *Journal of Fluency Disorders* 13 (6), 427–428.

Silverman, F.H. and Silverman, E. (1971) Stutter-like behavior in manual communication of the deaf. *Perceptual & Motor Skills* 33, 45–46.

Snyder, G. (2006) The existence of stuttering in sign language and other forms of expressive communication: Sufficient cause for the emergence of a new stuttering paradigm? Unpublished manuscript, University of Mississippi.

Sternberg, M. (1946) Auditory factors in stuttering. Masters thesis, University of Iowa.

Supalla, T. and Newport, E. (1978) How many seats in a chair? The derivation of nouns and verbs in American Sign Language. In P. Siple (ed.) *Understanding Language Through Sign Language Research* (pp. 91–133). New York: Academic Press.

Sussman, H.M. and MacNeilage, P.F. (1975) Hemispheric specialization for speech production and perception in stutterers. *Neuropsychologia* 13 (1), 19–26.

Van Beijsterveldt, C.I, Felsenfeld, S. and Boomsma, D.I. (2010) Bivariate genetic analyses of stuttering and nonfluency in a large sample of 5-year-old twins. *Journal of Speech, Language, and Hearing Research* 53, 609–619.

Van Borsel, J. and Pereira, M. (2005) Assessment of stuttering in a familiar versus unfamiliar language. *Journal of Fluency Disorders* 30 (2), 109–124.

Van Naarden, K., Decouflé, P. and Caldwell, K. (1999) Prevalence and characteristics of children with serious hearing impairment in metropolitan Atlanta, 1991–1993. *Pediatrics* 103 (3), 570–575.

Van Riper, C. (1971) *The Nature of Stuttering*. Englewood Cliffs, NJ: Prentice-Hall.

Van Riper, C. (1982) *The Nature of Stuttering* (2nd edn). Englewood Cliffs, NJ: Prentice-Hall.

Voelker, E. and Voelker, C. (1937) Spasmophemia in dyslalia cophotica – case report. *Annals of Otology, Rhinology and Laryngology* 46, 740–743.

Weber-Fox, C., Spencer, R., Spruill, J.E. and Smith, A. (2004) Phonologic processing in adults who stutter: Electrophysiological and behavioral evidence. *Journal of Speech, Language, and Hearing Research* 47, 1244–1258.

Whitebread, G. (2004) Stuck on the tip of my thumb: Stuttering in American Sign Language. Unpublished honors thesis, Gallaudet University.

WHO (2010) *The ICD-10 Classification of Mental and Behavioral Disorders*. Geneva: World Health Organization.

Wilber, R. (2011) Sign syllables. In M. van Oostendorp, C. Ewen, E. Hume and K. Rice (eds) *The Blackwell Companion to Phonology* (pp. 1309–1334). Malden, MA: Wiley-Blackwell.

Wingate, M.E. (1970) Effect on stuttering of changes in audition. *Journal of Speech and Hearing Research* 13, 861–873.

Yairi, E. (1983) The onset of stuttering in two- and three-year old children: A preliminary report. *Journal of Speech and Hearing Disorders* 48, 171–177.

Yairi, E. (1997) Disfluency characteristics of early childhood stuttering. In R.F. Curlee and G.M. Siegel (eds) *Nature and Treatment of Stuttering: New Directions* (2nd edn) (pp. 49–78). Boston, MA: Anllyn & Bacon.

Yairi, E. and Ambrose, N.G. (1999) Normative data for early childhood stuttering. *Journal of Speech and Hearing Research* 42, 895–909.

Yairi, E. and Ambrose, N.G. (2005) *Early Childhood Stuttering: For Clinicians by Clinicians.* Austin, TX: Pro-Ed.

Yairi, E. and Lewis, B. (1984) Disfluencies at the onset of stuttering. *Journal of Speech and Hearing Research* 27, 154–159.

Yairi, E., Ambrose, N.G. and Cox, N.C. (1996) Genetics of stuttering: A critical review. *Journal of Speech and Hearing Research* 39, 771–784.

7   Sign Dysarthria: A Speech Disorder in Signed Language

Martha E. Tyrone

Introduction

Sign production, like the production of speech, can be disrupted in instances where a language user develops a movement disorder. Many studies have investigated the structure of signed language by studying linguistic and cognitive disorders affecting individual signed language users. What has received less attention is the relationship between motor control and the structure of signed language. Disruption to speech resulting from an acquired neurogenic movement disorder is referred to as dysarthria, and it can take a variety of forms, depending on the nature of the movement disorder that underlies it. Dysarthria has traditionally been studied as a phenomenon specific to the speech mechanism, and it has only recently been explored in the sign modality.

The only signed languages that have been studied in the context of neurogenic motor deficits are American Sign Language (ASL) and British Sign Language (BSL). The earliest research on signed language and motor disorders examined small groups of ASL signers who acquired neurogenic disorders as adults (Brentari *et al.*, 1995; Loew *et al.*, 1995; Poizner, 1990; Poizner & Kegl, 1992). Later research on motor disorders and signed language grew out of the Deaf Stroke Project in the UK (cf. Atkinson *et al.*, 2005; Marshall *et al.*, 2004, 2005). That project collected data from BSL signers who had strokes as well as signers who developed other acquired neurogenic disorders, such as Parkinson's disease (PD) and progressive supranuclear palsy (PSP).

The Structure of Sign and Speech

Sign language and the brain

There is robust evidence that the same neural structures underlie language function for both signed and spoken language. Imaging and neurophysiological studies have demonstrated the role of traditional language areas in the inferior frontal and superior temporal lobes in sign language processing and production (Braun *et al.*, 2001; Levanen *et al.*, 2001; MacSweeney *et al.*, 2002; Neville *et al.*, 1998; Nishimura *et al.*, 1999; Petitto *et al.*, 2000). The superior temporal gyrus is typically associated with auditory function, but in Deaf signers it serves a role in the visual perception of signed language. In terms of sign production and the brain, Corina *et al.* (2003) found that secondary motor areas of the left hemisphere were active during the production of ASL signs. This was the case even when the signs were produced using only the left hand, whose movements are typically controlled by the right hemisphere. Thus, left hemisphere structures predominate in the production of signed language, even when the articulators involved are normally controlled by the right hemisphere.

Sign articulators and speech articulators

The clearest structural difference between sign and speech lies in the characteristics of the articulators for each modality. While spoken language uses the larynx and vocal tract, signed language uses the arms and hands as its primary articulators. The sign articulators are paired on opposite sides of the body, and some signs require the coordinated use of the two limbs. The speech articulators are located along the midline of the body, and they produce speech sounds by means of a source-filter mechanism, with an energy source (the vibrating vocal folds) that generates pulses that are modified by the filter that they pass through (the supralaryngeal vocal tract). Moreover, speech is powered by airflow through the vocal tract, while sign is not dependent on respiration patterns. This structural difference could affect utterance length or articulation/pause ratio differently in the two modalities.

The sign production mechanism is configured such that articulators that can perform small, rapid, precise movements (the hands) are attached at the ends of articulators that make only gross movements (the arms). Consequently, many signs are composed of precise movements superimposed on the gross movements of the same limb, and the two sets of movements are coordinated to partially overlap in time. When a typical signer produces a sign with an internal handshape change and a path movement of the arm, for example, the movement of the hand begins after arm movement has begun, and the two types of movement end at the same time (Brentari *et al.*, 1995). The tongue tip and tongue body serve roughly analogous roles in speech production, with the tongue tip making rapid, precise movements that are coordinated with the slower, larger movements of the tongue body. However, there is a much larger difference in the relative sizes of the large and small sign articulators than in the relative sizes of the small and large speech articulators.

Because its articulators and movement trajectories are large, the production rate for signed language tends to be slower than for spoken language. Bellugi and Fischer (1972) measured the durations of individual ASL signs and individual spoken English words, produced by hearing signers from Deaf households. Production rates for individual lexical items in that study were 4–5.2 words/second for English, and 2.3–2.5 signs/second for ASL. Despite this difference in production rate for individual words, signers are able to convey information as quickly and efficiently as users of spoken languages. Although producing a single sign takes longer than producing a single spoken word, signed languages employ fewer function words and they use the visual medium to present more information simultaneously (Bellugi & Fischer, 1972; Vermeerbergen *et al.*, 2007).

The role of sensory feedback

The sensory feedback that a language user receives is necessarily going to be different for spoken and signed language, since the former modality relies on acoustic output, while the latter does not. In addition to this, there is preliminary evidence that visual feedback is not very important for the production of signed language. Emmorey and colleagues (2009) carried out a study in which they modified visual feedback during signing, such that signers had a reduced view of the signing space or were completely blindfolded. The researchers found that signers did not alter their signing as an effect of either of these conditions, and they concluded that there is no sign equivalent to the Lombard effect, in which hearing people speak louder when they are wearing headphones and have reduced auditory feedback. This is perhaps not surprising, in light of the fact that many signs are produced outside the visual field of the signer, but spoken words are not usually produced outside the auditory perception of a hearing speaker. Moreover, there may be a different role for kinesthetic feedback in the two modalities, given that more joints are active during signing than during speech, and these provide feedback to the nervous system via nerve endings in the joint capsules. Researchers are not in agreement about the specific role of auditory feedback in speech production (cf. Nasir & Ostry, 2008; Villacorta *et al.*, 2007), but phenomena such as the Lombard effect and changes in speech production after hearing loss are well documented (Cowie *et al.*, 1982; Waldstein, 1990).

Dysarthria and Speech

Characteristics of dysarthria

Dysarthria describes a group of motor speech disorders resulting from neurogenic movement disorders (Darley *et al.*, 1969a, 1969b; Kent, 2000). It is broadly characterized by deficits in articulatory coordination, movement scaling, speech rate, prosody and weakness, independent of disruptions to language processing or production (such as those associated with aphasia). Nonetheless, cognitive or linguistic deficits can co-occur with dysarthria, for example, in conditions such as PD or Huntington's disease. Dysarthria can take a broad range of forms depending on the underlying movement disorder that is affecting speech production. For example, the characteristics of ataxic dysarthria (uncoordinated articulatory movements and exaggerated prosody) are distinct from the characteristics of dysarthria resulting from PD (rapid speech rate and reduced intensity and pitch range). The first researchers to describe dysarthria emphasized that it is a neurological symptom, unlike the speech motor deficits that result from nerve or muscle damage (Darley *et al.*, 1969a, 1969b). While the latter are likely to affect only individual articulators, dysarthria is more likely to affect multiple articulators simultaneously. Likewise, dysarthria is distinct from (oral or limb) apraxia, which disrupts representations of movements rather than affecting automatic movement execution. In both clinical and experimental research, dysarthria is typically assessed according to the components of speech laid out by Darley and colleagues: articulation, pitch, loudness, prosody, voice quality, nasality and respiration.

Neural basis of motor control and speech motor control

The human motor system comprises parts of the brain, brainstem, spinal cord and peripheral nerves controlling movement, and the muscles that execute movement. The areas of the cerebral cortex that control movement are located in the medial and posterior portions of the frontal lobe. The primary motor cortex generates movement commands that travel to the muscles, and the supplementary motor and premotor areas are activated before movement onset in order to facilitate movement planning. Motor areas of the cerebral cortex are organized somatotopically, so that specific cortical areas are associated with specific body parts.

The pathways that descend from the motor cortex are divided into the corticospinal and corticobulbar tracts. The corticospinal tract descends through the brainstem and terminates in the spinal cord. In the lower brainstem, most of the corticospinal fibers cross to the contralateral side of the nervous system. As a result, one cerebral hemisphere controls movements for the contralateral side of the body. The corticobulbar tract also originates in the motor cortex, but it terminates in the brainstem. The cranial nerves arise from the brainstem and control movements of the head, neck, eyes and speech articulators. The projections of the corticobulbar tract are largely bilateral, so that both sides of the brain control movements of both sides of most vocal tract structures.

Additional brain structures not located in the cerebral cortex are also involved in the control of voluntary movement, such as for speech or sign production. The most important of these are the cerebellum and basal ganglia. Neither is responsible for generating movements, but they both help shape voluntary movement so that it is accurate, well-timed and coordinated (Jueptner *et al.*, 1996; Lang & Bastian, 2002; Timmann *et al.*, 2001; VanGemmert *et al.*, 1999). In addition, the cerebellum and basal ganglia both modify muscle tone, balance and posture, and both have bidirectional connections with motor areas in the cerebral cortex.

Damage to cortical motor areas or to descending motor pathways that results from stroke may have different effects for sign and for speech, because those brain areas are laid out somatotopically. As a result, damage to them may affect particular articulators in isolation. By contrast, pathologies associated with basal ganglia or cerebellar damage are more likely to affect sign and speech production similarly. While portions of the basal ganglia and cerebellum are organized somatotopically, those discrete somatotopic regions are quite small and hence unlikely to be damaged selectively. Moreover, the most common basal ganglia pathologies disrupt the physiology of the entire basal ganglia motor circuit, and their effects are bilateral.

Types of dysarthria

Because dysarthria is caused by a number of different motor disorders, it can take a range of forms, each differing in symptomatology and severity (see Table 7.1). The most common variants of dysarthria are ataxic, hypokinetic, hyperkinetic, spastic-flaccid and unilateral upper motor neuron dysarthria (UUMN dysarthria). Ataxia is a motor disorder that results from damage to the cerebellum or its incoming projections. Ataxic dysarthria reflects incoordination and reduced muscle tone in the speech muscles. Speech is perceived to be slow and imprecise, with irregular variations in pitch and loudness (Kent *et al.*, 2000; Liss *et al.*, 2000). Ataxia affects multiple speech articulators together instead of individual articulators in isolation (Kent *et al.*, 1997; Murdoch & Theodoros, 1998; Sheard *et al.*, 1991). The other motor symptoms of ataxia parallel the symptoms of ataxic dysarthria. Qualitatively speaking, finger movements are slow and clumsy while proximal arm movements are jerky and imprecise. More specific symptoms include: reduced muscle tone, slowness, intention tremor, dysmetria, dysrhythmia and dysdiadochokinesia (i.e. disruption to alternating sequences of movements) (Darley *et al.*, 1975).

Hypokinetic dysarthria is characterized by speech that is monotonous, aprosodic and reduced in amplitude. Speakers with hypokinetic dysarthria also exhibit a harsh, breathy voice quality (Darley *et al.*, 1975; Weismer, 1984). The most common form of hypokinetic dysarthria results from PD (Theodoros & Murdoch, 1998b). It can also be caused by vascular or traumatic accident, or by a range of degenerative conditions affecting the brainstem. More general motor symptoms accompanying hypokinetic dysarthria

Table 7.1 Types of dysarthria in speech and sign

	Common etiologies	Effects on speech	Effects on signing
Ataxic dysarthria*	Cerebellar damage (from traumatic brain injury, stroke, genetic disorders)	Slow, imprecise speech, with irregular variations in pitch and loudness	Incoordination, difficulty with two-handed signs, movement overshoot
Hypokinetic dysarthria*	Parkinson's disease; progressive supranuclear palsy; corticobasal degeneration	Aprosodia, reduced intensity, reduced pitch range, articulatory imprecision and undershoot	Reduced signing space, laxed handshapes, slow signing
Hyperkinetic dysarthria	Huntington's disease; Tourette syndrome; cerebral palsy; essential tremor	Involuntary movements such as tics or tremors occur during speech	Involuntary limb movements occur during signing, incoordination on two-handed signs
Spastic-flaccid dysarthria	Multiple sclerosis; ALS	Slow, effortful, imprecise speech, hypernasality, low pitch and reduced pitch range, reduced intensity range, and harsh voice quality	Reduced signing space, imprecise handshapes, slow signing
UUMN dysarthria*	Cerebral stroke	Mild articulatory imprecision, mild hypernasality	Imprecise handshapes, mild articulatory undershoot

Note: *These types of sign dysarthria and their corresponding characteristics have been documented.

in PD include muscular rigidity, slowed movement, reduced movement size, stooped posture, postural instability and resting tremor.

Hyperkinetic dysarthria refers to speech that is disrupted by involuntary movements, such as tremors (Darley *et al.*, 1975; Theodoros & Murdoch, 1998a). Neurological pathologies that most often cause primary hyperkinetic dysarthria include Huntington's disease, Tourette's syndrome, cerebral palsy and essential tremor. Hyperkinetic dysarthria is often accompanied by uncontrolled limb movements in the form of tics, tremors or athetosis.

Spastic dysarthria reflects heightened muscle tone and loss of skilled movement, resulting from bilateral damage to the descending motor pathways. It most often occurs in conjunction with flaccid dysarthria, which is characterized by muscular weakness, reduced muscle tone and paralysis, resulting from damage to cranial and spinal nerves projecting to muscles. Spastic-flaccid dysarthria can be caused by traumatic brain injury or by diseases such as multiple sclerosis or amyotrophic lateral sclerosis. Speech is perceived to be slow, effortful and imprecise (Klasner & Yorkston, 2000; Nishio & Niimi, 2001). Other speech characteristics of spastic dysarthria include hypernasality (Enderby, 1986), low pitch and reduced pitch range, reduced intensity range and harsh/strained voice quality (Darley *et al.*, 1975). Spastic-flaccid dysarthria is often associated with impairments in both limbs, including reductions in movement range and force, and a loss of fine-grained, skilled movement (Enderby, 1986).

UUMN dysarthria is similar to spastic dysarthria, but it results from damage to only one side of the brain (Thompson-Ward, 1998), specifically to the fibers descending from the motor cortex. In general, UUMN dysarthric symptoms are mild, and they are often overshadowed by co-occurring apraxia, aphasia or aprosodia. Experimental research suggests that the symptoms of UUMN dysarthria include mild articulatory imprecision (Thompson-Ward, 1998), slow speech rate (Nishio & Niimi, 2001) and mild hypernasality (Thompson & Murdoch, 1995). Clinical research suggests that the common non-speech symptoms accompanying UUMN dysarthria are hemiplegia/paresis, tactile deficits, clumsy hand syndrome and unilateral weakness in the lower and central face (Duffy, 2005).

Research on Signed Language and Motor Disorders

Aphasia and apraxia

Although aphasia is qualitatively different from the motor disorders discussed here, early studies of motoric disruptions to signing were framed in terms of how the characteristics of aphasia and limb motor disorders differed in the sign modality (Brentari *et al.*, 1995; Loew *et al.*, 1995; Poizner & Kegl, 1992; Poizner *et al.*, 1987). In principle, a difference between the two types of disorders could provide evidence that signed languages were unlike pantomime or non-linguistic gesture – a point that was not universally agreed upon in linguistics or psychology at the time.

There have been several studies suggesting that aphasia patterns similarly in signed language and in spoken language. Moreover, the different types of aphasia correspond to similarly located lesions in the two modalities (Corina *et al.*, 1992; Hickok *et al.*, 1996; Marshall *et al.*, 2004; Poizner *et al.*, 1987). For both sign and speech, Broca's aphasia is characterized by limited and non-fluent language production, disrupted phonology and comparatively well-preserved language comprehension. Likewise, for sign and speech,

Wernicke's aphasia is characterized by severely disrupted comprehension and fluent production that lacks semantic content. To date, there have been no documented cases of conduction aphasia in a signed language.

While aphasia is qualitatively different from dysarthria, it often co-occurs with a different motor disorder, limb apraxia, in cases of anterior left hemisphere stroke. When a hearing speaker has a left hemisphere lesion, it is possible to differentiate aphasia from limb apraxia in part according to which body parts are affected. For sign language users, apraxia and aphasia could affect the same articulators. Similarly, for speech users, non-speech oral apraxia and apraxia of speech affect the same articulators as aphasia, but there is a larger literature outlining the distinctions among these disorders (Haley & Martin, 2011; Miller, 2002; Ziegler, 2002). Many studies have documented differences between sign aphasia and apraxia, but thus far there are no documented cases of apraxia occurring in the complete absence of aphasia in a signer.

In their early study on sign language and stroke, Poizner *et al.* (1987) showed that sign aphasia and apraxia could be differentiated in ASL users. The study included three signers with aphasia resulting from left hemisphere lesions. Only one of the signers with aphasia was impaired on pantomime production and imitation; none of them was impaired on pantomime recognition. In other words, gesture was not disrupted to the same extent as language in these signers. Corina *et al.* (1992) and Kegl and Poizner (1997) also reported dissociations between aphasia and apraxia in signers with left hemisphere damage. Corina *et al.* (1992) identified a signer with a left posterior lesion who had limited comprehension and fluent but non-grammatical production of ASL. Although his signing was disrupted, the signer could produce and understand non-linguistic gestures, and imitate sequences of gestures, which suggests that his representation of symbolic movements was preserved, and his deficit was clearly linguistic in nature. Kegl and Poizner (1997) described a signer who had a left parietal lobe lesion and exhibited severe comprehension deficits and mild production deficits. Despite his impaired signing, he performed normally on tests of ideomotor apraxia and pantomime recognition. In a similar study, Hickok *et al.* (1996) collected data from ASL signers with left hemisphere damage and found no correlation between their scores on aphasia and apraxia batteries. These findings contradict what had been predicted by Kimura (1993), who speculated that aphasia and apraxia would be indistinguishable in a signed language.

The findings from research in the UK are largely consistent with the earlier research on stroke and neurogenic disorders in sign language users in the USA. As part of their study on stroke in Deaf sign language users, Marshall *et al.* (2004, 2005) identified two BSL signers with aphasia who each showed differential impairment on sign and gesture tasks, indicating a dissociation between apraxia and aphasia. Marshall *et al.* (2005) described one Deaf signer with a left anterior lesion and severe aphasia; her comprehension deficits were

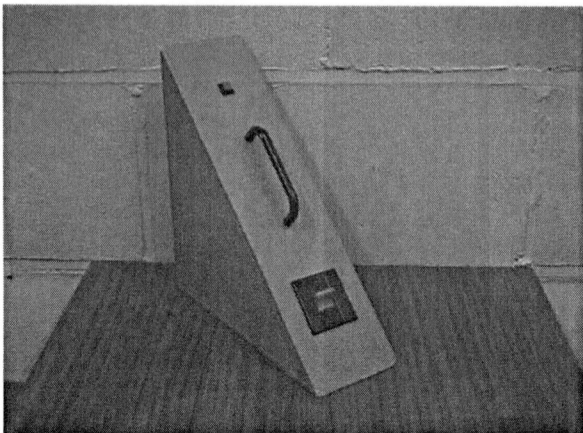

Figure 7.1 Kimura box

extensive and she had no spontaneous language production. That signer's performance on the Kimura box task (Figure 7.1) and the Kimura gesture task indicated that she was apraxic (Kimura, 1993), but her comprehension of gesture was better preserved than her comprehension of BSL signs. (The Kimura box is a mechanical device with three manipulanda that individuals are asked to handle, in a specific order, using specific hand configurations for each manipulandum.)

The same researchers identified another signer with aphasia who had good single-sign comprehension, but who experienced anomia and used non-linguistic gesture to communicate (Marshall *et al.*, 2004). He exhibited apraxia, like the first BSL signer with aphasia, but his gesture production and comprehension were more intact than his sign production and comprehension. It should be noted that these studies controlled for the possible role of iconicity in sign and gesture comprehension tasks. The researchers designed comprehension tasks that included visual distractors, so that if research participants were relying on iconicity, they would likely choose the distractor in place of the correct BSL sign. The two aphasic individuals described above both performed better on gesture comprehension than on sign comprehension, but neither of them mistook iconic gestures for real BSL signs. So although the signers used an iconic strategy to understand gestures, they did not seem to use this strategy for understanding signs.

Right hemisphere damage

In research on signed language and the brain, right hemisphere damage (RHD) has been studied mostly in the context of its effects on cognitive and sensory function and how they might affect the perception and production of signed language. Some well-known sensory deficits related to damage to the right cerebral cortex include perceptual neglect of one side of the visual space and a deficit in visually perceiving spatial relationships among objects. In terms of motor deficits, individuals with RHD often experience left-side paresis or paralysis, affecting both limb and facial movement. In addition, some individuals with RHD exhibit language-related deficits, such as aprosodia, pragmatic disorders and discourse processing deficits. These language deficits have been observed in signed as well as spoken language (Hickok et al., 1999; Loew et al., 1997).

Poizner et al. (1987) showed that despite their visuospatial processing deficits, ASL signers with RHD still had well-preserved language function. This was a noteworthy finding because signed languages use the spatial relationships among signs to mark those signs' grammatical and discourse relations. For example, signers can identify a referent in the discourse based on where the sign for that referent was placed initially. The two signers in the study who had RHD and visuospatial processing deficits could comprehend and produce complex sentences in ASL, in spite of the visuospatial demands of the task.

A few studies have specifically investigated the effects of RHD on motoric aspects of sign production. In one ASL study, Poizner and Kegl (1993) investigated a hearing signer with RHD who showed a mild sign production deficit. In particular, the signer had difficulty coordinating her arms during two-handed signs. When she produced two-handed signs, the movement of the left hand was delayed relative to movement of the right hand. The researchers described this coordination deficit as motor neglect – a disorder that is usually characterized as a spatial disorder, rather than a movement timing disorder (Heilman & Adams, 2003; Laurent-Vannier et al., 2003).

As part of their UK study on stroke in Deaf people, Marshall et al. (2003) compared signers with left hemisphere damage to signers with RHD. Study participants were tested on a range of linguistic processing tasks, which revealed that the signers with RHD retained good comprehension of BSL sentences and signs in isolation but were impaired in their processing of spatial information.

One signer with RHD from the same project was studied in terms of the motoric aspects of his signing (Tyrone, 2005). For that analysis, he was compared to an age-matched control signer on signing and fingerspelling tasks and on several non-linguistic motor control tasks. Compared to the control, the signer with RHD lowered signs that were high in the signing space. In addition, he produced laxed handshapes and showed difficulty with fine motor control. The fine motor control deficit manifested itself across tasks but was more apparent in sign production. It should be mentioned that this signer exhibited only minimal coordination deficits, consistent with what would be predicted for unilateral RHD.

Parkinson's disease

Several studies in the USA in the early 1990s investigated a group of signers with PD (Brentari & Poizner, 1994; Brentari *et al.*, 1995; Loew *et al.*, 1995; Poizner & Kegl, 1993). These studies were designed to determine how PD affected sign production in ASL and to contrast the motoric sign deficits of PD with language deficits that resulted from left hemisphere damage. ASL signers with PD were compared to healthy control signers and to signers with aphasia on sign production and on a few non-linguistic motor tasks. The results from these studies suggested that signers with PD produced signs with more distal articulators, used laxed handshapes and orientations, decreased the size of the signing space and showed reduced facial expression. In addition, these signers decoupled the coordinated movements of the hand and arm during signing. This last deficit was observed in signs that included a handshape change superimposed on an arm movement, in signs such as DRY in ASL (Figure 7.2). Loew *et al.* (1995) emphasized that signing in PD was reduced but that linguistic contrasts were preserved. The authors contrasted this with results from signers with aphasia, who produced phonological substitution errors and were often unable to preserve signs' linguistic contrastiveness.

Tyrone *et al.* (1999) carried out a similar study on ASL fingerspelling, and found that signers with PD showed incoordination, articulatory undershoot, and irregular hesitations in the production of fingerspelling. The researchers proposed that fingerspelling was especially difficult for signers with PD because of its rapid and sequential nature. All of these ASL studies highlighted the point that signing deficits in PD were phonetic rather than phonological and that incoordination in sign production was a fundamental characteristic of PD.

Tyrone and Woll (2008a) identified a fairly young BSL signer with PD – he was 54 years old during the testing sessions. This signer was different

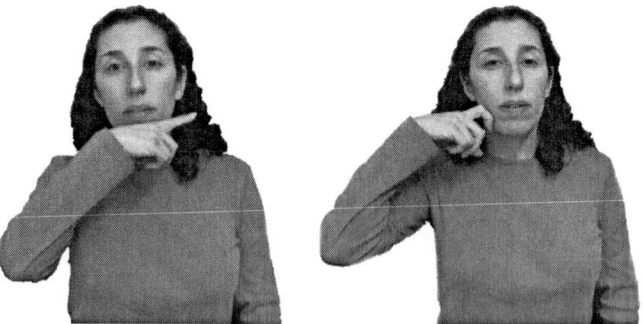

Figure 7.2 ASL sign DRY: The two interphalangeal joints of the index finger flex as the hand moves rightward along the chin

from the PD signers reported previously, in that he was a native signer. Given that his is the only reported case of a native signer with PD, it is unclear whether some aspects of sign production might have been better preserved as a result of his language background. This signer was tested on the production of fingerspelling, the production of signs in isolation, and a few standard non-linguistic movement tasks. Because his medication is known to cause motoric side effects, the signer with PD was tested on and off medication for all tasks.

The signer with PD exhibited some of the same dysarthria characteristics observed in hearing speakers with PD. The disease was at an early stage when he was tested, and his signing deficits were not severe, which is consistent with the progression of PD dysarthria in speech. In addition, this signer did not exhibit noticeable incoordination in signing or fingerspelling, either when he was on medication or off medication. This is consistent with findings from earlier speech research, suggesting that PD dysarthria does not greatly disrupt inter-articulator coordination (Tjaden & Wilding, 2005; Weismer et al., 2003). At the same time, this finding is in contrast to earlier findings on PD and ASL signing (Brentari et al., 1995; Poizner & Kegl, 1993), which suggested that coordination in particular was impaired in PD sign production. The BSL signer with PD also showed difficulty initiating movement and produced irregular movement hesitations, but less so in the signing task than in other movement tasks. Along similar lines, hearing speakers with PD do not show movement initiation problems as much in speech as in other movements.

This signer's productions in BSL broadly resembled the speech of individuals with PD, while his other limb movements were more similar to the non-linguistic limb movements produced by hearing speakers with PD. This suggests that the movement task was as important as the selected articulators in determining the nature of the movement deficit that was exhibited. Like ASL signers studied earlier, the BSL signer with PD often produced signs with laxed handshapes and sometimes with laxed orientations. In addition, his movements were slow both during signing and during other movement tasks. Unlike those signers, he did not produce signs at lowered locations, nor did he distalize his sign movements (Kegl et al., 1999). It should be noted that this was the only study to examine sign production in an individual with PD both on and off medication, so it is difficult to generalize about the effectiveness of PD medication for treating sign movements as opposed to non-linguistic limb movement.

Progressive supranuclear palsy

There has only been one case of hypokinetic dysarthria not resulting from PD identified in a sign language user. The individual was a 79-year-old British Deaf man who developed PSP (Tyrone & Woll, 2008b). He was not a native signer, but he was born deaf and learned BSL in school, and later it became his primary language. Following the onset of PSP, he exhibited slowed and reduced spontaneous movement, intention tremor and stooped posture.

Like PD, PSP is a hypokinetic disorder – it causes movements to be spatially reduced and slowed. PSP impacts the rostral brainstem and its connections to the cerebral cortex, cerebellum and basal ganglia. PSP differs from PD in that it results in limited eye movement and emergence of dysarthric symptoms early in the course of the disease. Speech production in PSP is characterized by articulatory undershoot, reduced loudness, limited pitch range and palilalia (Testa *et al.*, 2001). The last of these, palilalia, is defined as the repetition of entire words with decreasing amplitude across repetitions.

Movements produced by the signer with PSP were small, hypoarticulated and gradual. In producing individual signs, he often used laxed handshapes and palm orientations, and his signs were produced at lowered locations. The signer with PSP also showed incoordination in the production of two-handed signs. Unlike other signers with hypokinetic disorders, the signer with PSP produced involuntary movements and palilalia during signing. It is clear that what he exhibits is palilalia, because entire signs were repeated, and because repetitions decreased in movement amplitude. In contrast to what occurs in speech, individual signs were not repeated more than once.

The signer with PSP exhibited several sign deficits similar to those described earlier in signers with PD. For instance, he produced slow, small movements with laxed handshapes. Unlike signers with PD, he exhibited palilalia during the production of individual signs, but he had no similar type of movement anomaly during fingerspelling or non-linguistic movement tasks. Like hearing speakers with PSP, his palilalia was specific to the production of words and not a more general disorder of movement repetition. In summary, the signer with PSP had a production disorder that was slightly distinct from what has been reported for signers with PD, and similar to what has been reported for speakers with PSP.

Ataxia

Ataxia refers to the disruption to motor control that results from damage to the cerebellum. The mostly widely reported movement characteristics are dysmetria (movement undershoot or overshoot), dysrhythmia and dysdiadochokinesia (disturbance to rapidly alternating movements) (Bastian, 2002; Topka *et al.*, 1998). Only one case of ataxia in a sign language user has been documented (Tyrone *et al.*, 2009). He was a Deaf BSL signer who developed ataxia as the result of extensive hemorrhaging in the cerebellum during surgery for an arteriovenous malformation. The signer was 36 years old at the time of testing. He was born deaf in a hearing family, and he acquired BSL at age five when he went to an oral school for the deaf. After he developed

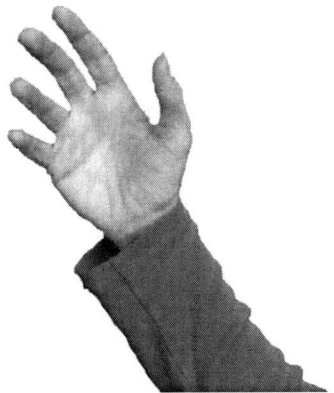

Figure 7.3 Lax handshape

ataxia, he was tested across multiple sessions on sign comprehension, sign production and fingerspelling tasks. He was also tested on non-linguistic movement tasks, such as pointing, reach and grasp, and the Kimura box (Kimura, 1993).

This signer differed notably from other reported cases of signers with movement disorders. Unlike signers with PD, who were reported to use laxed handshapes (Figure 7.3), the signer with ataxia used hyperextended handshapes during signing, so that his fingers extended backwards from the metacarpophalangeal joint (Figure 7.4). He also tended to use more proximal articulators for sign movements (for example, flexing the elbow instead of the wrist). This is in contrast to what was reported for ASL signers with PD,

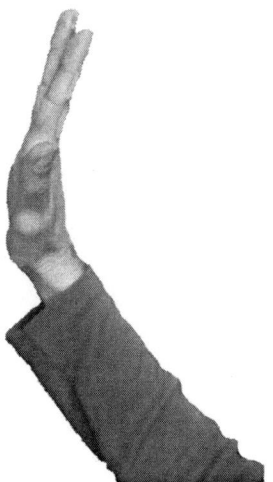

Figure 7.4 Hyperextended handshape

who often produced signs using distal articulators. In addition, the signer with ataxia showed bimanual incoordination and incoordination of proximal and distal articulators on the same limb during signing. In several cases, he added movements to signs where they were not required, for example, adding a handshape change to a sign that did not normally include it.

In both linguistic and non-linguistic tasks, the signer with ataxia often performed one-handed tasks with two hands. For example, during signing, he tended to produce one-handed BSL signs using two hands, mirroring the right hand's actions on his left hand. On the reach and grasp task, when this signer was asked to grasp a cylinder and move it a short distance forward, he would consistently use both hands to complete the task. It is unclear how he compares to other cases of ataxia in this respect – participants are not usually given the option of carrying out a standard motor control task with either one or two limbs.

One of the most widely reported characteristics of cerebellar ataxia is dysmetria (Bastian, 2002; Topka *et al.*, 1998). However, the signer with ataxia did not clearly exhibit dysmetria when he was signing. By contrast, he did produce dysmetric movements during a non-linguistic pointing task. This suggests that past findings on limb movements may have been influenced by the nature of the movement task as well as by which effectors were used for the tasks. The motor demands of signing are different from the motor demands of more standard movement tasks such as pointing; hence, signing may elicit a different pattern of deficits in individuals with cerebellar ataxia.

Discussion

Summary of findings

The studies reviewed here suggest that dysarthria is a disorder that occurs in signed language as well as spoken language. In addition, sign and non-sign movements may be affected in different ways by the same movement disorder, both in terms of which symptoms are present in which task and in terms of the severity of those symptoms. Dysarthria in the speech modality is often described with respect to the functions of individual articulators (Ackermann *et al.*, 1997; Yunusova *et al.*, 2008); however, since similar characteristics are observed in signed and spoken language dysarthria, the articulators used for production may not be the most relevant criterion for differentiating speech movement deficits from other movement deficits.

While dysarthria is not specific to the speech modality, it is also not a disorder of language function. Dysarthria occurs in both oral and manual languages because both modalities must use complex, rapid, coordinated movements. The complexity and fast movement speed shared by the two modalities facilitate the type of efficient information transfer needed for a linguistic system. However, this does not suggest that motoric disruption to language output is itself linguistic in nature. Speakers or signers with dysarthria would likely exhibit impairments in other tasks with similar motor demands, but few ordinary tasks require such speed and precision, so production deficits are more apparent in signed and spoken language.

The characteristics that have been reported for sign dysarthria follow patterns that would be expected, based what is known about the dysarthric characteristics of the same movement disorders in spoken language. For example, the signer with ataxia exhibited incoordination and large, exaggerated sign movements, which are similar to the dysarthric symptoms shown by hearing speakers with ataxic dysarthria. Similarly, the signer with PSP showed a severe form of dysarthria, partly characterized by palilalia. This is what would be predicted from the characteristics of dysarthria in hearing speakers with PSP. Given the variety of forms that dysarthria can take in sign as well as speech, research on signed language should move beyond broad comparisons of motor and linguistic disorders to consider more subtle analyses of individual disorders.

Comparing sign and speech

A few dysarthric symptoms arise in both sign and speech, while other symptoms do not appear in both modalities, which may highlight similarities and differences in the structure of signed and spoken language. Specific symptoms that occur across modalities include incoordination, reduced movement size, slowed movement and palilalia. The last of these, palilalia, is interesting, because the movement sequences that must be produced by the sign or speech articulators in a palilalic utterance are long and complex – they are the sequences necessary to repeat a word. Regarding reduced movement size in sign and speech, it should be noted that the size of articulatory movement in a signed language is typically described only in terms of the movement itself. By contrast, reduced movement size in a spoken language can alternatively be described in terms of its acoustic correlates (e.g., loudness or reduced vowel space).

In terms of symptoms that do not occur in both sign and speech, one difference is apparent from PD, which can cause speakers to produce rapid bursts of speech, even though voluntary limb movements are usually slow. By contrast, PD does not seem to induce rapid, brief bursts of signing. This difference in dysarthria across the two modalities may relate to the difference in production rate in typical speech and signing (Bellugi & Fischer, 1972). Language users may implement distinct production strategies, due to the difference in production rate.

There are aspects of sign and speech that cannot be easily compared, in individuals with motor disorders or in typical language users. For example, there is no clear equivalent to phonation, nasality or respiration in the sign modality. Similarly, while the primary sign articulators are positioned on opposite sides of the body and controlled by opposite sides of the brain, the speech articulators consist mostly of unitary structures positioned on the midline of the body; many of the speech articulators receive bilateral innervation. Hence, sign and speech are both likely to have some structural features, and by extension, some types of deficits, that are modality specific.

An important socio-cultural difference between signed and spoken language is that most sign language users do not acquire their language natively in the home. Most Deaf people are born into hearing families and do not acquire a signed language until they go to school or come in contact with other Deaf children. The effect of this is that most signers are non-native users of their primary language and, unlike hearing speakers, many Deaf signers do not have full exposure to any language in infancy. Along similar lines, signed languages are minority languages. They always co-exist with an ambient spoken language that is used by the majority of people in any given country or language region. As a result, sign language users are almost always bilingual, using a signed language in the Deaf community and a spoken or written language at work, with family and in other contexts. Almost all of the signers who have been studied in research on signed language and motor disorders were non-native signers, so very little attempt has been made to identify the effects of native versus non-native language acquisition on their production deficits. This is perhaps the biggest limitation to comparisons of language deficits across the sign and speech modalities.

Methodological issues in research on atypical signers

The study of sign dysarthria is limited by the small numbers of cases of signers with movement disorders, and the difficulty in collecting laboratory data on impaired sign production. Furthermore, there is an inadequate amount of normative data using precise, instrumented measures of sign production. A few early studies of ASL signers with movement disorders collected motion capture data during signing (Brentari et al., 1995; Poizner et al., 1987), but there is not a substantial amount of normative data to compare to these important early studies, whether from ASL or from another signed language. Moreover, the existing normative sign production data were collected primarily from young adult signers rather than from signers closer in age to most individuals with neurogenic disorders, such as stroke. As a result, there is a need for normative signing data that are collected from a broader range of the Deaf community.

With respect to comparisons of sign and speech production disorders, one limitation is that there has been only minimal research on limb movements in hearing speakers with dysarthria. Several studies have examined speech movements and non-linguistic limb movements in typical speakers (McNeill, 1992;

Meister *et al.*, 2009; Rochet-Capellan *et al.*, 2008) and in speakers who stutter (Max *et al.*, 2003; Olander *et al.*, 2010), but limb movement and gesture in individuals with dysarthria have received very little attention. It may be informative to analyze limb movements in isolation and the gestures that accompany speech in hearing speakers with dysarthria. This would provide researchers of signed and spoken language with useful information on how dysarthria can affect sign movements as opposed to limb movements that are coordinated with speech.

One serious challenge to the study of sign dysarthria is that there are no standard measurements or procedures for assessing phonetic variation in typical signers. The measurements currently used in sign phonetics are based on units that were identified from phonology, so there is no framework for describing aspects of production that do not involve linguistic contrasts. This makes it difficult to accurately describe motoric production disorders in a signed language. For example, several studies have suggested that signers with hypokinetic disorders, such as PD, tend to use handshapes that are laxed (e.g. Loew *et al.*, 1995; Tyrone & Woll, 2008b; Tyrone *et al.*, 1999). While multiple studies have reached this conclusion, there are no standardized measures and only limited normative data for articulatory laxing in signers who do not have motor disorders.

Quantitative measures of production in healthy signers are quite new (Cheek, 2001; Eccarius & Scheidt, 2010; Grosvald, 2009; Mauk *et al.*, 2008; Tyrone & Mauk, 2010), and they only describe a few aspects of sign language structure. Furthermore, in contrast to the field of speech research (Lisker & Abramson, 1964; Stevens & House, 1955), few studies of signed language have considered potential anatomical or physiological influences on language structure (Ann, 1996; Mandel, 1981). Similarly, there is currently only a limited understanding of phonetic and phonological differences between signed languages. This is problematic, because if it is unclear how languages themselves differ, then it becomes more difficult to distinguish disability from normal cross-linguistic variation. (For example, it could be difficult to disambiguate imprecise articulation of a location from variation in that location's realization across languages.)

The early, pioneering research on signed language and motor disorders was intended to address the question of whether signed languages were like other languages. Motor disorders such as PD served as the comparison case to aphasia in order to illustrate that signed languages could break down at a purely linguistic level. Now that there is a broader understanding of the equal status of signed and spoken languages, it should be possible to examine sign dysarthria in more detail to determine how distinct movement disorders affect signed language differently. Motor control, like language, is a multifaceted system that can break down in a variety of ways, some of them affecting linguistic communication. It would be informative to the fields of linguistics, psychology, neuroscience, and communication sciences and disorders to see how signing deficits relate to other deficits in limb movement, speech motor control and gesture.

Conclusions

In summary, while motor disorders can have different impacts on sign and speech, no motor disorder has been identified so far that has had a strong impact on one modality but not the other. Nor have there been language or motor disorders that are distinct in spoken language but indistinguishable in signed language, as had been predicted for aphasia and apraxia. Moreover, similar patterns tend to emerge across the two modalities with, for example, incoordination, movement undershoot and movement targeting errors occurring in both sign and speech as a result of the same movement disorders. Regarding the use of the term dysarthria for signed language, as with speech, what distinguishes sign dysarthria from other disruptions to limb movement is the differential impairment of signing. For example, some signers exhibited repetitive movement deficits in signing but not in non-linguistic movement tasks (Tyrone & Woll, 2008b). As such, sign dysarthria can most easily be identified in the realization of the phonological parameters of a sign (for example, laxed handshapes or lowered locations), rather than in movement aspects such as posture, which will likely be affected similarly across linguistic and non-linguistic tasks.

Given the small populations in signed language research and particularly in research on signing disorders, it is crucial that better methods of data sharing be developed. Just as useful databases have been developed for the analysis of large amounts of data on aphasia, child language and acoustic phonetics (Garofalo et al., 1993; MacWhinney, 2000), similar databases should be developed for the analysis of sign production data by typical signers and by signers with disorders. This includes consolidating and disseminating information about neurogenic sign deficits, so that disorders can be accurately diagnosed, based on the characteristics of particular cases of dysarthria. In addition, while many group comparisons have been made between signers with movement disorders and signers with linguistic disorders, it would be informative to carry out more within-group and within-subject comparisons of linguistic and non-linguistic limb movement. These types of comparisons would illuminate which deficits are sign specific and which deficits persist across movement tasks. One advantage of the collection of motion capture data for signing and for other limb movements is that these data can be anonymized and consequently shared easily by many researchers.

Research on sign dysarthria and other signing disorders would also be greatly enhanced by predictive models that could characterize typical and disordered sign production. Recent studies have begun to explore the explanatory value of articulatory phonology for signed language in healthy signers

(Tyrone *et al.*, 2010). It would be informative to pursue other types of models in the same way, and to attempt to apply them to disordered sign production. Testable models could then be compared against individual case studies as they are identified in future studies.

An explicit goal of future studies on signed language and motor disorders should be to improve diagnosis and therapy for individuals with sign dysarthria. There has been little research internationally on Deaf signers' access to language therapy for neurogenic communication disorders. However, research in the UK has suggested that clinical speech and language services for Deaf sign language users are extremely lacking (Atkinson *et al.*, 2002; Marshall *et al.*, 2003). With better insight into the sign production mechanism, it should be possible to improve future diagnosis and treatment for sign language users with motor disorders.

References

Ackermann, H., Hertrich, I., Daum, I., Scharf, G. and Spieker, S. (1997) Kinematic analysis of articulatory movements in central motor disorders. *Movement Disorders* 12, 1019–1027.

Ann, J. (1996) On the relation between the difficulty and the frequency of occurrence of handshapes in two sign languages. *Lingua* 98, 19–41.

Atkinson, J., Marshall, J., Thacker, A. and Woll, B. (2002) When sign language breaks down: Deaf people's access to language therapy in the UK. *Deaf Worlds* 18, 9–21.

Atkinson, J.R., Marshall, J., Woll, B. and Thacker, A. (2005) Testing comprehension abilities in users of British Sign Language following CVA. *Brain and Language* 94, 233–248.

Bastian, A.J. (2002) Cerebellar limb ataxia: Abnormal control of self-generated and external forces. *Annals of the New York Academy of Sciences* 978, 16–27.

Bellugi, U. and Fischer, S. (1972) A comparison of sign language and spoken language. *Cognition* 1, 173–200.

Braun, A.R., Guillemin, A., Hosey, L. and Varga, M. (2001) The neural organization of discourse: An H2O-PET study of narrative production in English and American sign language. *Brain* 124, 2028–2044.

Brentari, D. and Poizner, H. (1994) A phonological analysis of a Deaf Parkinsonian signer. *Language and Cognitive Processes* 9, 69–99.

Brentari, D., Poizner, H. and Kegl, J. (1995) Aphasic and Parkinsonian signing: Differences in phonological disruption. *Brain and Language* 48, 69–105.

Cheek, D.A. (2001) The phonetics and phonology of handshape in American Sign Language. PhD dissertation, Department of Linguistics, University of Texas at Austin.

Corina, D.P., Poizner, H., Bellugi, U., Feinberg, T. and O'Grady-Batch, L. (1992) Dissociation between linguistic and nonlinguistic gestural systems: A case for compositionality. *Brain and Language* 43, 414–447.

Corina, D.P., San Jose-Robertson, L., Guillemin, A., High, J. and Braun, A.R. (2003) Language lateralization in a bimanual language. *Journal of Cognitive Neuroscience* 15 (5), 718–730.

Cowie R., Douglas-Cowie, R.E. and Kerr, A.G. (1982) A study of speech deterioration in post-lingually deafened adults. *Journal of Laryngology & Otology* 96, 101–112.

Darley, F.L., Aronson, A.E. and Brown, J.R. (1969a) Clusters of deviant speech dimensions in the dysarthrias. *Journal of Speech and Hearing Research* 12, 462–496.

Darley, F.L., Aronson, A.E. and Brown, J.R. (1969b) Differential diagnostic patterns of dysarthria. *Journal of Speech and Hearing Research* 12, 246–269.

Darley, F.L., Aronson, A.E. and Brown, J.R. (1975) *Motor Speech Disorders*. Philadelphia, PA: Saunders.

Duffy, J.R. (2005) *Motor Speech Disorders: Substrates, Differential Diagnosis, and Management* (2nd edn). St. Louis, MO: C.V. Mosby.

Eccarius, P. and Scheidt, R. (2010) Defining an articulatory joint space for sign language handshapes. Paper presented at the 10th Conference on Theoretical Issues in Sign Language Research (TISLR 10), Purdue University, 30 September.

Emmorey, K., Gertsberg, N., Korpics, F. and Wright, C.E. (2009) The influence of visual feedback and register changes on sign language production: A kinematic study with deaf signers. *Applied Psycholinguistics* 30, 187–203.

Enderby, P. (1986) Relationships between dysarthric groups. *British Journal of Disorders of Communication* 21, 189–197.

Garofolo, J.S., Lamel, L.F., Fisher, W.M., Fiscus, J.G., Pallett, D.S., Dahlgren, N.L. and Zue, V. (1993) *TIMIT Acoustic-Phonetic Continuous Speech Corpus*. Philadelphia, PA: Linguistic Data Consortium.

Grosvald, M.A. (2009) Long-distance coarticulation: A production and perception study of English and American Sign Language. PhD dissertation, Department of Linguistics, University of California at Davis.

Haley, K.L. and Martin, G. (2011) Production variability and single word intelligibility in aphasia and apraxia of speech. *Journal of Communication Disorders* 44, 103–115.

Heilman, K.M. and Adams, D.J. (2003) Callosal neglect. *Archives of Neurology* 60 (2), 276–279.

Hickok, G., Bellugi, U. and Klima, E.S. (1996) The neurobiology of sign language and its implications for the neural basis of language. *Nature* 381, 699–702.

Hickok, G., Wilson, M., Clark, K., Klima, E.S., Kritchevsky, M. and Bellugi, U. (1999) Discourse deficits following right hemisphere damage in deaf signers. *Brain and Language* 66 (2), 233–248.

Jueptner, M., Jenkins, I.H., Brooks, D.J., Frackowiak, R.S.J. and Passingham, R.E. (1996) The sensory guidance of movement: A comparison of the cerebellum and basal ganglia. *Experimental Brain Research* 112, 462–474.

Kegl, J. and Poizner, H. (1997) Crosslinguistic/crossmodal syntactic consequences of left-hemisphere damage: Evidence from an aphasic signer and his identical twin. *Aphasiology* 11, 1–37.

Kegl, J., Cohen, H. and Poizner, H. (1999) Articulatory consequences of Parkinson's disease: Perspectives from two modalities. *Brain and Cognition* 40, 355–386.

Kent, R.D. (2000) Research on speech motor control and its disorders: A review and prospective. *Journal of Communication Disorders* 33, 391–428.

Kent, R.D., Kent, J.F., Rosenbek, J.C., Vorperian, H.K. and Weismer, G. (1997) A speaking task analysis of the dysarthria in cerebellar disease. *Folia Phoniatrica et Logopaedica* 49, 63–82.

Kent, R.D., Kent, J.F., Duffy, J.R., Thomas, J.E., Weismer, G. and Stuntebeck, S. (2000) Ataxic dysarthria. *Journal of Speech, Language, and Hearing Research* 43, 1275–1289.

Kimura, D. (1993) *Neuromotor Mechanisms in Human Communication*. Oxford: Oxford University Press.

Klasner, E.R. and Yorkston, K.M. (2000) Dysarthria in ALS: A method for obtaining the everyday listener's perception. *Journal of Medical Speech-Language Pathology* 8 (4), 261–264.

Lang, C.E. and Bastian, A.J. (2002) Cerebellar damage impairs automaticity of a recently practiced movement. *Journal of Neurophysiology* 87, 1336–1347.

Laurent-Vannier, A., Pradat-Diehl, P., Chevignard, M., Abada, G. and De Agostini, M. (2003) Spatial and motor neglect in children. *Neurology* 60, 202–207.

Levanen, S., Uutela, K., Salenius, S. and Hari, R. (2001) Cortical representation of sign language: Comparison of Deaf signers and hearing non-signers. *Cerebral Cortex* 11, 506–512.

Lisker, L. and Abramson, A.S. (1964) A cross-language study of voicing in initial stops: Acoustical measurements. *Word* 20, 384–422.

Liss, J.M., Spitzer, S.M., Caviness, J.N., Adler, C. and Edwards, B.W. (2000) Lexical boundary error analysis in hypokinetic and ataxic dysarthria. *Journal of the Acoustical Society of America* 107 (6), 3415–3424.

Loew, R.C., Kegl, J.A. and Poizner, H. (1995) Flattening of distinctions in a Parkinsonian signer. *Aphasiology* 9 (4), 381–396.

Loew, R.C., Kegl, J.A. and Poizner, H. (1997) Fractionation of the components of role play in a right-hemispheric lesioned signer. *Aphasiology* 11 (3), 263–281.

MacSweeney, M., Woll, B., Campbell, R., McGuire, P.K., David, A.S., Williams, S.C.R., Suckling, J., Calvert, G.A. and Brammer, M.J. (2002) Neural systems underlying British Sign Language and audiovisual English processing in native users. *Brain* 125, 1583–1593.

MacWhinney, B. (2000) *The CHILDES Project: Tools for Analyzing Talk. Vol. 2: The Database* (3rd edn). Mahwah, NJ: Lawrence Erlbaum.

Mandel, M.A. (1981) Phonotactics and morphophonology in ASL. PhD dissertation, Department of Linguistics, University of California, Berkeley.

Marshall, J., Atkinson, J., Thacker, A. and Woll, B. (2003) Is speech and language therapy meeting the needs of language minorities? The case of Deaf people with neurological impairments. *International Journal of Language and Communication Disorders* 38, 85–94.

Marshall, J., Atkinson, J., Smulovitch, E., Thacker, A. and Woll, B. (2004) Aphasia in a user of British Sign Language: Dissociation between sign and gesture. *Cognitive Neuropsychology* 21 (5), 537–554.

Marshall, J., Atkinson, J.R., Woll, B. and Thacker, A. (2005) Aphasia in a bilingual user of British Sign Language and English: Effects of cross-linguistic cues. *Cognitive Neuropsychology* 22, 719–736.

Mauk, C.E., Lindblom, B. and Meier, R.P. (2008) Undershoot of ASL locations in fast signing. In J. Quer (ed.) *Signs of the Time: Selected Papers from TISLR 2004* (pp. 3–24). Seedorf: Signum.

Max, L., Caruso, A.J. and Gracco, V.L. (2003) Kinematic analyses of speech, orofacial nonspeech, and finger movements in stuttering and nonstuttering adults. *Journal of Speech, Language, and Hearing Research* 46, 215–232.

McNeill, D. (1992) *Hand and Mind: What Gestures Reveal about Thought*. Chicago, IL: University of Chicago Press.

Meister, I.G., Buelte, D., Staedtgen, M., Boroojerdi, B. and Sparing, R. (2009) The dorsal premotor cortex orchestrates concurrent speech and fingertapping movements. *European Journal of Neuroscience* 29, 2074–2082.

Miller, N. (2002) The neurological bases of apraxia of speech. *Seminars in Speech and Language* 23, 223–230.

Murdoch, B.E. and Theodoros, D.G. (1998) Ataxic dysarthria. In B.E. Murdoch (ed.) *Dysarthria: A Physiological Approach to Assessment and Treatment* (pp. 242–265). Cheltenham: Stanley Thornes.

Nasir, S.M. and Ostry, D.J. (2008) Speech motor learning in profoundly deaf adults. *Nature Neuroscience* 11 (10), 1217–1222.

Neville, H., Bavelier, D., Corina, D., Rauschecker, J., Karni, A., Lalwani, A., Braun, A., Clark, V., Jezzard, P. and Turner, R. (1998) Cerebral organization for language in deaf and hearing subjects: Biological constraints and effects of experience. *Proceedings of the National Academy of Sciences* 95, 922–929.

Nishimura, H., Hashikawa, K., Doi, K., Iwaki, T., Watanabe, Y., Kusuoka, H., Nishimura, T. and Kubo, T. (1999) Sign language 'heard' in the auditory cortex. *Nature* 397, 116.

Nishio, M. and Niimi, S. (2001) Speaking rate and its components in dysarthric speakers. *Clinical Linguistics and Phonetics* 15 (4), 309–317.

Olander, L., Smith, A. and Zelaznik, H.N. (2010) Evidence that a motor timing deficit is a factor in the development of stuttering. *Journal of Speech, Language, and Hearing Research* 53, 876–886.

Petitto, L.A., Zatorre, R.J., Gauna, K., Nikelski, E.J., Dostie, D. and Evans, A.C. (2000) Speech-like cerebral activity in profoundly deaf people processing signed languages: Implications for the neural basis of human language. *Proceedings of the National Academy of Sciences* 97 (25), 13961–13966.

Poizner, H. (1990) Language and motor disorders in Deaf signers. In G.R. Hammond (ed.) *Cerebral Control of Speech and Limb Movements* (pp. 303–326). North-Holland, NY: Elsevier.

Poizner, H. and Kegl, J. (1992) Neural basis of language and motor behaviour: Perspectives from American Sign Language. *Aphasiology* 6 (3), 219–256.

Poizner, H. and Kegl, J. (1993) Neural disorders of the linguistic use of space and movement. In P. Tallal, A. Galaburda, R. Llinas and C. von Euler (eds) *Annals of the New York Academy of Science, Temporal Information Processing in the Nervous System*, Vol. 682 (pp. 192–213). New York: New York Academy of Sciences Press.

Poizner, H., Klima, E. and Bellugi, U. (1987) *What the Hands Reveal About the Brain.* Cambridge, MA: MIT Press.

Rochet-Capellan, A., Laboissiere, R., Galvan, A. and Schwartz, J.L. (2008) The speech focus position effect on jaw-finger coordination in a pointing task. *Journal of Speech, Language, and Hearing Research* 51, 1507–1521.

Sheard, C., Adams, R.D. and Davis, P.J. (1991) Reliability and agreement of ratings of ataxic dysarthric speech samples with varying intelligibility. *Journal of Speech and Hearing Research* 34, 285–293.

Stevens, K.N. and House, A.S. (1955) Development of a quantitative description of vowel articulation. *Journal of the Acoustical Society of America* 27, 484–493.

Testa, D., Monza, D., Ferrarini, M., Soliveri, P., Girotti, F. and Filippini, G. (2001) Comparison of natural histories of progressive supranuclear palsy and multiple system atrophy. *Neurological Sciences* 22 (3), 247–251.

Theodoros, D.G. and Murdoch, B.E. (1998a) Hyperkinetic dysarthria. In B.E. Murdoch (ed.) *Dysarthria: A Physiological Approach to Assessment and Treatment* (pp. 314–336). Cheltenham: Stanley Thornes.

Theodoros, D.G. and Murdoch, B.E. (1998b) Hypokinetic dysarthria. In B.E. Murdoch (ed.) *Dysarthria: A Physiological Approach to Assessment and Treatment* (pp. 266–313). Cheltenham: Stanley Thornes.

Thompson-Ward, E.C. (1998) Spastic dysarthria. In B.E. Murdoch (ed.) *Dysarthria: A Physiological Approach to Assessment and Treatment* (pp. 205–241). Cheltenham: Stanley Thornes.

Thompson, E.C. and Murdoch, B.E. (1995) Disorders of nasality in subjects with upper motor neuron type dysarthria following cerebrovascular accident. *Journal of Communication Disorders* 28, 261–276.

Timmann, D., Citron, R., Watts, S. and Hore, J. (2001) Increased variability in finger position occurs throughout overarm throws made by cerebellar and unskilled subjects. *Journal of Neurophysiology* 86, 2690–2702.

Tjaden, K. and Wilding, G.E. (2005) Effect of rate reduction and increased loudness on acoustic measures of anticipatory coarticulation in multiple sclerosis and Parkinson's disease. *Journal of Speech, Language and Hearing Research* 48, 261–277.

Topka, H., Konczak, J., Schneider, K., Boose, A. and Dichgans, J. (1998) Multijoint arm movements in cerebellar ataxia: Abnormal control of movement dynamics. *Experimental Brain Research* 119, 493–503.

Tyrone, M.E. (2005) Sign and speech articulation: Right and left. Paper at the Winter Meeting of the Linguistic Society of America, Oakland, CA.

Tyrone, M.E. and Mauk, C.E. (2010) Sign lowering and phonetic reduction in American Sign Language. *Journal of Phonetics* 38, 317–328.

Tyrone, M.E. and Woll, B. (2008a) Sign phonetics and the motor system: Implications from Parkinson's disease. In J. Quer (ed.) *Signs of the Time: Selected Papers from TISLR 2004* (pp. 43–68). Seedorf: Signum.

Tyrone, M.E. and Woll, B. (2008b) Palilalia in sign language. *Neurology* 70 (2), 155–156.

Tyrone, M.E., Kegl, J. and Poizner, H. (1999) Interarticulator co-ordination in Deaf signers with Parkinson's disease. *Neuropsychologia* 37, 1271–1283.

Tyrone, M.E., Atkinson, J.R., Marshall, J. and Woll, B. (2009) The effects of cerebellar ataxia on sign language production: A case study. *Neurocase* 15, 419–426.

Tyrone, M.E., Nam, H., Saltzman, E., Mathur, G. and Goldstein, L. (2010) Prosody and movement in American Sign Language: A task-dynamics approach. *Speech Prosody* 100957, 1–4. See http://www.speechprosody2010.illinois.edu/papers/100957.pdf.

VanGemmert, A.W.A., Teulings, H-L., Contreras-Vidal, J.L. and Stelmach, G.E. (1999) Parkinson's disease and the control of size and speed in handwriting. *Neuropsychologia* 37, 685–694.

Vermeerbergen, M., Leeson, L. and Crasborn, O. (2007) *Simultaneity in Signed Languages: Form and Function.* Amsterdam: John Benjamins.

Villacorta, V.M., Perkell, J.S. and Guenther, F.H. (2007) Sensorimotor adaptation to feedback perturbations of vowel acoustics and its relation to perception. *Journal of the Acoustical Society of America* 122, 2306–2319.

Waldstein, R.S. (1990) Effects of postlingual deafness on speech production: Implications for the role of auditory feedback. *Journal of the Acoustical Society of America* 88, 2099–2114.

Weismer, G., Yunusova, Y. and Westbury, J.R. (2003) Interarticulator coordination in dysarthria: An X-ray microbeam study. *Journal of Speech, Language, and Hearing Research* 46, 1247–1261.

Yunusova, Y., Weismer, G., Westbury, J.R. and Lindstrom, M.J. (2008) Articulatory movements during vowels in speakers with dysarthria and healthy controls. *Journal of Speech, Language, and Hearing Research* 51 (3), 596–611.

Ziegler, W. (2002) Task-related factors in oral motor control: Speech and oral diadochokinesis in dysarthria and apraxia of speech. *Brain and Language* 80, 556–575.

8 The Influence of Dementia on Language in a Signing Population

Patricia Spanjer, Mariëlle Fieret
and Anne Baker

Introduction

Older people with dementia reveal problems with language as the dementia progresses. In spoken languages these problems appear in various areas such word-finding problems, empty speech, grammatical errors and inadequate responses. In a sign language such problems can also be expected to appear. However, the situation is more complex since signers are usually bilingual. It may also be expected that signers with dementia will make the wrong language choice for the interaction partner. This chapter presents the results of an exploratory study of four signers with dementia in terms of such features compared to a control group of four older signers without dementia. It also discusses the problems of methodology and diagnosis.

Older deaf signers who are suffering from dementia have recently become the focus of attention for research, since practitioners are having to face the diagnosis, treatment and care of this group of deaf people. It is not possible to use existing diagnostic instruments in the elderly deaf population without considerable adaptation (Dean et al., 2009). The experiences of deaf signers with dementia and their family members also indicate quite clearly that more research is needed (Parker et al., 2010). Of course there have always been older signers with dementia, but they were apparently under the radar.

Dementia has a great impact in the older section of the hearing population. According to one study, it effects on average 6.4% of the population older than 55 years and prevalence increases with age. One in six men and one in three women suffer at some point from dementia (Breteler et al., 1998). In an American screening study it was found that almost 2% of the whole population older than 65 years of age had failed to be diagnosed with dementia (Boustani et al., 2003). In primary care almost 50% had been missed.

Dementia is usually diagnosed following the Diagnostic and Statistical Manual of Mental Disorders (DSM-IV-TR 2000). The clinical criteria as set out there consist of the following:

(1) Memory loss.
(2) Visible evidence of one of the following disorders: aphasia, apraxia, agnosia, problems with executive functions.
(3) Resulting in a clear restriction in functioning socially and at work as compared to previous levels.
(4) The problems are not only present during periods of acute delirium.

Dementia is often preceded by mild cognitive impairment and the borderline between the two is often difficult to trace (Reilly & Huang, 2013). It is also important to be aware that there are different kinds of dementia such as Alzheimer's disease, frontotemporal dementia, vascular dementia, semantic dementia or Wernicke–Korsikoff dementia, and that the cognitive profiles of the various types are different. Reilly and Huang (2013) emphasize the fact that different types of therapy are differentially effective according to the type of dementia.

As can be seen from the criteria listed above, language does not necessarily have to be affected for dementia to be diagnosed. This is, however, the case when the dementia affects cortical areas, as in dementia of the Alzheimer type or in forms of frontotemporal dementia such as semantic dementia. According to the study of Ott et al. (1995), these are the most frequent types of dementia and can account for about 85% of cases. The vascular type is also frequent. In the semantic type the language problems are the first symptoms to become visible and in Alzheimer's the language problems are initially most related to memory problems (Shinagawa et al., 2006). Most types of dementia develop some kind of language problems as the disease progresses. The language symptoms that occur differ according to the type and stage of the dementia, clearly being less severe in the beginning. Patients with Alzheimer's disease, for example, most often have initial problems with being relevant, later followed by problems with comprehension, and even later a loss of the ability to form sentences. In the final stages patients with dementia are often unable to speak or they only produce meaningless sounds or echolalic utterances.

The challenging question in this paper is whether it is possible to get an indication of the language problems that occur in the signed language of deaf older signers. The modality of the language used may impact on the sympto-mology so that characteristics observed in patients with dementia in spoken languages are different from those of signers. A second issue is the fact that most deaf people use two languages to a greater or lesser extent, namely a signed language and a spoken language. This bilingualism means that problems with language choice can arise. In deaf signers this bilingualism is of a special type, namely bimodal, adding a new dimension to the picture.

We will first give a brief overview of the language problems encountered in patients with dementia using spoken languages, and speculate on the implications for effects on a sign language. Secondly we will present the method of a small-scale empirical study examining language in older signers with dementia followed by the results and conclusions. This is an exploratory study both in terms of the methodology used and the interpretation of the results. It is hoped that it will stimulate further work on this group of signers to produce a more complete picture of their symptoms.

Symptoms of Dementia in Spoken Languages

Reilly and Huang (2013) and Reilly *et al.* (2010) provide a review of the symptoms of language and communication in a number of different types of dementia. These recent reviews will form the basis for the summary given here. The reviews discuss several different types of dementia, providing information on the types of language aspects affected in the individual types. The authors make it clear that their survey is by no means complete in terms of the types of dementia discussed. In this section we will give a brief, general overview of language symptoms, but organized around the language aspects affected. There will be slightly more detail given about Alzheimer's disease since this is the group involved in this particular study. We will conclude with a brief view on bilingualism and dementia, since it is our purpose to indicate the areas of language that it may be worthwhile investigating in elderly deaf signers. The types of dementia will be indicated per language aspect discussed using abbreviations as follows: Alzheimer's disease (AD); frontotemporal dementia (FTD), including the subtypes progressive non-fluent aphasia (PNFA) and semantic dementia (SD); vascular dementia (VaD); Parkinson's disease dementia (PDD); and Lewy body dementia (LBD). Again, research to date has been done only on spoken languages so the results pertain only to that modality.

Phonological problems mostly occur only in the later stages of dementia (PNFA, VaD, PDD) and consist of phonological paraphasias such as *ripamid* instead of *pyramid*. Fluency can also be affected. Prosody production and comprehension is noted as occurring in PDD.[1] In the final stages of dementia, speech is often unintelligible. In SD, phonology is quite clearly spared (Jefferies *et al.*, 2005). Since the phonological problems in speech seem to arise in relation to a deterioration of fine motor control, it could be expected that in a sign language phonological problems will arise at the point when motor control of the manual articulators will be affected. Fine motor control deteriorates earlier than gross motor control in dementia (Kluger *et al.*, 1997) and since speech involves finer motor control than manual signs, it might be expected that phonological problems will occur at an earlier stage of dementia in the spoken language of individuals with dementia.

In the morphology and syntax of spoken languages, the symptoms of dementia are often similar to those of aphasia. Agrammatism is mentioned as occurring frequently in patients with PNFA and PDD. Murdoch *et al.* (1987) studied patients with AD and found a highly significant difference from controls on sentence repetition and sentence construction. Studying verb agreement in AD and FTD patients, it was found that there was insensitivity to violations of the argument structure of verbs (Price & Grossman, 2005). A study of patients with AD (Blanken *et al.*, 1987) found that they were in fact capable of producing long and complex utterances in an elicitation task, but that in spontaneous speech their utterances were often shorter than age-matched controls. The syntax of sign languages contains many (surface) features that are quite different from those of spoken languages, but the underlying structures are quite similar (for an overview of syntax in sign languages, see Pfau *et al.*, 2012: 245–387). Sign languages contain considerable simultaneity, but it might still be expected that utterances will become shorter as measured in signs in patients with dementia. Grammatical problems can also be expected, but it is not clear which areas might be affected. In many sign languages verb agreement is optional (Mathur & Rathman, 2012: 145–146) so that differences here may be difficult to observe. The use of spatial grammar, classifiers and non-manual markers may also be affected since these can be affected in aphasic signers (Campbell *et al.*, 2008).

Difficulties with naming (anomia) form a core problem in AD, but occur also in several other types (PNFA, SD, PDD, LBD). Nouns seem to be particularly difficult to find for patients with AD (Bucks *et al.*, 2000). Semantic paraphasias are particularly common in SD patients. Empty speech, that is with impoverished semantic content and an increased use of fillers, also occurs in several types of dementia (AD, FTD, LBD). Snowden *et al.* (1996) report considerable use of fillers as an example of empty speech. Word recognition and comprehension is particularly a problem for SD patients. It is known that word-finding difficulties as indicated by the tip-of-the-tongue phenomenon are more common in bilinguals, and since signers are usually bimodal bilinguals, this phenomenon has been found to occur more often in signers than in monolingual non-signers (Pyers *et al.*, 2009). It is therefore highly likely that similar symptoms can be expected in signers with dementia. The control needs to be, however, with deaf signers without dementia.

Patients with AD are also reported as having problems with keeping to the topic and maintaining coherence in a narration (Dijkstra *et al.*, 2004), but also in spontaneous conversation (Ripich & Terrel, 1988). They also had more problems with turn-taking, producing shorter turns and using more non-verbal responses (Ripich *et al.*, 1991). It is likely that similar problems will arise in signers with dementia.

In sum, we see that language problems occur in most areas of language, albeit in different types of dementia. The symptoms identified in the earliest stages are generally in the area of word finding, semantics and pragmatics. It is likely that this will also be the case in signers with dementia.

When an older person is bilingual, they can of course also suffer from dementia, although recent research has indicated that they will possibly show the symptoms later than monolingual individuals (Bialystok *et al.*, 2007; Craik *et al.*, 2010; Luk *et al.*, 2011; Schweizer *et al.*, 2012). It is suggested that this is due to improved cognitive control in bilinguals. This improved cognitive control has been shown in bilinguals generally in spoken languages due to the practice in inhibiting the other language (e.g. Bialystok, 2001; Bialystok *et al.*, 2004; Carlson & Meltzoff, 2008). However, this advantage has not been found in bimodal bilinguals (Emmorey *et al.*, 2008), possibly because, the authors argue, bimodal bilinguals have far less practice in inhibiting since the modalities allow simultaneous production. This result might imply that bimodal bilinguals will not have the advantage in showing symptoms of dementia later.

The language symptoms discussed above also occur in bilingual patients with dementia, but in addition bilingual patients indicate problems with language choice; that is, they make an incorrect choice with respect to their conversation partner. It is not necessarily the case that patients always show a preference in terms of language choice for the language first learned (Hyltenstam & Stroud, 1989; Luderus, 1995). With respect to errors, the picture is also not clear: Mendez *et al.* (1999) found that patients made more errors in their non-dominant language, but in a picture-naming task Gollan *et al.* (2010) found that it was not clear which language would be most affected. In deaf patients with dementia problems with language choice can also be expected and may be dependent on the dominance of the two modalities.

In this first exploratory study of the possible language symptoms of dementia in deaf older signers we will consider a restricted number of variables. They will be taken from semantics including lexical problems and word-finding difficulties, pragmatics and grammar, since it is unlikely that phonology will be severely affected until the later stages.[2] Furthermore, since most deaf signers are bimodal bilinguals to some extent, learning both a signed and a spoken language, we will consider the aspect of language choice. Since deaf adults use bimodal mixing in their communication, we will also explore what types occur in the individuals we will study. The methods used for exploring these aspects will be set out in the next section.

Methodology

This exploratory study is based on the spontaneous language collected in conversations with four deaf patients suffering from dementia. These patients will be compared to four older deaf signers without dementia. The data collected will also be compared to norms from other populations related to the instruments used. The informants and the data collection will be described in the following two sections. General points of analysis will then be discussed as used to examine semantic and grammatical aspects, pragmatic aspects and aspects of bilingualism.

The informants

Spontaneous conversation was collected from four female informants aged between 84 and 94 years of age living in residential care in The Netherlands. Diagnosis is usually carried out using a combination of sources of information such as behavioral testing, neuroimaging, family history, and other biomarkers like cerebrospinal fluid proteins (Reilly & Huang, 2013). The diagnosis of dementia in this case was done by the medical staff of the residential care home where the informants were living. The diagnosis was based on the functional criteria of the DSM-IV and several memory tests. No instruments were available for diagnosis with deaf signers in The Netherlands at that time. The Mini-Mental State Exam has been adapted for use with American deaf signers in a signed form (Dean et al., 2009), but this instrument contains few items related to language. Work is currently being done to develop a battery of cognitive and language and communication tests in the UK, but this is still in development (Atkinson et al., 2011a; DCAL, 2012). The focus in that project is on developing such tests as can be easily and reliably be used with deaf signers. It will include language tests on picture naming, sentence repetition, picture description and verbal working memory in BSL. For non-verbal cognition there are tests for working memory and visual-spatial skills (Atkinson et al., 2011b).

Table 8.1 provides details of the four informants, including hearing status, language background, type of education and diagnosis. The point at which the diagnosis was made relative to the recording is given as a possible indication of the severity of the dementia. On the basis of such information it would appear that the dementia was the least advanced in D3. In terms of the other background variables the four informants are fairly similar.

The four deaf informants with dementia were compared to four older signers with no diagnosis of dementia as a control group (see Table 8.2). All four informants were female and were residents of the same care home as the informants with dementia. One of the informants, C3, was considerably younger than the other three; it was unfortunately not possible to find another informant of a similar age to the other three and to the group with dementia. On the other background variables the four control informants were fairly similar to the other group: all had hearing parents, but a deaf partner.

Table 8.1 Details of the four deaf informants suffering from dementia

Name	D1	D2	D3	D4
Age	94	81	84	88
Onset deafness	Before age 3	Before age 3	Before age 3	Before age 3
Hearing status of parents and siblings	Parents hearing, two hearing siblings, one deaf sibling	Parents hearing, no siblings	Parents hearing, one hearing sibling, one deaf sibling	Parents hearing, no siblings
Hearing status of partner and children	Deaf partner, 2 deaf children, 1 hard-of-hearing	Deaf partner, 2 hearing children	Deaf partner, 2 deaf children	Deaf partner, 2 hearing children
Education	Residential school for the deaf	School for the deaf and foster home	Residential school for the deaf	Residential school for the deaf
Diagnosis including time prior to data collection	Advanced dementia (diagnosed 3 years earlier)	Advanced dementia of Alzheimer type (diagnosed ca. 4 years earlier)	Dementia of Alzheimer type (diagnosed 2 years earlier)	Probable dementia of Alzheimer type (diagnosed 1 year earlier)

Table 8.2 Details of the four older deaf informants not suffering from dementia (control group)

Name	C1	C2	C3	C4
Age	84	88	66	83
Onset deafness	Before age 3	Before age 3	Before age 3	Before age 3
Hearing status of parents and siblings	Parents hearing, 10 hearing siblings	Parents hearing, no siblings	Parents hearing, nine hearing siblings	Parents hearing, one hearing sibling
Hearing status of partner and children	Deaf partner, no children	Deaf partner, no children	Deaf partner, one hearing child	Deaf partner, no children
Education	School for the deaf	School for the deaf	School for the deaf	Residential school for the deaf

All the informants grew up in The Netherlands at a time when deaf education in Europe was still strongly influenced by the Milan Convention of 1880. In the period from 1930 to 1950 deaf children were sent to residential schools in The Netherlands and the emphasis was on learning to speak and speech-read. Little information was obtainable from (the families of) the informants about their early education, but it appears that they spent most of their time as children away from their families and in a predominantly oral educational setting. It is known that deaf children communicated among themselves using signs, but this was not encouraged (Rietveld-van Wingerden & Tijsseling, 2010). As mentioned above, all informants had a deaf partner and used signing at home in their own families. It was not possible to ascertain whether this was a formed of signed speech or Sign Language of the Netherlands (NGT). It was also not possible to establish what the level of signing or spoken language was in the four informants with dementia prior to onset or what their language preference was if they had one. This is a general problem in studying bilingual informants with dementia.

Data collection

All the informants were residents of the same care center for the deaf in the central region of The Netherlands. They were recorded in spontaneous interaction with a deaf member of the care staff.[3] For the informants with dementia this was a person with whom they had daily contact and who was therefore very familiar to them. For the control group the person was known to them but they did not have daily contact. Each interaction partner used NGT in conversation with the informants. Approximately 20 minutes of interaction were filmed in order to obtain around 150 signs. A hearing researcher was also present but she kept in the background and out of the interaction as much as possible. For three of the group with dementia a hearing camerawoman was also present. The camera was set up long before recording began so that all were used to the situation.

Analysis

The conversations were transcribed using the ELAN software.[4] All words, mouth movements and signs were transcribed by one of the first two authors. Two interpreters who permanently work at the residential care home assisted with the transcription since they were familiar with some lexical signs used by residents. Signs that were unclear or which could not be glossed were excluded from the analysis. The recorded material available for the informants with dementia varied from 13 minutes to 19 minutes, whereby the goal was to obtain at least 300 signs. The material used for the control group was about 10 minutes and had to include at least 300 signs. The analysis procedures used for each aspect studied will be described together with the results in the following section. The measures used were applied to spoken forms on the one hand and to signs on the other, where the latter was possible. To provide a general impression of the interviews with one of the informants with dementia, an excerpt from the transcript from D2 is provided in Example 8.1.[5]

Example 8.1 Example from the recorded conversation between an informant with dementia (D2) and a deaf staff member (I)

I:		_____y/n
	sign	MIDDAY NICE EAT
	translation	Did you have a nice meal at midday?
D2:		headnod
	spoken	jaja gewoon
	translation	yes, yes, as usual
I:		____wh
	sign	WHAT?
D2:	spoken	gewoon dus
	translation	just as usual
I:		_____wh
	sign	WHAT EAT MIDDAY?
D2:	sign	FORGOTTEN
	spoken	weet niet meer vergeten
	translation	I don't remember, forgotten
I:	sign	PANCAKES EAT
D2:	spoken	lust wel pannenkoek maar niet altijd
	translation	(I) like pancakes but not always.
I:	sign	MIDDAY OUT GO BENNEKOM INDEX 3B
D2:		head nod
I:		_____y/n
	sign	PANCAKES EAT INDEX2 NICE?
D2:	spoken	slagroom slagroom
	translation	whipped cream whipped cream
I:		_____y/n
	sign	PANCAKES WITH WHIPPED-CREAM?
D2:	spoken	lekker
	translation	Nice.

The results of the two groups on all measures used were tested for statistical significance using non-parametrical statistics, namely chi-square due to the small sample size.

Results

Pragmatic aspects

As discussed in the first section, patients with dementia can have problems with keeping to the topic and with giving adequate responses to questions. Here responses to questions in the interview were categorized as being adequate or non-adequate. In this last category there were two types of inadequacy. Firstly the information provided was judged to be not appropriate as in Example 8.2. Here D2 is asked where she is currently, and instead of answering that she is in the care home, she answers as if she were still a child. Echolalic answers, that is, the mere repetition of a word or sign from the interviewer, were for example counted as non-adequate as in Example 8.4. Answers could also be a combination of the two as in Example 8.5. Secondly, if no response was given or an answer was given such as *I can't remember*, this was also considered inadequate. Minimal answers such as *yes* or *no* were counted as adequate if they fitted the context. Often they did not as in Example 8.3, since D1 agreed to all the suggestions of food that she had eaten for lunch.

Example 8.2 Inadequate response on the basis of content (D2)

I:	sign		_____wh	
		WHERE INDEX2 NOW?		
D2:	sign	INDEX-3B INDEX-3B		INDEX-3B
	spoken	pleegmoeder pleegouders Spagen, Spagen voetbalveld		
	translation	(With my) foster-mother, foster-parents in Spagen,		
		(close to a) soccerfield.		

Example 8.3 Inadequate response on the basis of content (D1)

I:		_____y/n
	sign	INDEX2 EAT MIDDAY SPINACH?
D1:	spoken	spinazie
	translation	spinach
I:		_____y/n
	sign	POTATOES?
D1:	spoken	zo (with headnod)
	translation	yes
I:		___y/n
	sign	FISH?
D1:	spoken	ja
	translation	yes

Example 8.4 Inadequate response on the basis of echolalia (D1)

I: _____y/n
     sign   INDEX-here GOOD CARE؟
     translation   (do they) take good care of you in here؟

D1:   ___hn
     sign   CARE
     spoken   zorgen
     translation   care, yes.

Example 8.5 Inadequate response on the basis of content and echolalia (D1)

I: _____y/n
     sign   TOGETHER GO HOLIDAY؟
D1: sign   TOGETHER GO
     spoken   samen vakantie
     gloss   together holiday
     translation   (We) went together on holiday
I: sign   _____wh
                       WHERE؟
D1: sign   TOGETHER SIGN INDEX-B3 TOGETHER
     spoken   samen gebaren daar naartoe samen
     translation   together signing to there together

The data were not split out into words and signs for this analysis. The results are presented in Table 8.3.

The group with dementia have significantly fewer adequate responses ($\chi^2 = 4.02$, df = 1, $p < 0.05$) and more non-adequate responses in

Table 8.3 Percentage of answer types according to adequacy in the group with dementia and the control group

	D1 (80)	D2 (129)	D3 (70)	D4 (80)	Mean	C1 (40)	C2 (23)	C3 (28)	C4 (20)	Mean
Adequate response	61	82	76	66	71	97	100	96	95	97
Non-adequate response (content)	13	13	21	13	15	0	0	4	0	1
Non-adequate response: no response or *I can't remember*	26	5	3	21	14	3	0	0	5	2

Note: Numbers in brackets indicate the number of possible answer points.

both categories (non-adequate content: $\chi^2 = 12.25$, df = 1, $p < 0.001$; no response: $\chi^2 = 9$, df = 1, $p < 0.01$). Of the informants with dementia, informant D1 has the most problems in this respect.

Semantic aspects

The measures used here were derived from analysis procedures for spontaneous language developed for use with samples from patients with aphasia in The Netherlands (Boxum *et al.*, 2010). The three aspects that were considered were word-finding difficulties, empty speech and semantic paraphasia.

Word-finding difficulties were established by considering a type-token ratio (TTR) in terms of words and signs based on a count of full nouns. Excluded were echolalic or imitated forms, numbers and neologisms. The results for TTR in words could also be compared to ranges found for older adult hearing controls with no dementia, measured using the same procedure as in research by Boxum *et al.* (2010).

As is evident from Table 8.4, there were no significant differences between the groups on either measure. All of the informants in the control group fell within the normal range for word TTR found by Boxum *et al.* (2010): 0.53–0.89. In that study, adults in the age range 17–78 were studied and no age effect was found. Of the informants with dementia, only the word TTR of D2 was outside this range, indicative of repetition of the same words and possibly word-finding difficulties. There is a considerable range in the sign TTR in both groups. Informant D3 has a lower sign TTR than the other informants with dementia but is similar to informant C1 from the control group. This variation may be due to a language dominance for speech (see below in this section).

Empty speech was operationalized by counting the number of fillers in both modalities. These were then calculated as a proportion of the total number of words or signs in the sample. Minimal answers such as *yes, no* or *don't know* or their equivalents in NGT were excluded. Examples of fillers in Dutch are *gewoon* 'like you do' or *nou ja* 'now yes'. In NGT these are elements such as Palm Up (PU) where it is used without any syntactic function. Example 8.6 comes from an informant with dementia, D4.

Table 8.4 Type-token ration based on nouns in the group with dementia and the control group

	D1	D2	D3	D4	Mean	C1	C2	C3	C4	Mean
Sign TTR	0.8 (20)	0.58 (62)	0.44 (55)	0.64 (53)	0.62	0.46 (52)	0.80 (25)	0.61 (54)	0.63 (48)	0.63
Word TTR	0.70 (47)	0.49 (148)	0.64 (44)	0.60 (102)	0.61	0.70 (46)	0.78 (37)	0.57 (69)	0.57 (51)	0.65

Note: Number in brackets indicates the total number of tokens.

Example 8.6 Use of palms up as a filler (D4)
D4 had just related where she had met her husband:

D4:	sign	THEN	PU
	spoken	then begins you know	
	translation	then it began	
I:	sign	IN-LOVE	
	translation	you were in love	
		hk	
D4:	sign	PU	
	translation	yes, you know	

The results (Table 8.5) suggest differences between the two groups, the informants with dementia producing more fillers in both words and signs. However, these group difference were not significant. The group with dementia compared favorably with a small sample of Dutch hearing patients with AD where an average of 8% of fillers were found (van Rhee-Temme, 2002). There is considerable variation in the number of sign fillers. One of the control group informants had in fact the highest number of fillers in NGT (C2), so it is questionable whether this variable as operationalized here is adequate for distinguishing informants with dementia.

No examples of semantic paraphasia were found in any of the four informants with dementia. It could be the case that the dementia was not yet so advanced in any of the informants that these might be expected.

Grammatical aspects

The first variable to be considered here is the mean length of utterance (MLU) in both modalities. The segmentation of the signed parts of the transcripts into utterances was done using the conventions usual in sign linguistic analyses and the MLU calculated on the basis of signs (Baker *et al.*, 2008: 24, 33). The guidelines set up by Boxum *et al.* (2010) were used for the segmentation and MLU calculation for Dutch which was based on words, not morphemes. That work also provides some comparison data from the spoken language of older Dutch controls without dementia. This calculation was

Table 8.5 Percentage of fillers in the group with dementia and the control group

	D1	D2	D3	D4	*Mean*	C1	C2	C3	C4	*Mean*
Sign fillers	8	10	2	12	8	4	13	1	4	5.3
	(233)	(302)	(266)	(292)		(292)	(291)	(299)	(313)	
Word fillers	7	3	1	0	3.5	2	2	1	1	1.5
	(307)	(618)	(111)	(261)		(333)	(173)	(253)	(193)	

Note: Number in brackets indicates the total number of tokens in that modality.

done on the utterances in NGT only and the NGT signs used in bimodal utterances on the one hand, and on the other on the Dutch only utterances and the Dutch words used in bimodal utterances. Minimal responses and inaudible or incomprehensible utterances were excluded.

As can be seen from Table 8.6, the MLU in signs is longer for all informants in the control group than the informants in the group with dementia. The group difference is, however, not significant. The utterances produced in NGT are quite short, even in the control group, in fact comparable to the input from deaf mothers to their young deaf children at age three years (van den Bogaerde, 2000). The group means of MLU of spoken Dutch are also not significantly different. There is overlap between the two groups: informant D2 has a longer MLU than C4. The MLU in words is lower in the control group than the hearing Dutch group studied by Boxum *et al.* (2010): 5.71–13.05. It is also lower than the MLU measured in the Dutch and Frisian of bilingual patients with AD (Stastra, 2010) where it was about 4. It is likely that this short MLU is a reflection of the fact that Dutch is the second language of these deaf signers and that some of the Dutch utterances produced are accompanied by signs forming a bimodal utterance. This point will be returned to in the concluding section.

The spoken utterances were also analyzed for grammatical correctness and then further for correct verbal inflection. Inaudible or incomprehensible spoken utterances and minimal responses were again excluded. Analyses for correctness were not done for the NGT utterances since there is considerable optionality involved in the grammar of NGT making it difficult to make clear decisions on correctness or incorrectness. Again the guidelines of Boxum *et al.* (2010) were used for the analysis of the Dutch utterances. According to their procedure, as used for aphasia data, grammatical errors were noted in sentences where the lexical verb or compulsory arguments were omitted from obligatory contexts resulting in an ungrammatical sentence. Ellipsis was considered correct if it was used in a correct context. The phonology of individual words could be non-target as long as the words were recognizable. In this exploratory study it was decided not to include omitted or incorrect articles in the analysis. All participants, including the control group, rarely used articles in their spoken utterances, and analyzing these omissions as incorrect would have resulted in a very high number of ungrammatical utterances. Their limited use is possibly due to the fact that their Dutch is influenced by NGT which has no articles, especially in the context of bimodal utterances.

Table 8.6 The MLU in signs and words of the group with dementia and the control group

	D1	D2	D3	D4	Mean	C1	C2	C3	C4	Mean
Sign MLU	1.8	2.5	1.8	2.3	2.1	3.3	3.2	4.0	3.4	3.5
Word MLU	2.1	3.2	1.7	2.4	2.4	4.1	3.0	3.5	2.4	3.3

In the sentences in Example 8.7, examples are provided of the errors involving the omission of compulsory arguments. These examples are taken from the data collected in this study.

Example 8.7 Examples of grammatically incorrect sentences (omitted compulsory arguments or lexical verbs)
(a)   Omitted subject (D4)
          Amersfoort gaan
          'go Amersfoort'
      Target: toen ging ik naar Amersfoort
                         'then I went to Amersfoort'
(b)   Omitted subject (C1)
          gaan met de bus of met auto
          'going by bus or by car'
      Target: we gingen met de bus of met de auto
                         'we went by bus or by car'

The verb form was also analyzed for the correctness and realization of inflection. Tense errors were not included here. Thus the utterances in Example 8.8 were marked as incorrect for inflection.

Example 8.8 Examples of incorrect or missing verbal inflection
(a)   Missing auxiliary (D4)
          broer verdronken
          'brother drowned'
      Target: mijn broer is verdronken
                         'my brother was drowned'
(b)   Incorrect inflection (D2)
          Ik koken zelf
          'I cook by myself'
      Target: Ik kook zelf
                         'I cook by myself'

Where a lexical verb is missing, then automatically the inflection is missing. This is illustrated in Example 8.9.

Example 8.9 Example of missing lexical verb, and thus missing inflection (D2)
          pleegmoeder, pleegouders Spagen voetbalveld
          'foster mother, foster parents Spagen soccerfield'
      Target: mijn pleegmoeder, pleegouders wonen in Spagen (naast) een voetbalveld
                      'my foster mother, foster parents live in Spagen next to a soccerfield'

Table 8.7 Percentage of incorrect Dutch utterances expressed over all spoken utterances (in brackets) and percentage of incorrect or missing verbal inflection expressed over all finite verb forms (in brackets)

	D1	D2	D3	D4	Mean	C1	C2	C3	C4	Mean
Incorrect Dutch utterances	59 (113)	56 (178)	49 (69)	41 (80)	51.2	35 (78)	33 (48)	30 (63)	30 (63)	32.0
Incorrect or missing verbal inflection	68 (82)	49 (118)	69 (29)	87 (38)	68.2	37 (49)	71 (24)	55 (42)	85 (42)	62.0

The percentages of incorrect utterances as defined above as shown in Table 8.7 are significantly higher than the percentages of the control group ($\chi^2 = 17.8$, df = 1, $p < 0.001$). In comparison to the results from Boxum *et al.* (2010) the control group perform just outside the range of adult Dutch speakers: 0–33%. There is considerable variation in the number of verbs produced with incorrect or missing inflection. The group difference is not significant. In Boxum *et al.* (2010) the range was 0–22% correct and the control group here are far below that. All informants have a lower accuracy than the bilingual patients with AD studied by Stastra (2010) where the percentage ranged from 0% to 17%. The results are suggestive that the informants with dementia are becoming weaker in Dutch, but there is a confound with the fact that spoken Dutch is being produced in a bimodal bilingual context which can affect the correctness of the Dutch forms produced, as will be discussed in the concluding section.

Bilingualism and bimodality

As mentioned in the previous section, deaf signers produce many bimodal utterances in their spontaneous language. The informants with dementia were no exception. The use of bimodality is not seen as an indicator of dementia since this form of language mixing is very common in deaf people with no dementia. It indicates, however, the orientation of the informants to one modality or the other. This variable may be of value in seeing whether there is a language shift in preference across the course of dementia, although that analysis is only possible with longitudinal data.

The definitions of bimodality as set out by Baker and van den Bogaerde (2005, 2008) were used to identify the bimodal utterances and then to divide the bimodal utterances into their four types: Full, Sign bimodal, Spoken bimodal and Mixed. Briefly, the utterances are categorized as Full when the full proposition is expressed in both modalities, as Sign bimodal when the proposition is fully expressed in sign with some spoken words added, as

Spoken bimodal when with proposition is expressed fully in spoken language with some signs added, and as Mixed when the proposition can only be formed by combining both modalities. Examples in (6) to (9) below are taken from the three informants.

(6) Full bimodal: (D1)
      sign   BALL THROW
      spoken   bal gooien
                       ball throw
      translation   (I) threw a ball

(7) Sign bimodal: (D3)
      sign   ZEELAND STAY INDEX1 GROW-UP
      spoken   Zeeland
      translation   I stayed all the time in Zeeland while growing up.

(8) Spoken bimodal: (D2)
      sign   BAKE
      spoken   gebakken aardappelen gebakken
                       baked   potatoes   baked
      translation   Baked potatoes

(9) Mixed bimodal: (D3)
      sign   FOOD GOOD FOOD
      spoken   pap   pap
                       porridge   porridge
      translation   I like porridge

Minimal responses and incomprehensible utterances were excluded from this analysis.

From Figure 8.1 we can see that bimodal utterances are very common in all informants, being more than 60% of all utterances (n) and even as much as 100% in informant C3. There is, however, considerable variation within

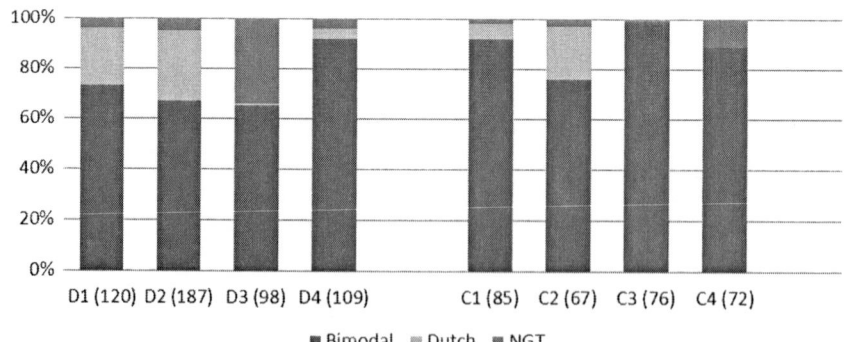

Figure 8.1 Frequency of bimodality in the group with dementia and the control group

the two groups. In the group with dementia, D3 uses a fair number of NGT utterances in contrast to the other informants who produce very few. Two, D1 and D2, have on the other hand more Dutch utterances. In the control group there are very few NGT utterances and only C2 has a considerable proportion of Dutch utterances.

These findings suggest that some of the informants are more sign oriented and others more spoken language oriented, but that there is no clear distinction between the two groups. This picture is confirmed by an analysis of the bimodal types as shown in Figure 8.2. Here we see again that informant D3 in the group with dementia is the most oriented towards the sign modality, producing far more Sign bimodal utterances than the other informants. In the control group C2 and C4 have a larger proportion of Sign bimodal utterances. There are no comparative figures for younger adult deaf signers. The only data we have come from three deaf mothers in interaction with their deaf children at age 6;0 (Baker & van den Bogaerde, 2008). All three mothers used bimodal utterances, between 40% and 70%, but primarily within these Sign bimodal utterances. That is, these deaf mothers are primarily oriented to signing.

As was discussed in the previous section with respect to grammaticality, the use of Dutch in bimodal utterances may be affected by NGT. An examination of the percentages of accuracy from Table 8.7 does not indicate a clear relationship between the choice for NGT, full or sign bimodal utterances and a lower score on correctness. This aspect needs further exploration in later work.

In sum, this analysis of bimodality does not indicate group differences between the informants with dementia and the informants in the control group. It does indicate the individual's preference in language choice, but

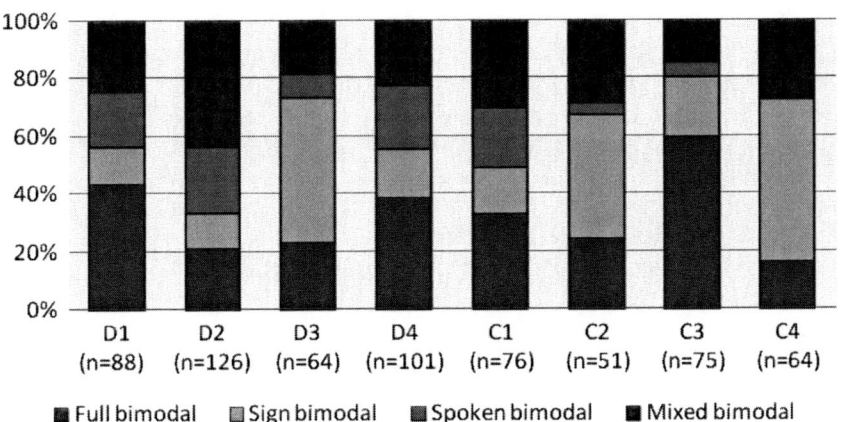

Figure 8.2 Bimodal utterance types from the group with dementia and the control group expressed as percentages of all bimodal utterances (*n*)

Table 8.8 Percentage of appropriate language choice by group with dementia and the control group for responses to questions from the deaf interviewer

	D1 (54)	D2 (50)	D3 (80)	D4 (60)	Mean	C1 (40)	C2 (36)	C3 (61)	C4 (55)	Mean
% Appropriate language choice	45	27	82	55	52	47	54	80	76	64

Note: Figures in brackets indicate the total number of utterances in the analysis.

since the conversations were recorded at one point in time, this variable as operationalized here cannot indicate if there is any shift within individual language choice.

The analysis of bimodality does, however, give an indication as to whether the informants are making a correct language choice for the conversation with the deaf carer. An appropriate language choice was defined as one in which the full proposition was accessible to the deaf interviewer, that is, when the utterance was either in NGT only, Full or Sign bimodal. Table 8.8 shows the result of this analysis based on the language choice per utterance produced by the informant, again excluding minimal responses and incomprehensible utterances.

There is a significant difference between the means of the two groups ($\chi^2 = 4.9$, df $= 1$, $p < 0.05$), indicating that the controls show more appropriate language choice. However, it must be pointed out that the variation is great, so the group difference has to be taken with some caution. There is overlap between the two groups, with informant D3 having a higher percentage appropriate language choice than any of the informants in the control group. This could also be the result of her overall preference for the sign modality rather than a correct control of language choice. On the other hand, she is in the least advanced stages of dementia compared to the other two informants. Without comparing language choice between two different conversation partners, one deaf, and one hearing and non-signing, it is not possible to have real insight into their control of language choice. This variable needs to be investigated with a far larger group.

Discussion and Conclusions

As stated at the outset, this is a highly exploratory piece of research into the language symptoms of deaf signers with dementia. We can find some indications of where to look further and also some evidence for methodological issues that need to be considered.

In terms of the areas of language affected by dementia, there seemed to be little evidence that particular aspects of grammar were affected, since it could not be ruled out that the lower MLU and lower percentages of correct utterances in Dutch were due to the type of bilingualism in deaf signers where the spoken language is clearly the less dominant language. It was not possible to investigate NGT with respect to grammar in this study but this needs to be explored further using other kinds of observation and tests before we can get clarity on the effects on grammar. The semantic aspects examined provided only some data for fillers and word-finding problems, none for semantic paraphasia. For fillers and TTR, the data were not clear due to a lack of directly comparable data, but D2 appeared to perform the lowest. D1, on the other hand, performed the worst in terms of the number of appropriate responses to questions, with D2 performing the best. On language choice for a conversation with the deaf carer, however, D2 performed far and away the worst and D3 the best. It is not clear that any one of the informants was in a more advanced stage of dementia than the other two on the basis of the language variables examined. D2, for example, was worst on three variables but best on two. D3, who had the diagnosis of the mildest form of dementia, performed best on the number of fillers (having the least); she also had the highest number of correct Dutch utterances and the highest appropriate number of language choices but, on the other hand, the lowest MLU in both signs and words.

The variables selected for the analysis of spontaneous language offer possibilities for further research, but it is necessary to have comparable data from older deaf signers without dementia. Hopefully, this will be available soon for this age group. It is also necessary to have access to larger groups. In a small country like The Netherlands the number of signers available for this kind of research is limited. International collaboration is necessary to compare results for this important group of signers.

Notes

(1) Some work has been done on signers with Parkinson's Disease but none with PDD. This work indicates articulatory problems due to motor difficulties (Kegl *et al.*, 1999) and adjustments in pragmatics (Kegl & Poizner, 1998).
(2) A dissertation is in preparation comparing five signers with dementia and five control subjects, but the results are not yet available (DiBlasi, 2011).
(3) Permission to record was obtained from the informants themselves (control group) or from the family member who had legal authority to grant this (group with dementia).
(4) Available for the Max Planck Institute Nijmegen at http://tla.mpi.nl/tools/tla-tools/elan/
(5) The usual conventions for sign transcription are used here; that is, in the first line signs in small capitals glossed in English, spoken words in Dutch lower case and then translated, and finally an English free translation. Non-verbal responses accompanying speech or occurring on their own are described in terms of head gestures.

References

Atkinson, J., Denmark, T., Woll, B., Ferguson-Coleman, E., Rogers, K., Young, A., Keady, J., Burns, A., Geall, R. and Marshall, J. (2011a) Deaf with Dementia: Towards better recognition and services. *Journal of Dementia Care* 19 (3), 38–39.

Atkinson, J., Denmark, T., Marshall, C. and Woll, B. (2011b) Cognitive norms in healthy older Deaf people and the development of a dementia screening tool for Deaf BSL users. Presentation to IMPRS NeuroCom Summer School, London, June 2011.

Baker, A. and van den Bogaerde, B. (2005) Code mixing in mother–child interaction in deaf families. *Sign Language & Linguistics* 8, 151–174.

Baker A. and van den Bogaerde, B. (2008) Codemixing in signs and words in input to and output from children. In C. Plaza-Pust and E. Morales Lopéz (eds) *Sign Bilingualism: Language Development, Interaction, and Maintenance in Sign Language Contact Situations*. Studies in Bilingualism No. 38 (pp. 1–27). Amsterdam: John Benjamins.

Baker, A.E., van den Bogaerde, B. and Woll, B. (2008) Methods and procedures in sign language acquisition studies. In A.E. Baker and B. Woll (eds) *Sign Language Acquisition* (pp. 1–50). Amsterdam: John Benjamins.

Bialystock, E. (2001) *Bilingualism in Development: Language, Literacy, and Cognition*. Cambridge: Cambridge University Press.

Bialystock, E., Craik, F.I.M., Klein, R. and Viswanathan, M. (2004) Bilingualism, aging, and cognitive control: Evidence from the Simon Task. *Psychology and Aging* 19 (2), 290–303.

Bialystok, E., Craik, F.I.M. and Freedman, M. (2007) Bilingualism as a protection against the onset of symptoms of dementia. *Neuropsychologia* 45 (2), 459–464.

Blanken, G., Dittmann, J., Haas, J.C. and Wallesch, C-W. (1987) Spontaneous speech in senile dementia. *Cognition* 27, 247–274.

Boustani, M., Peterson, B., Hanson, L., Harris, R. and Lohr, K.N. (2003) Screening for dementia in primary care: A summary of the evidence for the U.S. Preventive Services Task Force. *Annals of Internal Medicine* 138, 927–937.

Boxum, E., van der Scheer, F. and Zwaga, M. (2010) *ASTA: Analyse voor Spontane Taal bij Afasie* [Analysis for Spontaneous Language for Aphasia]. Vereniging Klinische Linguistiek.

Breteler, M., Ott, A. and Hofman, A. (1998) The new epidemic: Frequency of dementia in the Rotterdam study. *Haemostasis* 28, 117–123.

Bucks, R.S., Singh, S., Cuerden, J.M. and Wilcock, G.K. (2000) Analysis of spontaneous conversational speech in dementia of Alzheimer type: Evaluation of an objective technique for analyzing lexical performance. *Aphasiology* 14, 71–91.

Campbell, R., MacSweeney, M. and Waters, D. (2008) Sign language and the brain: A review. *Deaf Studies and Deaf Education* 13 (1), 3–20.

Carlson, S.M. and Meltzoff, A.N. (2008) Bilingual experience and executive functioning in young children. *Developmental Science* 11 (2), 282–298.

Craik, F.I.M., Bialystok, E. and Freedman, M. (2010) Delaying the onset of Alzheimer disease. Bilingualism as a form of cognitive reserve. *Neurology* 75, 1726–1729.

DCAL (2012) DCAL Briefing Sheet: Summer 2012. See http://www.ucl.ac.uk/dcal.

Dean, P., Feldman, D., Morere, D. and Morton, D. (2009) Clinical evaluation of the Mini-Mental State Exam with culturally deaf senior citizens. *Archives of Clinical Neuropsychology* 24 (8), 753–760.

DiBlasi, A. (2011) Evaluating the effects of aging on American Sign Language users. MA thesis, Ohio. https://etd.ohiolink.edu/ap:10:0::NO:10:P10_ETD_SUBID:74672

Dijkstra, K., Bougeois, M.S., Allen, R.S. and Burgio, L.D. (2004) Conversational coherence: Discourse analysis of older adults with and without dementia. *Journal of Neurolinguistics* 17, 263–283.

Emmorey, K., Luk, G., Pyers, J.E. and Bialystok, E. (2008) The source of enhanced cognitive control in bilinguals: Evidence from bimodal bilinguals. *Psychology of Science* 19 (12), 1201–1206.

Gollan, T.H., Salmon, D.P., Montoya, R.I. and da Pena, E. (2010) Accessibility of the nondominant language in picture naming: A counterintuitive effect of dementia on bilingual language production. *Neuropsychologia* 48 (5), 1356–1366.

Hyltenstam, K. and C. Stroud (1989) Bilingualism in Alzheimer's dementia: Two case studies. In K. Hyltenstam and L.K. Obler (eds) *Bilingualism across the Lifespan* (pp. 23–52) Cambridge: Cambridge University Press.

Jefferies, E., Jones, R.W., Bateman, D. and Lambon Ralph, M.A. (2005) A semantic contribution to nonword recall? Evidence for intact phonological processes in semantic dementia. *Cognitive Neuropsychology* 22 (2), 183–212.

Kegl, J. and Poizner, H. (1998) Shifting the burden to the interlocutor: Compensation for pragmatic deficits in signers with Parkinson's disease. *Journal of Neurolinguistics* 11 (1–2), 137–152.

Kegl, J., Cohen, H. and Poizner, H. (1999) Articulatory consequences of Parkinson's disease: Perspectives from two modalities. *Brain and Cognition* 40, 355–386.

Kluger, A., Gianutsos, J.G., Golomb, J., Ferris, S.H., George, A.G., Franssen, E. and Reisberg, B. (1997) Patterns of motor impairment in normal aging, mild cognitive decline, and early Alzheimer's disease. *Journal of Gerontology* 52B (1), 28–39.

Luderus, S.W.B. (1995) Language choice and language separation in bilingual Alzheimer patients. PhD thesis, University of Amsterdam. Studies in Language and Language Use IFOTT No. 35. Amsterdam.

Luk, G., Bialystok, E., Craik, F.I.M. and Grady, C.L. (2011) Lifelong bilingualism maintains white matter integrity in older adults. *Journal of Neuroscience* 31 (46), 16808–16813.

Mathur, G. and Rathmann, C. (2012) Verb agreement. In R. Pfau, M. Steinbach and B. Woll (eds) *Sign Language: An International Handbook* (pp. 136–157). Berlin and Boston, MA: De Gruyter Mouton.

Mendez, M.F., Perryman, K.M., Pontón, M.O. and Cummings, J.L. (2009) Bilingualism and dementia. *The Journal of Neuropsychiatry and Clinical Neurosciences* 11: 411–412.

Murdoch, B.E., Chenery, H., Wilks, V. and Boyle, R.S. (1987) Language disorders in dementia of the Alzheimer type. *Brain and Language* 31 (1), 122–137.

Ott, A., Breteler, M.M.B., van Harskamp, F., Claus, J.J., van der Cammen, T.J.M., Grobbee, D.E. and Hoffmann, A. (1995) Prevalence of Alzheimer's disease and vascular dementia: Association with education. The Rotterdam Study. *British Medical Journal* 310, 970–973.

Parker, J., Young, A.M. and Rogers, K. (2010) My mum's story. A deaf daughter discusses her Deaf mother's experience of dementia. *Dementia: The International Journal of Social Research and Practice* 9 (1), 5–20.

Pfau, R., Steinbach, M. and Woll, B. (eds) (2012) *Sign Language: An International Handbook.* Berlin and Boston, MA: De Gruyter Mouton.

Price, C. and Grossman, M. (2005) Verb agreements during on-line sentence processing in Alzheimer's disease and frontotemporal dementia. *Brain and Language* 94, 217–232.

Pyers, P.E., Gollan, T.H. and Emmorey, K. (2009) Bimodal bilinguals reveal the source of tip-of-the-tongue. *Cognition* 112 (2), 323–329.

Reilly, J. and Huang, J. (2013) Dementia and communication. In L. Cummings (ed.) *The Cambridge Handbook of Communication Disorders.* Cambridge: Cambridge University Press.

Reilly, J., Rodriguez, A.D., Lamy, A. and Neils-Strunjas, J. (2010) Cognition, language, and clinical pathological features of non-Alzheimer's dementias: An overview. *Journal of Communication Disorders* 43, 438–452.

Rietveld-van Wingerden, M. and Tijsseling, C. (2010) *Ontplooing door communicatie. Geschiedenis van het onderwijs aan doven en slechthorenden in Nederland* [Development through communication. A history of education for the deaf and hard-of-hearing in the Netherlands]. Antwerp: Garant.

Ripich, D. and Terrell, D. (1988) Patterns of discourse cohesion in Alzheimer's disease. *Journal of Speech and Hearing Disorders* 53, 8–15.

Ripich, D.N., Vertes, D., Whitehouse, P., Fulton, S. and Ekelman, B. (1991) Turn-taking and speech act patterns in the discourse of senile dementia of the Alzheimer's type patients. *Brain and Language* 40 (3), 330–343.

Schweizer, T.A., Ware, J., Fischer, C.E., Craik, F.I.M. and Bialystok, E. (2012) Bilingualism as a contributor to cognitive reserve: Evidence from the brain atrophy in Alzheimer's disease. *Cortex* 48 (8), 991–996. doi:10.1016/j.cortex.2011.04.009.

Shinagawa, S., Ikeda, M., Fukuhara, R. and Tanabe, H. (2006) Initial symptoms in frontotemporal dementia and semantic dementia compared with Alzheimer's disease. *Dementia and Geriatric Cognitive Disorders* 21, 74–80.

Snowden, J.S., Neary, D. and Mann, D.M.A. (1996) *Frontotemporal Lobar Degeneration: Frontotemporal Dementia, Progressive Aphasia, Semantic Dementia.* New York: Churchill Livingstone.

Stastra, S. (2010) Tweetaligheid bij de ziekte van Alzheimer [Bilingualism in Alzheimer's disease]. MA thesis, University of Groningen.

Van den Bogaerde, B. (2000) Input and interaction in deaf families. PhD thesis, University of Amsterdam.

Van Rhee-Temme, W. (2002) Spontane taalanalyse bij patienten met AD: methodiek en follow up [Spontaneous language analysis in patients with Alzheimer's disease and follow-up]. Unpublished MA thesis, University of Nijmegen.

Part 3

Hearing Children from Signing Households

9 KODAs: A Special Form of Bilingualism

Anne E. Baker and Beppie van den Bogaerde

Introduction

The purpose of this chapter is to consider the special position of hearing children of deaf adults (kodas = kids of deaf adults).[1] In particular we will focus on kodas who grow up being exposed to both a signed language and a spoken language; it must be remembered that not all kodas are exposed to a sign language.

It is important to state from the outset that various researchers have found that the interaction between Deaf parents and their hearing children seems effortless and natural, in whatever mode it is conducted (e.g. Griffith, 1990; Mallory et al., 1993; Prinz & Prinz, 1979, 1981), even though identity issues might develop over the years (Preston, 1995). On the other hand, as Singleton and Tittle (2000) point out in their review article, Deaf parents are 'essentially raising foreign children', since the parents do not share all the same experiences and culture. The question is whether this affects their language acquisition and in what ways.

If the deaf parents of a hearing child have both been raised in a hearing family or have chosen to avoid signed language, there might be no sign language in the home at all; then of course the children are unlikely to be bilingual. However, if both a signed language and a spoken language are offered, kodas will, at least to some extent, resemble other bilingual children who grow up with two languages and two cultures. The variety in input can be as great for kodas as for hearing children reared in a bilingual home. For example, both parents can offer a signed language and/or a spoken language, or there might be a one-person-one-language situation: one parent signs, the other speaks. One language may be confined to the home; the other may be used outside. The input may be balanced across the two languages, or one language may be dominant. Interesting issues related to all bilingual children and thus also to the group of kodas are, for example, how much input is necessary to develop both languages well or whether specific periods for exposure to input exist. Where relevant and possible, we will make the comparison with bilingual children learning two spoken languages.

For kodas, this is, however, also a special form of bilingualism and in more than one way. Firstly, these hearing children are learning a signed language in the visual-spatial modality. Preston (1994) maintains that 60% of kodas are offered sign language and may become fluent sign language users. They also are learning a spoken language in the oral/aural modality. Modality has an impact on the form of the language used (Emmorey, 2002); thus specific features such as verb inflection are learned later in most sign languages than in the spoken languages that have that feature. The acquisition of the language pair in this kind of bilingualism has therefore specific features. It is relevant to examine whether the milestones reached in monolingual spoken language development are reached at the same time, and whether the sign language is acquired at the same rate as deaf children of deaf parents. Secondly, because the languages are in different modalities, they can be combined in ways that are not possible with two spoken languages. They can be produced simultaneously, which leads to a phenomenon called code-blending (Emmorey *et al.*, 2005a). This form of language mixing has a different dimension from the mixing of spoken languages common in bilingual children, namely the simultaneity. We will discuss how code-blending affects language acquisition in kodas. Thirdly, sign languages are always a language of a minority. Learning a minority language places a child socially in a special position and this can have an effect on acquisition. Since Deaf people form a specific kind of cultural minority, it is of relevance to know how kodas are affected in their linguistic preference.

All babies start their linguistic journey by producing vocalizations and hand and body movements that initially have no meaning (Iverson & Goldin-Meadow, 2005). Later, when exposed to both a spoken language and sign language, the modalities become more distinct. Here we will consider first the path of acquisition of both languages in this group: in Section 1 the spoken language and in Section 2 the signed language. In these sections we will consider aspects such as the source and influence of the input, and the speed of acquisition compared to other groups. In Section 3 we will consider the special features of the simultaneous combination of the two languages, code-blending, as mentioned above. Finally in Section 4 the influence of social aspects will be discussed, leading to a general summary and conclusion in Section 5.

Spoken Language Development

Children growing up bilingually can be exposed to both languages from the beginning. This is called simultaneous bilingualism or bilingual first language acquisition (2L1). One language may be introduced later than the other, resulting in sequential bilingualism as discussed in Genessee *et al.* (2004) with respect to spoken languages. The nature of the bilingualism affects the way the languages are acquired since the later a child is exposed to the second language, the more their development resembles that in second language acquisition. This is in contrast to the first language acquisition of two languages in parallel (2L1) as is found in simultaneous bilinguals (see for a discussion Meisel, 2004). Clearly there is also a gradation of exposure to the two languages so that one language may be or become more dominant than the other, even in simultaneous bilinguals (e.g. Genessee *et al.*, 1995). The preference of the child can also be a factor in determining dominance (Kasuya, 1998). Bilinguals also switch from one language to another and also mix their languages, as mentioned in the Introduction. In the case of hearing children of Deaf parents being exposed to both a spoken and signed language, all these aspects are also relevant and will be mentioned in the discussion below as appropriate. In this section we will consider the data on reported speech and language problems in this group of children. Then we will consider the various areas of spoken language acquisition and discuss the evidence for any unusual patterns of acquisition. The comparison group, as stated above, will be children who are growing up bilingual in two spoken languages.

It must be first stated that there are in fact very few studies on the spoken language acquisition of kodas. The most extensive studies are summarized in Schiff-Meyers (1993) and this will be the main source of the information presented here. Other studies are often single case studies from which no general conclusions can be drawn.

Schiff and Ventry (1976) studied 52 American-English children between the ages of six months and 12 years, coming from 34 families; they used general speech and language measures. Of these, 23 (44%) had clear problems but in 12 cases these problems could be clearly related to factors which had nothing to do with the deafness of the parents, for example, articulatory problems. The remaining 11 children came from only seven families and their language problems did not disappear once exposed to spoken language in the classroom environment. The authors tentatively suggest that an undiagnosed familial clustering of problems is responsible and that these problems are not clearly related to the quantity and/or quality of the spoken language input from the deaf parents. When the factors other than the parents' deafness were factored in, there was no significant difference between the expected proportion of speech and language problems in the population as a whole and the proportion in this group (Schiff-Meyers, 1993: 49).

There have been a few cases reported on kodas receiving very little exposure to spoken language up to the age of three (Sachs *et al.*, 1981, reported in Schiff-Meyers, 1993; Todd, 1975). As might be expected, these children did have delays in their spoken language development. Schiff-Meyers concludes from the studies in which she had been involved that normal development is possible with a minimum of five hours' exposure per week (Schiff-Meyers, 1993: 60). Although the scientific evidence is not conclusive, general findings on children bilingual in two spoken languages clearly suggest a correlation between exposure and ability. It is generally thought that exposure for less than 20% of a young child's waking time may lead to a delay in that language (Genessee, 2012).

It might be expected that the acquisition of the phonology of a spoken language may be different in some ways for kodas. Some Deaf parents do not seem to use their voice at all with their children but others do, albeit with variation. This can vary also per Deaf community; the figures for the United States appear to indicate less use of voice compared to The Netherlands, for instance (compare Petitto *et al.*, 2001 with van den Bogaerde, 2000). The hearing child is then dependent on spoken language input from other sources. There is, however, no indication in the literature that this generally affects their acquisition of spoken language phonology, as long as they are exposed to some spoken language input as discussed above.

If their parents do provide spoken language input, then that input is often phonologically different in terms of articulation of individual segments, stress patterns and intonation. In Schiff-Meyers' (1993) survey there are, however, few cases where the hearing child demonstrated a different articulation or intonation. In one case where this was reported as being quite frequent, the child in question had spent much less time with hearing speakers (Schiff-Meyers & Klein, 1985); however, Schiff-Meyers concludes in her summary that there is no strong evidence for the input being a primary factor in determining phonological ability. The same conclusion is drawn in a more recent study of three kodas by Toohey (2003).

Some hearing children will use whispering in interaction with their deaf parents, as Schiff-Meyers (1993) reports from her own studies. This was also reported in van den Bogaerde (2000) and van den Bogaerde and Baker (2008) for the three Dutch hearing children studied (Jonas, Alex and Sander). This whispering seems to reflect awareness in the child of the fact that the parent cannot hear. It is not clear whether it is an imitation of their voice behavior. Bishop and Hicks (2008) do report the use of 'deaf voice' in codas, which they define as the imitation of the speaking voice of deaf people, or lowering their voice when they took the role of a hearing person conversing with a Deaf person (Bishop & Hicks, 2008: 86). This occurred frequently when talking about themselves as a child in conversation with their parents.

Vocabulary is an area that is often reported as being affected in the non-dominant language in spoken bilinguals (Thordardottir, 2011). In her own study, Schiff-Meyers (1993: 55) found that two of the three children were well within age range on receptive vocabulary tests and all were normal on productive vocabulary. All three children had a good amount of input.

In terms of morphology and syntax, an early study by Schiff, reported in Schiff-Meyers (1993), found that the five children aged between two and three years who were exposed also to ASL were not performing statistically differently on grammatical aspects of English from hearing children in hearing families. Her analysis was done on the basis of spontaneous language samples and looked at MLU, word order, plural formation and verb inflection. It is relevant that only two of the five mothers were producing obligatory morphemes in more than 90% of the obligatory contexts. Nevertheless, the children's development did not seem to be affected. Three of the five children were later examined at age seven to eight and were found to be performing within the norms on standardized language tests. In the study by van den Bogaerde (2000: 206) the three hearing children produced a variety of word orders in their spoken Dutch, but these are typical for Dutch children in the same age range who are gradually acquiring the verb-second rule.

In terms of MLU, the three hearing Dutch children followed by van den Bogaerde (2000) had an MLU at age 3;0 that, although below the mean found for hearing children in non-deaf families, was still within the normal range of three-year-olds in Dutch. It is important to remember that this was not necessarily a reflection of their MLU when in a conversation with only hearing participants. The children were in interaction with their deaf mothers who are producing predominantly code-blended utterances. In a combination of sign and speech the MLU can be reduced, especially if the main types of blends have signed language as the Base language (see Section 3 for a fuller discussion). Other studies (Schiff-Meyers, 1993) also report a shorter MLU from hearing children in interaction with their deaf parent than when interacting with hearing adults. The Dutch deaf mothers (van den Bogaerde, 2000) also produced a low MLU in spoken language in interaction with their children at age three years, lower in fact than the MLU of their hearing children.

In some bilingual children there are reports of one language negatively affecting the other in the sense that structures from one language are then used incorrectly in the other, a phenomenon called negative transfer (Gottardo, 2008). For simultaneous bilingual children there is more evidence that the grammars are acquired independently (Paradis & Genesee, 1996). From the reports on children learning both a signed and a spoken language there is very little evidence that the children are experiencing negative transfer from the signed language (Schiff-Meyers, 1993). Negative transfer might be expected, for example, in aspects such as the omission of determiners where the spoken language has these and the sign language not, or in word order where these are different in the signed and spoken language. Mayberry (1976), describing two young children who were communicating primarily with their parents in ASL, reported that they showed no detrimental effects in their spoken English at age three.

There is, however, some evidence of transfer, but this cannot be termed negative since it does not impact on the functionality of the spoken language. Work on adult bimodal bilinguals (codas) indicates that they do use co-speech gesture differently from non-signers (Casey & Emmorey, 2008). In a task of re-telling a cartoon in English, where they were asked to speak rather than sign, codas produced more iconic gestures, more gestures from a character perspective and fewer beat gestures. The gestures also have a greater variety of handshapes than in non-signers. This all indicates the influence of ASL. It was also the case that all participants produced at least one ASL sign, displaying failure to completely inhibit their other language.

Further evidence of transfer comes from the study of Pyers and Emmorey (2008). In this study codas were asked to produce English sentences in contexts in which hypothetical clauses and questions were the targets. In such situations ASL grammar marks the structures using raised and furrowed eyebrows respectively. It was found that all 12 participants produced these facial grammatical markers while articulating the structure in English, and to a larger extent than non-signers. Complete inhibition of the second language appears therefore to be very difficult when the articulation mode does not prevent simultaneous production.

Bilinguals in interaction with other bilinguals who know the same languages commonly use a form of code switching. It is very common, for example, between Spanish and English in the southern United States or parts of South America, both in spoken and written language (Callahan, 2004), and between Dutch and French in Belgium (Treffers, 1994). Interestingly, in the latter case code-switching is decreasing due to social acceptability (Treffers-Daller, 1992). Observations have only been made of adult bimodal bilinguals to date, but these codas, in conversation among themselves, do have some special features of their speech specific to that context (Bishop & Hicks, 2008). One such feature is word reversals – for example, *King Lion* for *Lion King* or *blue and black* for *black and blue*. These orders are taken from ASL, and are generally unacceptable in English. ASL expressions can be 'translated' into English, such as *fork in the throat*, which is in fact a description of the ASL sign STUCK. Another feature is the use of their deaf parents' mispronunciations in English; for example, a vowel is inserted in *chapasticks* 'chopsticks' or in *napikin* 'napkin'. Some idiosyncratic expressions are also used such as *you call me shut up?* meaning 'did you tell me to shut up?' (Bishop & Hicks, 2008: 91). Interestingly, these are not viewed as negative by this group of codas themselves but as a way of identifying with their Deaf background (see Section 4).

In sum, the spoken language of kodas does not seem to be greatly under the influence of the signed language they are exposed to and does not indicate that they are delayed. There is evidence that a minimum exposure to a spoken language is necessary but it is not clear precisely how much this needs to be. The spoken language used by Deaf parents in their code-blending does not seem to negatively affect the children's acquisition. The spoken language acquisition of kodas appears to be under the influence of the same factors as any spoken language in bilingual acquisition.

Sign Language Development

There are few studies that have examined the sign language acquisition of hearing children in Deaf families, i.e. families where a signed language is used. The main focus has always been on the sign language acquisition of deaf children in Deaf families. Although deaf children are in the minority by far among the children born to deaf parents, they are seen as the most reliable source of information on the acquisition of a sign language.

This section will draw primarily on the data used in the study by van den Bogaerde (2000) and later papers based on the same three children mentioned in the previous section – Jonas, Alex and Sander. These children were born into families in which NGT (Sign Language of the Netherlands) was used and Dutch. In one case, the child had two deaf younger siblings, his mother was deaf and used NGT, but his father was a coda and signed and spoke in the home. The two other children both had deaf or severely hard-of-hearing parents who signed but both also had hearing siblings. In this section we will discuss what is known of the sign language acquisition of this group of children from this study and including other studies where possible. The kodas will be compared to deaf children of deaf parents.

First we would like to point out that visual attention for signed input is crucial for learning a sign language for either deaf or hearing children. Research has indicated that hearing children learn to look for input (van den Bogaerde, 2000) just as deaf children do, that is, around two years of age. A difference between the two groups of children is that the deaf mothers will also use voice to gain the attention of the hearing children, as well as visual strategies such as signing within the visual field of the child, waving the hand. Mather and Andrews (2008), after studying young children in daycare situations, indicate that some kodas grow up being so used to using such visual strategies that they apply them and expect them in all hearing environments. They will therefore sometimes fail to respond to a vocal summons. The authors state that such behaviors can lead to some misunderstandings in their hearing conversation partners since hearing adults do not know how to interpret their apparently uncooperative behavior. However, for signed language communication, hearing children of deaf parents acquire appropriate interactive visual behavior just as deaf children do, with the exception that they can also respond to sounds or spoken language.

All babies, whether deaf or hearing, generally start (0–7 months) by producing vocalizations and hand and body movements that initially have no meaning (Iverson & Goldin-Meadow, 2005). Babies, whether hearing or deaf, if exposed to a signed language, try to imitate the movements of the signs that are offered to them (babbling, from 7 to 12 months). Deaf parents also have been shown to respond to their babies' hand movements as if they were intentional communication on the part of their child (see, for an overview, Volterra & Erting, 1990). Manual babbling thus provides a motivation for both infant and parent to engage in conversations in the same way as vocal babbling does (Petitto & Marentette, 1991). In the study by van den Bogaerde (2000: 58) two of the three hearing children produced hand movements similar to babbling in the recordings up to age 2;0, even though they had already produced their first meaningful sign around 12 months. The data here were not recorded early enough, i.e. before age 1;0, to capture the real sign babbling phase.

In deaf children from deaf families the first referential signs, with truly symbolic meaning, appear around the first birthday, even though proto-productions may have been interpretable in context for the parents at an earlier age (Baker et al., 2008; Schick, 2003; see Spencer & Harris, 2006 for a review). The three kodas studied by van den Bogaerde (2000) also produced their first signs between 12 and 14 months of age, not significantly later than the deaf children in the same study. Combinations of signs, that is two-sign utterances, usually occur in deaf children around 1;6–1;11 (Bonvillian et al., 1983; Folven & Bonvillian, 1991; Pizzuto, 1990). van den Bogaerde (2000: 118) reports that combinations of NGT signs could be observed at 2;0 in two children, Jonas and Sander. Alex did not produce these, however, until age 3;0. The input also contained very few NGT utterances, that is, utterances in which there was no spoken language used. It is therefore not surprising that the MLU of the children's NGT output remained low (less than 1.4 signs up to 3;0).

Early signs usually differ phonologically from the adult forms. From previous research (e.g. Boyes Braem, 1990) a seemingly universal pattern of handshape development has emerged for deaf children, with maximally visually contrasting handshapes (e.g. fist, pointing hand and flat hand) appearing first. There has been less research on location and movement, but it appears that children substitute simple for more complex move-ments, tend to proximalize movement (e.g. Meier et al., 2008), and often exhibit perseveration. This development is predominantly directed by the development of articulatory control. There are as yet no reported findings on this aspect of sign acquisition in kodas, although Chen Pichler et al. (2010) have looked at perseveration, or in their terms, cyclicity. There seems to be no reason, however, why any different order or delayed acquisi-tion in comparison to deaf children should occur, unless insufficient input is provided.

It has been found in several sign languages that deaf children produce signed verbs between 1;6 and 1;11, but up to 3;0 no productive verb morphol-ogy appears; that is, only citation forms of verbs are used comparable to uninflected verb forms in spoken languages (Baker et al., 2008). Full acquisi-tion of verb morphology seems to take considerable time in deaf children (Newport & Meier, 1985). It has also been observed that few examples of inflection are offered in the early input (Newport & Meier, 1985; van den Bogaerde, 2000). In the NGT study, the kodas also produced mainly uninflected verbs under three years of age, as did the deaf children. Use of verb agreement starts to appear around three years of age as in deaf children, but unfortunately we have no quantitative data to chart detailed development for the kodas after three years.

In sum, there are few data on the sign language acquisition of kodas, too little to conclude whether they are different from deaf children offered a signed input. In many aspects they appear to be similar but the main difference may lie in the fact that the kodas produce above all bimodal bilingual language in contexts where signing is required, as will be discussed in the following section. In two studies reporting accuracy on a signed language task slightly lower scores are reported for adult bimodal bilinguals, codas, compared to native signers (MacSweeney et al., 2002; Neville et al., 1997). It may well be that with time the signed language will become the less dominant language. We will return to the issue of dominance in Section 4.

Bimodal Bilingual Production

As mentioned in the Introduction, a very interesting aspect of bimodal bilingual language production is that words and signs can be uttered *simultaneously*. This is of course quite different for spoken language bilinguals, who cannot produce two words from different languages at the same time. Since neither the terms code-switch nor code-mix cover the phenomenon, and the terminology is problematic anyway in the contact literature, Emmorey et al. (2005a) coined the term 'code-blend' for such simultaneous combinations of words and signs. Code-blends are thus different from code-switches and code-mixes that occur sequentially (Emmorey et al. 2005a: 665). An example of an adult coda's code-blending (ASL/English) is taken from the study by Emmorey et al. (2005a: 668, Example 6), see (1).

(1)
P2: '(he) [goes in] and [tries] [to get] [the bird] [but] [the old] [woman]
GO-IN TRY CATCH BIRD BUT OLD WOMAN
[who] [owns] [the bird] [whacks him over the head]
WHO #OWNS BIRD BEAT-OVER-HEAD_{[repeat]}
[and he falls out of the building]
Classifier construction: 'animal falls from flat surface'

According to the authors, this and other examples illustrate that the coda signer 'is skilled at ASL-English code-blending and at simultaneously producing grammatical English and ASL' (Emmorey et al., 2005a: 268).

In (1) we see that the order of words and signs are the same but that certain functional elements such as determiners and conjunctions present in the English are not present in ASL. The combinatorial possibilities in code-blending are in fact large. The basic structure of the mixed utterance can be that of the spoken language or that of the signed language, but can also be shared by the two languages as in (1). This makes it hard to establish the base language (Donati & Branchini, 2009; Lillo-Martin *et al.*, 2010; van den Bogaerde & Nortier, 2006). It has been proposed that skilled bimodal bilinguals may actually use a 'third language' (Emmorey *et al.*, 2005a: 668; Romaine, 1995), consisting of grammatical elements of both languages. This is what is called language mixing on the continuum, as discussed for spoken languages by Auer (1999) and more recently as examples for language synthesis by Lillo-Martin *et al.* (2012). This bimodal form never seems to become fixed in a fused lect, however. Bishop and Hicks (2008: 88) propose that blending words with signs is similar to the unified system of spoken language and gestures, suggesting that code-blending should also be seen as a unified system.

However, so far there is no firm evidence that *two languages* are produced at the same time. As has been shown for spoken language processing and production in bilinguals (Grosjean, 2010), both languages are activated in bimodal bilinguals (Emmorey *et al.*, 2005b). The psycholinguistic status of the combined production in code-blending is unclear, though.

The reason for examining this code-blending in kodas is that this type of language production is unique to bimodal bilinguals and may well have specific features in acquisition. To date very little is known about code-blending in children.

As we described in Section 2, the vast majority of children start communicating with gestures and communicative facial expressions before they are actually able to produce symbolic words or signs (Capirci *et al.*, 1996; Volterra & Erting, 1990). Kodas also start with vocalizations, and reaching and pointing gestures, and gradually will start to simultaneously produce, for instance, a demonstrative 'that' or a noun 'book' together with the pointing gesture, a deictic determiner. Such utterances are also produced by monolingual hearing children.

Kodas, however, also start combining lexical items from both modalities early on, that is, code-blending. It is important to note that in such code-blended utterances, voice is often used. Some kodas may, however, omit sounds in such utterances, and only mouth the words (i.e. articulate the sounds but without any voicing) while producing the sign(s). As discussed in Section 1, this appears to have little effect on their acquisition of spoken language phonology. In our own research we made no distinction between mouthed or voiced words, but other researchers, for instance Petitto *et al.* (2001), only analyze utterances as bimodal productions if voice is used.[2] This methodological decision has an impact on the amount of code-blending reported in different studies; that is, far less code-blending is reported in deaf children since they tend to use less voice.

The code-blends were categorized in our studies into four types, on the basis of the semantics of the utterances (van den Bogaerde & Baker, 2008: 108). Using semantics is common in work on code-mixing in spoken languages; there the notion of semantic congruence is often used (Muysken, 2000). In these studies, the proposition is crucial in determining the *base language* (BL) (Baker & van den Bogaerde, 2006; Bishop, 2006, for adult codas; van den Bogaerde, 2000: 108; van den Bogaerde & Baker, 2008).

The four types of code-blending are:

(a) Code-blended Dutch Base Language (Dutch BL), e.g.
    spoken   where is the horse¿
    signed   HORSE¿
    Translation   'Where is the horse¿'
(b) Code-blended NGT Base Language (NGT BL), e.g.
    spoken   outside
    signed   BICYCLE RED OUTSIDE
    Translation   'The red bicycle is outside.'
(c) Code-blended Mixed, e.g.
    spoken   big
    signed   HORSE
    Translation   'a big horse'
(d) Code-blended Full, e.g.
    spoken   that is a horse
    signed $POINT_{to-horse}$ HORSE
    Translation   'That is a horse.'

Code-blended utterances of these four types were found in the input of the three deaf mothers to the kodas prior to three years of age (van den Bogaerde & Baker, 2008: 113). In fact the bulk of their utterances are code-blended. Two of the three children, Jonas and Alex, also produce some code-blends but Alex does not until age 3;0. This may have to do with his slower development in NGT as mentioned in Section 2.

At ages 3;0 and 6;0 (Figures 9.1 and 9.2, respectively), we see that there is considerable variation between the three kodas studied and their deaf mothers. At age 3;0 there were NGT utterances, Dutch utterances and code-blends in the input, code-blended utterances forming the largest proportion of the input for Sander and Alex, but slightly less for Jonas. The kodas produce 30–40% code-blends at this age, Jonas the least. At age 6;0 all three kodas show an increase in code-blends (Figure 9.2). This goes together with a decrease in Dutch utterances and an increase in NGT. The input also shows the same tendency. The ability to produce code-blending may be related to an increasing ability in the signed language, or the influence of the input, or both.

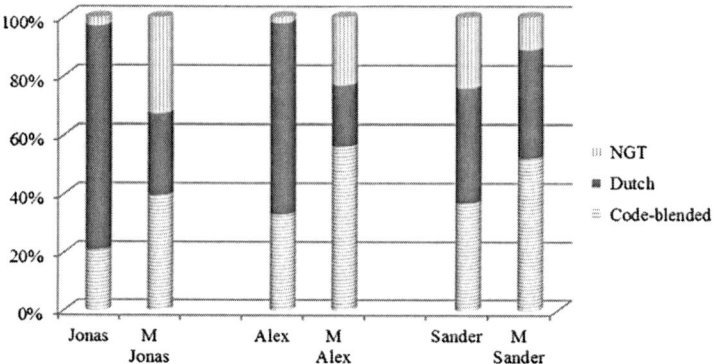

Figure 9.1 The types of languages produced by the hearing children and their deaf mothers (input) at age 3;0

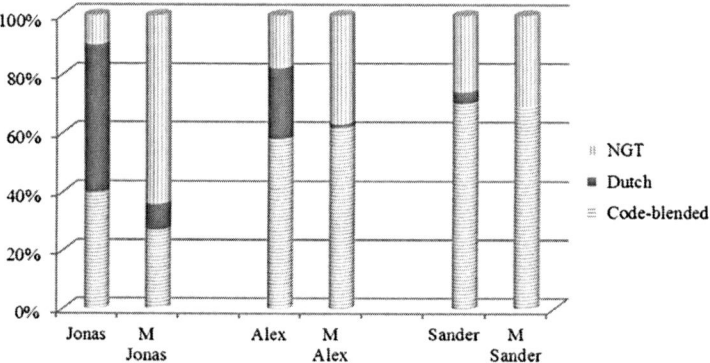

Figure 9.2 The types of languages produced by the hearing children and their deaf mothers (input) at age 6;0

There was a considerable difference in code-blending between the kodas and the deaf children in our study. At age 3;0 the kodas use far more code-blending with their mothers than the deaf children, although in the input we find very similar amounts of code-blends (Baker & van den Bogaerde, 2008: 10).

In sum, our studies show that all three Dutch deaf mothers used code-blends in the interaction with their hearing children at all ages, but it must be remembered that this is using our definition, including utterances both with and without voice. That deaf mothers all use code-blending may very well be the case in other countries, but there is scarcely any literature on this aspect.

When we further analyzed the blended input using the four categories described above, differences in the quality of the input to the kodas and the deaf children became clearly apparent. These differences were also reflected in the output of the three kodas. At a young age (one to two years) many Full blends were offered but these decreased over time. The Full blends consisted usually of short, simple utterances. At age three the three kodas were being offered more Full-blended utterances (around 40%) than the deaf children (Baker & van den Bogaerde, 2008: 14–16). Quite long utterances can be Full-blends. Jonas' mother produced a four-word/sign utterance with him at age 6;0:

spoken	police	motorbike	can	too
signed	POLICE MOTORBIKE CAN TOO			
Translation	'A police motorbike is also possible.'			

On the other hand, at age 3;0 the input contained far fewer code-blended NGT BL utterances: 6–20%, compared to more than 60% offered to the deaf children. The categories Dutch Base Language and Mixed were also well represented in the input to the kodas, whereas they were quite infrequent for the deaf children. Overall this suggests a more Dutch-influenced input offered to the kodas.

The kodas also used all four types of code-blending but produced more Dutch BL than their mothers and slightly more Mixed blends such as Jonas' utterance:

spoken	blue jacket, blue
signed	COLOUR
Translation	'The color of the jacket is blue.'

Their NGT BL utterances were less frequent, although they did occur, such as from Alex at age 6;0:

spoken	face		trousers	shoes	gloves
signed	FACE CLOTHES TROUSERS INDEXshoes GLOVES			
Translation	[I see:] 'A face, and clothes, like trousers, shoes, gloves.'			

There were some individual differences between the three children, with the mother of Sander producing fewer NGT BL utterances and more Mixed than the other two mothers; this was also reflected in Sander's output.

The kodas changed language modes casually and naturally, as did the deaf mothers. The interaction is smooth. Interestingly, our data show that the different language choices and the different types of code-blending occurred all within the same period of interaction. The fact that the kodas used a considerable amount of Dutch and Dutch BL code-blends, that is, utterances that do not provide the full proposition in signs, did not seem to lead to many misunderstandings. The mothers seemed to be good at speech-reading in this context. It was, however, clear that the kodas could adapt their language choice to the conversation partner, since from observation in interaction with only a hearing adult they used predominantly spoken Dutch.

Griffith (1990) also described the natural way of mode-finding behavior of a young child, David, who switches between speaking, signing or code-blended output at ages 1;7–1;9, to match the mode most frequently used by his conversational partner of the moment (Griffith, 1990: 241). At 20 months he was quite skillful at applying the 'person-to-language' principle even with strangers. This behavior is also described by Mallory *et al.* (1993). Language choice according to conversation partner and situation is a typical development of all bilingual children (Genesee, 2006), and the kodas fit into this pattern.

In adult discourse, bimodal bilinguals or codas also use the four types of code-blended utterance described above. Bishop and Hicks (2008) studied the natural bimodal interaction of codas in interaction with each other ($n = 19$). They found 59% English Base Language, 7% ASL Base Language, 28% Full and 6% Mixed. Compared to the Dutch child kodas at 6;0 reported above, the adult codas had far more code-blending based on the spoken language. It is highly likely that this difference has primarily to do with the hearing status of the conversational partners. In interaction with a deaf conversational partner kodas and codas will probably choose fewer spoken language-based blends, but this has as yet not been studied.

An intriguing aspect of code-blending that emerges from our own studies is that the complexity of the code-blends in terms of MLU is greater than in Dutch-only utterances (see Table 9.1). This is true of both the input to the kodas and the kodas' own production with their mothers. For an extensive description of how we calculated MLU for blended utterances, see van den Bogaerde (2000: 168, 286–289), but in short we divided the number of words/signs by the number of utterances. Signs and words that occurred simultaneously were counted in two ways. If the semantic content of the sign and the word was the same (e.g. HOUSE + house) the combination is counted as one element; if the content was not the same (e.g. HOUSE + big),

Table 9.1 Overview of MLU in Dutch and code-blends, averaged across the three deaf mothers and three kodas at ages 3;0 and 6;0

	MLU Dutch	MLU Code-blended
3 Deaf mothers at 3;0	1.83	3.13
3 Deaf mothers at 6;0	–[a]	3.47
3 Kodas at 3;0	1.76	3.30
3 Kodas at 6;0	2.63	3.77

Notes: [a]Mother Jonas 1;7; Mother Alex only 1 utt; Mother Sander none.

the sign and the word were counted separately, thus counting as two elements in that sentence.

The MLU of code blends in the input was at least 2.7 at 3;0 with a maximum of 4.07 at 6;0 (van den Bogaerde & Baker, 2008: 121). In the kodas' own production the MLU was 2.7 at 3;0 with a maximum of 4.2. At age 6;0 the three kodas differed considerably: in the code-blends Alex's MLU was 2.04, compared to 4.5 and 4.76 in Jonas and Sander respectively. The higher MLU of the kodas in code-blends is mainly due to a longer MLU of the word parts (van den Bogaerde & Baker, 2008: 121–122). It is not the case that the category Mixed-blends causes this longer MLU in the code-blends. The Dutch utterances contain a fair number of short elliptical utterances such as *in there* or *don't know*. It might be the case that the children judge their mothers' lip-reading skills as good enough so that they can understand these less complex utterances without any signing.

In sum, the kodas in our studies produce a considerable amount of code-blended utterances and these are predominantly Dutch Base Language. This suggests a dominance of the spoken language for this group of bilinguals (see Section 4). There are so few data on kodas, however, that it is difficult to draw general conclusions, but since kodas increasingly have to function in a hearing world as they move through schooling and then into work, it may well be the case that the spoken language becomes dominant.

Social Attitudes

As stated at the end of Section 2, for kodas the signed language is liable to become the non-dominant language, as is the case for all minority languages with low status in bilingual children. This can occur not only because signing is commonly not used in regular schools and the hearing society, but also because social attitudes and peer pressure can exert influence on the developing child. Wilhelm (2008: 169), for instance, reports on a coda who, out of shame, kept her Deaf parents a secret while growing up.

If we reconsider Figures 9.1 and 9.2 from Section 3, we see that one child from our own studies, Sander, is behaving slightly differently from the other two Dutch kodas since he consistently has the fewest Dutch utterances and the most NGT utterances of the three. The input to the children cannot be the reason for this. Sander's family in fact contained many Deaf members, providing him with a Deaf environment in his early years. This influenced not only his language development but also his cultural and social identity development (see van den Bogaerde & Baker, 2008: 126). He was strongly oriented towards the Deaf community and his linguistic and cultural attitude as expressed when he was approximately 16 years old reflected this identity. He wrote: 'When I was small I started out with signing, it was so normal for me. And now, still, signing comes very natural to me. I know no better than that NGT is my second mother tongue.' The other two kodas showed a less strong identification with the Deaf community.

This variation in attitude is noticeable in the literature on codas. Napier (2008: 220) describes herself as a 'double A'[3] bilingual interpreter, using the terminology of Pöchhacker (2004: 114), since she has native-like proficiency in both BSL and English. In fact she is a multilingual, since she speaks several other languages, and considers herself a polyglot (Napier, 2008: 221). She has a strong association with the deaf community.

Shield (2004), on the other hand, posits that being raised in a Deaf family is no guarantee that you are raised bilingually or biculturally. Wilhelm (2008) provides some examples of kodas who have faced serious communication challenges with their Deaf parents (Wilhelm, 2008: 185). On the basis of interviews she concludes that communication problems in the form of language barriers are common. There can be lack of competence in the sign language (German Sign Language: DGS) and asymmetric language use in the family, with the Deaf parents using DGS and the children predominantly German. Furthermore, she claims that Deaf parents may have information deficits and that:

> familial misunderstandings follow partially from the behavior of Deaf parents who have internalized the majority of negative attitudes toward Deaf people and sign language. They try to integrate their hearing children into the hearing world and prevent them from fully acquiring the stigmatized culture and language of Deaf people. (Wilhelm, 2008: 186)

Even when this is not the case, kodas are aware of their bicultural heritage and the gap that exists between a deaf and a hearing member of the Deaf community. This is confirmed by Napier (2008), who trained and works, among other things, as an interpreter. She formulates this as follows:

> I grew up as a member of the deaf community, enculturated to the deaf way of life, and I am a person whose first (and sometimes preferred) language is a signed language. When I am with deaf people, I behave as they do, use the language they do, and share their beliefs. But ultimately, I am not deaf or Deaf. I do not have the majority of the (positive or negative) shared experiences that most deaf people have – in relation to education, access, communication, discrimination etc. Although I could be considered a member of the deaf community, do I really belong? (Napier, 2008: 228)

She concludes that she does not relate to the coda identity. She does not partake in coda activities and prefers the term HMFD (Hearing, Mother Father Deaf) to describe herself (Napier, 2008: 232).

Her story is corroborated by Hoffmeister, who wrote about the 'One Generation Thick' phenomenon. He explains (Hoffmeister, 2008: 212):

[...] Probably 90 percent of all children of Deaf people are hearing. And coda children tend to be Hearing.[4] Codas grow up and marry hearing people, have hearing kids, and lose the connection to the Deaf community [...].

This implies that there is usually only one generation of codas, since codas typically go on to have hearing children who do not learn the sign language. Hoffmeister compares this process to bicultural immigrant people, where it typically takes three generations to become fully acculturated (Hoffmeister, 2008: 191). He states 'In the Deaf world for many codas it is completed in one generation'. Going back to the three Dutch kodas, and Sander in particular, we see that he is a third-generation koda: his parents and grandparents were deaf, and he has several deaf uncles and aunts. Hoffmeister also says that usually firstborn kodas learn the sign language, whereas the rest of the siblings may learn some sign language but are not always fluent (Hoffmeister, 2008: 192). This may be important for the two other children in our study: Jonas as the oldest of three children became reasonably fluent but was more oriented towards Dutch (Baker & van den Bogaerde, 2008: 124). The number of Deaf relatives is the same for Jonas as for Sander, except that Jonas is a second-generation koda: his father is also a coda. Alex, who showed the least proficiency in sign language, is a third child, with two older siblings, and no deaf relatives besides his parents. This fits the pattern Hoffmeister described.

The number of 'borders' one has to cross as a koda obviously is related to the 'deafness' of the family, or the degree of 'Deafhood', as Ladd (2003) calls it. Adams (2008) distinguishes four types of kodas, viz. koda as a misfit, as foreigner, as middleman or go-between, and a fourth category 'glass-ceiling'; these categories are not mutually exclusive. The codas as 'misfits' are 'aware early on that they are not the same as everyone else. In contrast, when they are young, they do feel they fit in at home. As they get older, they fit in less in both Deaf and hearing situations' (Adams, 2008: 272). Codas as 'foreigners' feel different from other Hearing people, that is, as if they are a foreigner in another country (Adams, 2008: 280). 'Middleman' codas feel like a go-between between the Deaf world of their parents and the Hearing world they live in (Adams, 2008: 281). The glass ceiling metaphor is used for the idea that there is a glass ceiling preventing codas from progressing beyond a certain point, consisting of preconceived views of what a hearing child born to Deaf parents might become as an adult (Adams, 2008: 282). Adams believes that 'the four categories [...] confirm codas' status as a separate and autonomous group with an identity of its own beyond their position as members of both Deaf and hearing culture' (Adams, 2008: 289).

Kodas do not feel the same as others in the hearing world and, while wanting to belong, experience a gap between themselves and both the Deaf world and the hearing (misfit). They balance on the borders between deaf and hearing, and are often the 'middleman' between the Deaf world of their parents and the Hearing world they also live in (Adams, 2008: 281). Many kodas feel that both deaf and hearing people have specific expectations of them, for example to function as communication support workers, or interpreters, and to be gatekeepers, which sometimes inhibited their ambitions for possible careers (glass ceiling; Adams, 2008: 282). The attitude taken towards the use of sign language and spoken language with hearing children, and the degree of enculturation in both the Deaf and the Hearing culture play an important role in the choices that are made in raising kodas. Wilhelm (2008), for instance, explains the use of code-blending as follows:

> Some [Deaf] parents choose to communicate using a mixture of spoken language and sign language, instead of using merely sign language with their own child. This is especially true for Deaf parents of hearing children who must feel under pressure to provide their children with a linguistic model that is as much adapted as possible to the spoken language of the society's majority to which hearing children also belong. (Wilhelm, 2008: 168–169).

Like Hoffmeister (2008), she compares such an attitude to the attitudes in bilingual migrant families. It must be pointed out here that it appears that all Deaf parents studied thus far use a mixture of spoken language and sign language both with their deaf children and their hearing children (see Section 3), so that it is the question whether this is a really a choice that is consciously made.

Singleton and Tittle (2000) end their review article with a list of recommendations for the support of kodas. All of these recommendations focus on the social situation, the importance of developing a good sense of identity in the two cultures and the importance of good communication between parents and children. All these recommendations are in fact equally applicable to children growing up with two spoken languages.

In sum, we find that the degree to which kodas become bimodal bilingual and bicultural is shaped by many external (society) and internal (family) factors, comparable to the way hearing children may or may not become bilingual and bicultural in (unimodal) spoken languages. Language choice in the family, the frequency and quality of input of either language, the social settings in which the languages are encountered and the status of the languages all play a role in the linguistic, social, emotional and cultural development of kodas.

Discussion and Conclusions

As became clear in the previous section, being bilingual does not mean that an individual functions as a monolingual but in two languages. There is clearly a great deal of variation within the group of bimodal bilinguals related to the identification with the linguistic and cultural community and these in turn related to the dominance of the spoken language.

It must be pointed out that bimodal bilinguals are not the same neuro-linguistically as deaf native signers. Evidence shows that whereas in deaf native signers areas of the brain have been recruited for visual processing, this does not happen for codas since they are exposed to auditory information (e.g. MacSweeney et al., 2002: 1588). Deaf signers are thus better than codas at paying visual attention to the periphery (Bavelier et al., 2001), in haptic orientation processing ability (Van Dijk et al., 2012), and recognition of facial expressions (Emmorey & McCullough, 2008).

Bimodal bilinguals are in fact similar to unimodal bilinguals in many respects. They can learn their two languages to a very high level, but this is dependent on the input and exposure they get to both, as the discussion in Sections 1 and 2 showed. Just as bilinguals in two spoken languages they will suffer more from the tip-of-the tongue phenomenon (TOT) than mono-linguals (Pyers et al., 2009). This is due to the competing lexicons, even though for bimodal bilinguals the two lexicons are in different modalities.

On the other hand, bimodal bilinguals are also different from unimodal bilinguals. Learning a sign language has an effect on some non-linguistic skills. Thus codas, together with deaf signers, are better than non-signers at generating and transforming mental images (Emmorey et al., 1993), and com-pleting spatial arrays (Keehner & Gathercole, 2007). However, the advantage that unimodal bilinguals have been reported to have in cognitive control (e.g. Bialystok, 2001; Bialystok et al., 2004; Carlson & Meltzoff, 2008) has not been found in bimodal bilinguals (Emmorey et al., 2008). The explanation offered is that unimodal bilinguals have practice in inhibiting the other lan-guage, whereas bimodal bilinguals have far less, since the modalities allow simultaneous production.

The bimodal bilingual circumstances that many kodas are raised in pro-vide a very special linguistic environment, in which they acquire the spoken language of the majority of their community as well as the signed language used by their parent(s). The acquisition of the two languages as first lan-guages does not necessarily pose any problems. The aspects that are different for kodas have to do with bilingualism. The input in both languages must be sufficient and have native-like quality for it to be possible for full acquisition to take place. Being bilingual and bimodal also means that interesting forms of code-mixing are used.

Even being provided with enough input in two languages does not always imply that a child will become fully bilingual. Social and psycho-logical factors also play a role; identification with the language group is an important prerequisite. Such factors determine to what extent a koda will acquire and use the spoken and signed languages, and to what extent s/he may feel free and able to use the two languages and combine them. Being raised in a Deaf family also means that kodas are raised in two cultures, viz. the Deaf culture at home and the Hearing culture 'outside'. How they cross this border and to what extent they identify with their two worlds and can move to and fro between them is highly individual and needs further study.

Notes

(1) In earlier literature, kodas are also called codas (children of deaf adults). Here we will systematically refer to kodas when referring to children in development. Where we are talking about adults, we will use the term codas.
(2) For the role of mouthed words in different sign languages, see Boyes Braem and Sutton-Spence (2001).
(3) Pöchhacker (2004: 21) defines A-languages as 'native or best active language'.
(4) Hoffmeister explains the use of Hearing (capital H) as follows: 'I use the capitalized version of *Deaf* for all Deaf people who identify themselves as being Deaf, which makes them a member of the culture. I capitalize Hearing because this is the cultural contrast group. [...] Codas [...] do not have a hearing loss; however, I would not include them as part of Hearing' (Hoffmeister, 2008: 213, his endnote 1).

References

Adams, S. (2008) Characteristics of the coda-experience in the 21st century. In M. Bishop and S.L. Hicks (eds) *Hearing Mother, Father Deaf: Hearing People in Deaf Families* (pp. 261–292). Washington, DC: Gallaudet University Press.

Auer, P. (1999) From code-switching via language mixing to fused lects: Towards a dynamic typology of bilingual speech. *International Journal of Bilingualism* 3 (4), 309–332.

Baker A. and Van den Bogaerde B. (2008) Codemixing in signs and words in input to and output from children. In C. Plaza-Pust and E. Morales López (eds) *Sign Bilingualism: Language Development, Interaction, and Maintenance in Sign Language Contact Situations* (pp. 1–27). Amsterdam: John Benjamins.

Bavelier, D., Brozinsky, C., Tomann, A., Mitchell, T., Neville, H. and Liu G. (2001) Impact of early deafness and early exposure to sign language on the cerebral organization for motion processing. *Journal of Neuroscience* 21, 8931–8942.

Bialystok, E. (2001) *Bilingualism in Development: Language, Literacy, and Cognition.* Cambridge: Cambridge University Press.

Bialystok, E., Craik, F.I.M., Klein, R. and Viswanathan, M. (2004) Bilingualism, aging, and cognitive control: Evidence from the Simon task. *Psychology and Aging* 19 (2), 290–303.

Bishop, M. (2006) Bimodal bilingualism in hearing native signers. Unpublished dissertation, Gallaudet University.

Bishop, M. and Hicks, S.L. (2008) Coda talk: Bimodal discourse among hearing native signers. In M. Bishop and S.L. Hicks (eds) *Hearing Mother, Father Deaf: Hearing People in Deaf Families* (pp. 54–99). Washington, DC: Gallaudet University Press.

Bonvillian, J.D., Orlansky, M.D. and Novack, L.L. (1983) Developmental milestones: Sign language acquisition and motor development. *Child Development* 54, 1435–1445.

Boyes Braem, P. (1990) Acquisition of the handshape in American Sign Language: A preliminary analysis. In V. Volterra and C.J. Erting (eds) *From Gesture to Language in Deaf and Hearing Children* (pp. 107–127). Berlin: Springer Verlag.

Boyes Braem, P. and Sutton-Spence, R. (2001) *The Hands are the Head of the Mouth. The Mouth as Articulator in Sign Languages.* Seedorf: Signum-Verlag.

Callahan, L. (2004) *Spanish/English Codeswitching in a Written Corpus.* Amsterdam: John Benjamins.

Capirci, O., Iverson, J.M., Pizzuto, E. and Volterra, V. (1996) Gestures and words during the transition to two-word speech. *Journal of Child Language* 23, 645–673.

Carlson, S.M. and Meltzoff, A.N. (2008) Bilingual experience and executive functioning in young children. *Developmental Science* 11 (2), 282–298.

Casey, S. and Emmorey, K.E. (2008) Cospeech gesture in bimodal bilinguals. *Language and Cognitive Processing* 24 (2), 290–312.

Chen Pichler, D., Quadros, R.M. and Lillo-Martin, D. (2010) Effects of bimodal production on multi-cyclicity in early ASL and LSB. *Supplement to the Proceedings of the 34th Boston University Conference on Language Development (BUCL).* Somerville, MA: Cascadilla Press.

Donati, C. and Branchini, C. (2009) Simultaneous Grammars: Two Word Orders but only One Morphology. Paper presented at the 21st European Summer School in Logic, Language and Information. Bordeaux, France, July 20–31.

Emmorey, K. (2002) *Language, Cognition, and the Brain. Insights from Sign Language Research.* Mahwah, NJ: Lawrence Erlbaum.

Emmorey, K. and McCullough, S. (2008) The bimodal bilingual brain: Effects of sign language experience. *Brain and Language,* doi:10.1016/j.bandl.2008.03.005.

Emmorey,. K., Kosslyn, S.M. and Bellugi, U. (1993) Visual imagery and visual-spatial language: Enhanced imagery abilities in deaf and hearing ASL signers. *Cognition* 46, 139–181.

Emmorey K., Borinstein H. and Thompson R. (2005a) Bimodal bilingualism: Code-blending between spoken English and American Sign Language. In J. Cohen, K.T. McAlister, K. Rolstad and J. MacSwan (eds) *Proceedings of the 4th International Symposium on Bilingualism* (pp. 663–374). Somerville, MA: Cascadilla Press.

Emmorey, K., Grabowski, T., McCullough, S.M., Ponto, L.L., Hichwa, R.D. and Damasio, H. (2005b) Neural correlates of spatial language in English and American Sign Language. A PET study with hearing bilinguals. *NeuroImage* 24 (3), 832–840.

Emmorey, K., Luk, G., Pyers, J.E. and Bialystok, E. (2008) The source of enhanced cognitive control in bilinguals: Evidence from bimodal bilinguals. *Psychology of Science* 19 (12), 1201–1206.

Folven, R.J. and Bonvillian, J. (1991) The transition from nonreferential to referential language in children acquiring American Sign Language. *Developmental Psychology* 27 (5), 806–816.

Genesee, F. (2006) Bilingual first language acquisition in perspective. In P. McCardle and E. Hoff (eds) *Childhood Bilingualism: Research on Infancy through School Age* (pp. 45–67). Clevedon: Multilingual Matters.

Genesee, F. (2012) Simultaneous bilingual acquisition. *Encyclopedia of Language and Literacy Development* (online publication). See http://literacyencyclopedia.ca/index.php?fa=items.show&topicId=305.

Genessee, F., Nicoladis, E. and Paradis, J. (1995) Language differentiation in early bilingual development. *Journal of Child Language* 22, 611–631.

Genessee, F., Paradis, J. and Crago, M. (2004) *Dual Language Development and Disorders: A Handbook of Bilingualism and Second Language Learning.* Baltimore, MD: Brookes.

Gottardo, A. (2008) Defining bilingualism. *Encyclopedia of Language and Literacy Development* (online publication). See http://literacyencyclopedia.ca/index.php?fa=items.show&topicId=236.

Griffith, P.L. (1990) Emergence of mode-finding and mode-switching in a hearing child of deaf parents. In V. Volterra and C.J. Erting (eds) *From Gesture to Language in Hearing and Deaf Children* (2nd edn) (pp. 223–245). Washington, DC: Gallaudet University Press.

Grosjean, F. (2010) *Bilingual. Life and Reality.* Cambridge, MA and London: Harvard University Press.

Hoffmeister, R. (2008) Border crossings by hearing children of deaf parents: the lost history of codas. In H-Dirksen L. Bauman (ed.) *Open Your Eyes: Deaf Studies Talking* (pp. 88–215). Minneapolis, MN: University of Minnesota Press.

Iverson, J. and Goldin Meadow, S. (2005) Gesture paves the way for language development. *Psychological Science* 16 (5), 367–371.

Keehner, M. and Gathercole, S.E. (2007) Cognitive adaptations arising from nonnative experience of sign language in hearing adults. *Memory & Cognition* 35 (4), 752–761.

Kasuya, H. (1998) Determinants of language choice in bilingual children: The role of input. *International Journal of Bilingualism* 2, 327–346.

Ladd, P. (2003) *Understanding Deaf Culture: In Search of Deafhood.* Clevedon: Multilingual Matters.

Lillo-Martin, D., Müller de Quadros, R., Koulidobrova, H. and Chen Pichler, D. (2010) Bimodal bilingual cross-language influence in unexpected domains. In J. Costa, A. Lobo and F. Pratas (eds) *Language Acquisition and Development: Proceedings of GALA 2009.* Newcastle: Cambridge Scholars Publishing.

Lillo-Martin, D., Müller de Quadros, R., Koulidobrova, H. and Chen Pichler, D. (2012) Bilingual language synthesis: Evidence from WH-questions in bimodal bilinguals. In A.K. Biller, E.Y. Chung and A.E. Kimball (eds) *Proceedings of the 36th Annual Boston University Conference on Language Development* (pp. 302–314). Somerville, MA: Cascadilla Press.

MacSweeney, M., Woll, B., Campbell R., *et al.* (2002) Neural systems underlying British Sign Language and audio-visual processing in native users. *Brain* 125, 1583–1593.

Mallory, B.L., Zingle, H.W. and Schein, J.D. (1993) Intergenerational communication modes in Deaf-parented families. *Sign Language Studies* 78, 73–92.

Mather, S.M. and Andrews, J.F. (2008) Eyes over ears: The development of visual strategies by hearing children of deaf parents. In M. Bishop and S.L. Hicks (eds) *Hearing Mother, Father Deaf: Hearing People in Deaf Families* (pp. 132–161). Washington, DC: Gallaudet University Press.

Mayberry, R. (1976) An assessment of some oral and manual skills of hearing children of deaf parents. *American Annals of the Deaf* 121, 507–512.

Meier, R.P., Mauk, C.E., Cheek, A. and Moreland, C.J. (2008) The form of children's early signs: Iconic or motoric determinants? *Language Learning and Development* 4 (1), 1–36.

Meisel, J. (2004) The bilingual child. In T.K. Bhatia and W.C. Ritchie (eds) *The Handbook of Bilingualism* (pp. 91–113). Oxford: Blackwell.

Muysken, P. (2000) *Bilingual Speech: A Typology of Code Mixing.* Cambridge: Cambridge University Press.

Napier, J. (2008) Exploring linguistic and cultural identity: My personal experience. In M. Bishop and S.L. Hicks (eds) *Hearing Mother, Father Deaf: Hearing People in Deaf Families* (pp. 219–243). Washington, DC: Gallaudet University Press.

Neville, H.J., Coffey, S.A. and Lawson, D.S., *et al.* (1997) Neural systems mediating American Sign Language. *Brain and Language* 57, 285–308.

Newport, E. and Meier, R. (1985) The acquisition of American Sign Language. In D.I. Slobin (ed.) *The Crosslinguistic Study of Language Acquisition, Vol. 1: The Data* (pp. 881–998). Hillsdale, NJ: Lawrence Erlbaum.

Paradis, J. and Genessee, F. (1996) Syntactic acquisition in bilingual children. Autonomous or interdependent? *Studies in Second Language Acquisition* 18, 1–25.

Petitto, L.A. and Marentette, P.F. (1991) Babbling in the manual mode: Evidence for the ontogeny of language. *Science* 251, 1493–1496.

Petitto, L.A., Katerelos M., Levy B.G., Gauna K., Tetreault, K. and Ferraro V. (2001) Bilingual signed and spoken language acquisition from birth: Implications for the mechanisms underlying early bilingual language acquisition. *Journal of Child Language* 28 (2), 453–496.

Pizzuto, E. (1990) The early development of deixis in American Sign Language: What is the point? In V. Volterra and C.J. Erting (eds) *From Gesture to Language in Hearing and Deaf Children* (pp. 142–161). New York, Springer-Verlag.

Pöchhacker, F. (2004) *Introducing Interpreting Studies.* London: Routledge.

Preston, P.M. (1994) *Mother, Father Deaf. Living Between Sound and Silence.* Cambridge, MA: Harvard University Press.

Preston, P.M. (1995) Mother, father deaf: The heritage of difference. *Social Science & Medicine* 40 (1 I), 461–1467.

Prinz, P. and Prinz, E. (1979) Acquisition of ASL and spoken English by a hearing child of a deaf mother and a hearing father: Phase I. Early lexical development. *Papers and Reports on Child Language Development* 17, 139–146.

Prinz, P. and Prinz, E. (1981) Acquisition of ASL and spoken English by a hearing child of a deaf mothers and a hearing father: Phase II. Early combinatorial patterns. *Sign Language Studies* 30, 78–88.

Pyers, J.E. and Emmorey, K. (2008) The face of bimodal bilingualism: ASL grammatical markers are produced when bilinguals speak to English monolinguals. In M. Bishop and S.L. Hicks (eds) *Hearing Mother, Father Deaf: Hearing People in Deaf Families* (pp. 44–53). Washington, DC: Gallaudet University Press.

Pyers, P.E., Gollan, T.H. and Emmorey, K. (2009) Bimodal bilinguals reveal the source of Tip-of-the-Tongue. *Cognition* 112 (2), 323–329.

Romaine, S. (1995) *Bilingualism* (2nd edn). Oxford: Blackwell.

Schick, B. (2003) The development of American Sign Language and manually coded English systems. In M. Marschark and P.E. Spencer (eds) *Deaf Studies, Language, and Education* (pp. 219–231). Oxford: Oxford University Press.

Schiff-Meyers, N. (1993) Hearing children of deaf parents. In D. Bishop and K. Mogford (eds) *Language Development in Exceptional Circumstances* (2nd edn) (pp. 47–61). Hillsdale, NJ: Lawrence Erlbaum.

Schiff-Meyers, N. and Klein, H.B. (1985) Some phonological characteristics of the speech of normal-hearing children of deaf parents. *Journal of Speech and Hearing Research* 28, 466–474.

Schiff, N. and Ventry, I. (1979) Communication problems in hearing children of deaf parents. *Journal of Speech and Hearing Disorders* 41, 348–358.

Shield, A. (2004) Ideological conflict at group boundaries: The hearing children of deaf adults. Manuscript from University of Texas at Austin. See http://studentorgs.utexas.edu/salsa/proceedings/2004/Shield.pdf.

Singleton, J.L. and Tittle, M.D. (2000) Deaf parents and their hearing children. *Journal of Deaf Studies and Deaf Education* 5 (3), 221–235.

Spencer, P.E. and Harris, M. (2006) Patterns and effects of language input to deaf infants and toddlers from deaf and hearing mothers. In B. Schick, M. Marschark and P.E. Spencer (eds) *Advances in the Sign Language Development of Deaf Children* (pp. 71–101). Oxford: Oxford University Press.

Thordardottir, E. (2011) The relationship between bilingual exposure and vocabulary development. *International Journal of Bilingualism* 15 (4), 426–445.

Todd, P.H. (1975) A case of structural interference across sensory modalities in second language learning. *Word* 27, 102–118.

Toohey, E.N. (2003) Phonological development in hearing children of deaf parents. Honors scholar thesis, University of Connecticut.

Treffers, J. (1994) *Mixing Two Languages: French–Dutch Contact in a Comparative Perspective.* Amsterdam: de Gruyter.

Treffers-Daller, J. (1992) French–Dutch codeswitching in Brussels: Social factors explaining its disappearance. *Journal of Multilingual and Multicultural Development* 13 (1–2), 143–156.

van den Bogaerde, B. (2000) Input and interaction in deaf families. PhD dissertation, University of Amsterdam. LOT series No. 35. Utrecht: LOT.

van den Bogaerde, B. and Baker, A.E. (2008) Bimodal language acquisition in Kodas. In M. Bishop and S.L. Hicks (eds) *Hearing Mother, Father Deaf: Hearing People in Deaf Families* (pp. 99–131). Washington, DC: Gallaudet University Press.

van den Bogaerde, B. and Nortier, J. (2006) Bimodaal codewisselen: Simultaan spreken en gebaren [Bimodal codeswitching: Simultaneously speaking and signing]. *Toegepaste Taalwetenschap in Artikelen* 75 (1), 79–88.

Van Dijk, R, Kapper, M. and Postma, A. (2012) Superior spatial touch: Improved haptic orientation processing in deaf individuals (doctoral dissertation). In R. Van Dijk (ed.) *Cognitive Perspectives on Deafness* (pp. 49–59). Baarn: De Weijer.

Volterra, V. and Erting, C.J. (1990) *From Gesture to Language in Hearing and Deaf Children.* Berlin: Springer Verlag.

Wilhelm, A. (2008) Aspects of the communication between hearing children and deaf parents. In M. Bishop and S.L. Hicks (eds) *Hearing Mother, Father Deaf: Hearing People in Deaf Families* (pp. 162–196). Washington, DC: Gallaudet University Press.

10 Language Development in ASL–English Bimodal Bilinguals

Deborah Chen Pichler, James Lee and Diane Lillo-Martin

Introduction

Recently, simultaneous bilingualism has enjoyed a surge in public interest, as researchers uncover unsuspected cognitive benefits associated with knowledge of two languages (Bialystock *et al.*, 2009). At the same time, bilingualism continues to be regarded with suspicion by many, as a perturbation of 'normal' language development that leads to 'language handicap' and delays, particularly for school-aged children (Darcy, 1953; Rossell & Baker, 1996). This is particularly true with respect to the simultaneous acquisition of one sign language and one spoken language, which we will refer to as *bimodal bilingualism* (Emmorey *et al.*, 2008). In this chapter, we will focus our discussion on hearing children of deaf parents, also known as *codas* or *kodas* (the latter term used specifically for young coda children). These children have often been diagnosed as language delayed or disordered, due to deviations in their development of spoken English with respect to their monolingual hearing peers. At the same time, there is a widespread view that kodas' ASL development is often weak compared to that of Deaf children. Yet we argue that, as bilinguals, kodas can be expected to display different developmental patterns from those of their typical comparison groups, due to influence from their other language. This is the usual situation for bilinguals, whether children or adults – both languages are mentally active and interactions between the languages are to be expected. Such interactions are more a sign of language skill than language problems (e.g. Poplack, 1980). Deviations from monolingual English norms, then, should not automatically be considered evidence of language disorder. Neither should deviations from

Deaf sign language norms be automatically interpreted as poor sign language skills. In this sense, the koda development patterns discussed in this chapter are typical, in that they do not seem to indicate any language disorder. At the same time, studies of koda development are still few and too new for us to claim that the patterns observed so far are typical of koda populations in general.

This chapter begins with an overview of a research project currently being conducted by co-authors Chen Pichler and Lillo-Martin, investigating koda language development in the US. This project targets specific aspects of phonological, morphological and syntactic development in kodas' spoken English and signed ASL, and investigates divergences from monolingual[1] patterns as possible bilingual effects. The general finding that has emerged so far from our early analyses of koda participants is that they have productive use of both English and ASL, but with some cross-linguistic influence, or language synthesis effects. For the youngest kodas, from two to four years old, these effects tend to be from ASL to English, while the older koda children, who have entered school, display influence from English to ASL. Not surprisingly, a major factor affecting ASL development is the quantity and quality of input that children receive in that language (see the previous chapter for discussion of input effects among Dutch codas). It is not surprising that we should see an increase in cross-linguistic effects from English to ASL once kodas enter school and begin to speak English all day. For Deaf families, this raises the practical concern of whether ASL exposure limited to one's parents is sufficient for kodas to continue developing their ASL grammar beyond early childhood. We make several suggestions for maintenance and continued development of the home language, based on reports from the spoken bilingual literature.

Many of these same suggestions for the maintenance and continued development of ASL were integrated by the second author of this chapter (Lee) into the services provided to kodas by the Hearing and Speech Center (HSC) at Gallaudet University, in response to concerns from Deaf parents that their children's ASL development was stagnating. Charged with the task of assessing the English development of koda clients, but recognizing the insufficiency of using static English tests to evaluate ASL–English bilinguals, the Gallaudet HSC developed dynamic assessment techniques taking into consideration the effects of bimodal bilingualism. These techniques, discussed in more detail below, were designed to provide as comprehensive a picture as possible of a child's developing bilingual competency, with the goal of distinguishing true language *disorder* from language *difference* caused by ASL–English bilingualism. Lee draws on observations from his 20-plus years of interaction with kodas and their parents as a speech pathologist, noting that although kodas vary widely in their English development, they display a number of 'typical differences' in early koda English that indicate important areas to investigate through targeted linguistic research.

Varying Levels of Input for Bilinguals

Speech language pathologists (SLPs) not familiar with Deaf culture and ASL may find the notion of evaluating kodas to be daunting. SLPs in the mainstream often have limited professional experience with bilingualism and even fewer have experience with ASL. A demographic profile of American Speech Language Hearing Association (ASHA) member and non-member Certificate holders who self-identified as bilingual service providers from 1 January through 31 December 2009 revealed that out of 6248 providers, only 5.1% identified themselves as bilingual. This very low percentage of bilingualism among SLPs, combined with their unfamiliarity with ASL and Deaf culture, often leads to the mistaken belief that kodas are inherently input deprived in terms of language, which can lead to unwarranted diagnoses of language disorder. For instance, non-target use of pronoun gender, number and/or case has been anecdotally observed for many koda children. While such errors are also common among monolingual English learners and unimodal bilinguals, they are more likely to be interpreted as signs of disorder for koda children, on the assumption that Deaf parents provide insufficient English input to their children (see Sachs *et al.*, 1981; Schiff & Ventry, 1976, for some early research articles supporting this view). Language professionals may also see ASL as an obstacle to English development, dismissing the importance of a strong early ASL foundation for koda spoken English development. As a result, well-meaning SLPs err on the side of paternalism and automatically assume that kodas are language deprived.

Indeed, characterizing typical development for bilingual children is always challenging, given the wide variation in exposure that children receive in their two languages. This variation is due to many factors, including the context of bilingualism, and the quality and quantity of language input that the child receives. For instance, our research project on koda bilingual development includes children with the varied profiles listed in Table 10.1. These profiles trigger very different concerns for both 'lay professionals,' or language specialists who are unfamiliar with ASL, and the children's Deaf parents.

All of these children are considered ASL–English bilinguals, yet they can display very different developmental patterns. Furthermore, comparisons with 'baseline' early ASL patterns observed for Deaf children exposed primarily to ASL (before entering school) may not be appropriate for children whose ASL input falls below some threshold level, although it is difficult at this time to determine where that threshold lies. With so many factors potentially affecting koda children's language acquisition, we cannot currently define the limits of what is 'normal' for bilingual ASL and English development. This is especially true given the small number of children under investigation. Nevertheless, we feel that it is still useful to report the

Table 10.1 Koda input profiles, expectations and typical reactions from professionals and parents

Koda input profile	Typical expectations	Typical reactions
Receive substantial ASL exposure from parents and other sources, e.g. at a bilingual ASL–English school with koda and Deaf classmates and teachers; English input from other relatives and friends.	Have strong ASL skills, comparable to that of Deaf children, and may even be ASL-dominant early on; English development may appear somewhat delayed.	• Professionals: concerns that dominant ASL and relatively lower input in English will lead to delays in English development.
Are immersed in English at a hearing daycare or school, but are also part of a larger Deaf community and have regular contact with signing children and adults.	Have strong ASL skills, as well as strong English skills.	• Professionals: less concern about delayed English development than for the group described above.
Use not only ASL, but also a foreign spoken language and/or a foreign sign language at home and in their community.	Have weak skills in both ASL and English.	• Professionals: serious concerns about language delays in English; • Parents: concerns that child's home languages are not developing well.
Immersed in English at a hearing daycare or school, and do not have regular contact with ASL signers other than their parents.	Have strong English skills, but weak ASL skills.	• Professionals: less concern about delayed English; • Parents: concerns that child's ASL is not developing well.

patterns that we are seeing, particularly non-target patterns that are potentially effects of bimodal bilingualism, to demonstrate the range of structures that we note in our data. Since none of the children in our current study has any identified language disorder, this information should be helpful for professionals charged with the task of evaluating koda children for bona fide language disorders.

Throughout, it must be kept in mind that knowledge of two languages does not imply equal control of both. Bilingual adults and children are rarely *balanced bilinguals*; they are more likely to be dominant in one language, and weaker in the other (Grosjean, 2010). More importantly, bilinguals are not simply two monolinguals in a single body; the grammars of their two languages influence each other, and as such can diverge quite noticeably from that of monolingual speakers of either language (De Houwer, 2009; Grosjean, 2010; Romaine, 1999). With respect to child bilinguals, this divergence can manifest in a number of ways. Some are striking and immediately noticeable. For instance, bilingual children often engage in *code mixing* of their two languages, either *code switching* from one language to the other, or inserting words from one language into the grammatical structures of the other. Bimodal bilinguals also make frequent use of *code blending*,[2] or bimodal production of overlapping sign and speech, a unique type of code mixing not observed in spoken language bilinguals (Emmorey *et al.*, 2008). Other divergences from monolingual development are more subtle. For example, acquisition of specific structures may be protracted for bilingual children compared to their monolingual counterparts, or certain error patterns may persist longer than usual, due to reinforcement from the other language (Hulk & Müller, 2000). Identifying developmental patterns that result specifically from bilingualism is of major interest to acquisition researchers: how does the development of a bilingual child's grammar of a given language diverge from developmental patterns that have been established for monolingual learners of that language? Are there recognizable patterns for bilingual development for particular pairs of languages that could eventually constitute 'baseline' norms specific to bilingual ASL–English acquisition?

Research on the Development of Bimodal Bilingualism

Beyond the clinical applications to be discussed in this chapter, bimodal bilingual research offers insight on a number of interesting research questions regarding bilingualism and language acquisition in general. These questions include (but are by no means limited to) the following:

- What are the typical developmental milestones for bimodal-bilingual development, and how do they compare with those of unimodal bilingual development?
- How is bimodal bilingual acquisition different for hearing children who are born with access to both speech and sign (kodas) and Deaf children who access speech through a cochlear implant?
- Are there 'critical' ages when exposure to a spoken language is more important than at other ages?
- How much exposure to a language does a child need to achieve 'typical' phonological, morphological, syntactic and pragmatic competence? Do these thresholds vary depending on the modality of the target language(s)?

- Do bimodal bilinguals exhibit phonological transfer between their two languages and, if so, do they exhibit less than unimodal bilinguals due to the modality differences of their two phonological systems?
- What unique insights to bilingual development do code blending behaviors offer that cannot be learned from observing unimodal bilingualism?

Our research project focuses on the first two items in the list above, studying ASL–English kodas as part of a larger, binational project comparing bimodal bilingual development by kodas and Deaf children with cochlear implants in the US and Brazil. All of the koda children in this study (currently 30 in the US) are acquiring sign language from signing families where one or both parents are Deaf. The data for the project are collected using a combination of longitudinal and experimental methodologies (Chen Pichler et al., 2010a; Quadros et al., in press). A select few participants are filmed on a weekly-to-biweekly basis in naturalistic play with experimenters and family members, beginning around age 1;06 and continuing for two or more years. This practice has generated a large corpus of naturalistic data that offers us a picture of the overall linguistic development of bimodal bilinguals. We have also assembled a battery of language tests for both signed and spoken language, targeting kodas between 4;0 and 8;0 years. These tests focus on specific aspects of language development, such as early phonology, WH-questions and word order.

Although we have collected a substantial amount of data, particularly from the longitudinal participants, the transcription process is slow and painstaking, so only a subset of our videotaped data is fully transcribed and available to us for analysis. We have, however, made some preliminary findings, which we summarize in the following section.

Preliminary Findings

At the early ages, we find that the children are quite productive in both sign and speech. They distinguish between the languages, although they do sometimes show a preference for the spoken language, even when conversing with their Deaf parents or Deaf researchers whom they know are Deaf (cf. Petitto et al., 2001; Pizer, 2008). We see clear development of lexicon, phonology and syntax in both languages (Chen Pichler et al., 2010b; Lillo-Martin et al., 2010, 2012). As mentioned earlier, we also see several examples of bimodal bilingualism effects, including code blending and language synthesis, or the use of structures from the sign language in their speech. We expand on each of these below. Because the focus of this chapter is koda children, we restrict our discussion to the data from our koda subjects only, and report on our data for Deaf children with cochlear implants only very briefly at the end of this subsection.

Code blending

Overall, in the data we have coded so far, the children use code blending anywhere from a very small portion to 50% of the time during filmed sessions (Quadros *et al.*, 2010; Lillo-Martin *et al.*, 2010). Previous studies of adult codas in the US (Emmorey *et al.*, 2008) and child codas in the Netherlands (van den Bogaerde, this volume) and Canada (Petitto *et al.*, 2001) have all noted the prevalence of code blended utterances in coda production, so this should be considered a common and normal feature of bimodal bilingualism. Van den Bogaerde (2000) reported that overall rates of koda code blending by young (under 3;0) Dutch kodas closely mirror the rates of code blending in the input from their Deaf parents. These rates diverge as the same koda children grow older (between 3;0 and 6;0) and increase their use of code blending, while their Deaf mothers' use of code blending decreases. The use of voiced English by Deaf parents (with or without accompanying signing) with their hearing children has been documented among American families (Mallorey *et al.*, 1993; Pizer, 2008) and is an important factor to consider when studying the use of koda code blending. However, we have anecdotally noted an interesting generational shift in the use of spoken English reported by Deaf parents at the Gallaudet University HSC over the last 20 years. In the early 1990s most families reported that at least one of the Deaf parents used code blending or spoken English with their koda children. In more recent years, parents have explicitly stated that they do not use their voices when signing with their children, so as to maintain a 'purer' form of ASL than would result from mixing with voiced English. It is not clear at this time how widely this perception is shared among Deaf families outside Gallaudet and the greater Washington, DC area.

In terms of koda production, we have not yet carried out any analysis of the factors that trigger specific instances of code blending in our data, but we have observed many varied contexts that are potential factors affecting language choice. These include whether or not the koda's interlocutor is also bimodal bilingual, whether the filming location is a place where code blending frequently occurs (such as Gallaudet University), the type of discourse the child is producing (e.g. narratives frequently lend themselves to depiction and code blending), and even the topic of conversation (e.g. shifting a speech-only discussion to a topic related to the child's Deaf parent may trigger code blending).

The form of code blended utterances also varies, including those in which the complete utterance is expressed in both sign and speech, those which are primarily spoken utterances with some signs included, and those which are primarily signed utterances with some speech included. Finally, code blended utterances vary in the level of phonation of the spoken language. Our use of the term code blending includes utterances in which the spoken language is fully voiced or whispered (Guerrera *et al.*, 2013), but not signed utterances with mouthed English only (in contrast to van den Bogaerde & Baker (2005), who count signing and mouthing as instances of code blending).

One important observation we have made about the code-blended utterances is that it is always the case that the spoken portion and the signed portion contribute to a single proposition (Quadros *et al.*, 2010). The children do not produce one proposition on the hands while a different proposition is produced vocally, and in this they are like bimodal bilingual adults (Emmorey *et al.*, 2008). The children's code blends differ from adults in one respect, however. We found numerous cases where the children attempt to produce a sign together with a spoken element, but the timing of their utterances is not coincident. As an example, consider the diagram in Figure 10.1.

The diagram shows a portion of the coding screen using ELAN software (Crasborn & Sloetjes, 2008) developed at the Max Planck Institute for Psycholinguistics in Nijmegen, The Netherlands (http://www.lat-mpi.eu/tools/elan/). The top line is the tier on which the child's ASL utterances are transcribed, while the second line shows the tier on which the child's English utterances are transcribed. Annotations in ELAN reflect the timing and duration of the child's utterances. As the figure demonstrates, the child BEN (age 2;01) produces the spoken word 'snake' before the signed utterance, then again after the signed utterance has started. During this part of the utterance, the speech and sign are not coordinated. BEN then repeats the signed/spoken pair, and this time the coordination is accurate (the sign annotation starts just before the speech annotation, taking into consideration the transition time needed to move the hand into position for the sign; the lexical movement of the sign and the spoken word are completely coordinated). Thus, children seem to still be developing their ability to coordinate the timing of code-blended utterances, but the structure and nature of these utterances appear adult-like.

Language synthesis effects

In addition to code blending, our koda data feature language mixing in the form of language synthesis, or the interaction of the vocabulary and grammatical rules for ASL and English. Although it is widely agreed that bilingual children develop two autonomous grammars from the very beginning of language development (Genessee, 1989), language synthesis effects are widely documented in the production of bilingual children (and adults).

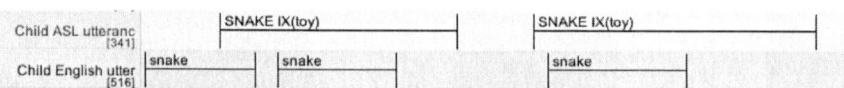

Figure 10.1 Code-blended utterance with timing mismatch

Like other children developing in two languages – and in fact, like adult bimodal bilinguals (Bishop & Hicks, 2005) – bimodal bilingual children sometimes produce utterances which appear to be composed of words from one language, using a grammatical structure from the other. We have found numerous examples of such cross-linguistic influence, including the ones illustrated below (Koulidobrova, 2012; Lillo-Martin *et al.*, 2010). In all of these examples, the English word order is non-standard (a preverbal object in (1); doubled verb in (2); post-verbal subject (Padden, 1988 [1983]) in (3); and WH-question word in final position in (4)), and appears ungrammatical. However, closer examination reveals that these are all word order variations that are permitted in ASL. Such ASL-to-English effects are most common in the longitudinal data from our youngest koda participants, at a time in their lives when they tend to have relatively strong input in ASL compared to English.

(1) O-V order
  Ben (2;01)   Eng: chocolate   eat
          ASL: HOT CHOCOLATE IX EAT
          'He's eating hot chocolate.'
(2) Doubling
  Ben (2;01)   Eng: sleeping mouse sleeping
          'The mouse is sleeping.'
(3) Subject Pronoun Copy (a subject pronoun appears sentence-finally)
  Ben (2;03)   Eng: stuck it
          'It's stuck.'
(4) WH *in situ* (WH element fails to raise to sentence-initial position)
  Tom (2;04)   Eng: bug go where
          'Where did the bug go?'

Other researchers have also noticed cross-linguistic influence in coda production (e.g. Johnson *et al.*, 1992; Todd, 1971) and we regard it as a normal aspect of bilingual development, parallel to what is documented for unimodal bilingual children (Cantone, 2007). Quinn (2004) argued that English–ASL code mixing in koda production is frequently misinterpreted by SLPs as language deviance according to monolingual English standards, leading to unwarranted diagnoses of language disorder among kodas. In her examination of naturalistic ASL and English production by four koda subjects, Quinn documented recurring patterns of code mixing at all levels (syntax, semantics, morphology, phonology and pragmatics) of her koda subjects' English production, accounting for 27% of their non-target-like English constructions. Her thesis highlighted the most common types of code mixes she observed and pursued the hypothesis that some of these mixing behaviors were potentially attributable to natural mixing in the input (cf. a similar discussion in the previous chapter), rather than linguistic insufficiency or disorder. Overall,

Quinn concluded that most of her subjects' non-target English production was best characterized as bilingual difference, not disorder. Parents, teachers and therapists need to recognize that such structures emerge naturally in bilingual children and are not necessarily signs of language disorder, despite the fact that they may diverge from standard English word order.

Turning now to the older koda participants in our project (ages four to seven), we have noticed two other general patterns. First, the spoken language skills of these older kodas are largely age-equivalent in comparison to monolingual English speakers, based on results from our test battery (Davidson *et al.*, in press). Second, their ASL skills, while still fluent, display noticeable influence from their spoken language. We will address each of these general patterns in turn.

We administered several standard spoken English tests to the participants in our experimental studies, including the Preschool Language Scales (PLS; an overall language measure) and the Goldman–Fristoe Test of Articulation. On these tests, the koda children in our study all scored at or above the age-equivalent level. We also administered a number of tests designed by our research group targeting specific morphosyntactic structures, such as verbal morphology, adjective-noun word order, and WH-questions. On all of these tests, the children produced target-like structures for English (e.g. WH-questions with the WH-word in the initial position, and Adjective + Noun combinations), as well as non-target structures that are also observed in monolingual English-speaking children (e.g. failure to invert the subject and auxiliary verb in 'why' questions; see Quadros *et al.*, 2013; Lillo-Martin *et al.*, 2012, for details.)

Standardized tests for sign languages are far less common than for spoken languages, so most of the tests we used for assessing aspects of koda children's phonology, morphology and syntax were adapted from spoken language tests or created by our research team specifically for our project. The results from these tests indicate that the children's signing is fluent, but on some of the tests their signing is notably influenced by English. For example, although ASL permits WH-elements to appear in initial position or final position or both, the 5–6-year-old kodas in our study overwhelmingly preferred to use sentence-initial WH-questions, the order that is also used in English (Lillo-Martin *et al.*, 2012), as shown in Figure 10.2. This contrasts with results from Deaf signing children on a similar experimental task, for whom sentence-initial WH-structures were only one of a variety of ASL question structures that they produced (Lillo-Martin, 2000), as shown in Figure 10.3.

The contrast between Deaf and koda WH-questions in our experimental data is so striking that the Deaf experimenters administering the test expressed concern that some koda participants were essentially performing the WH-task 'in signed English'. The WH-task is cognitively more demanding than the other tests in our battery, and the experimenters' assessment was that some children were simply unable to perform it in ASL. Alternatively,

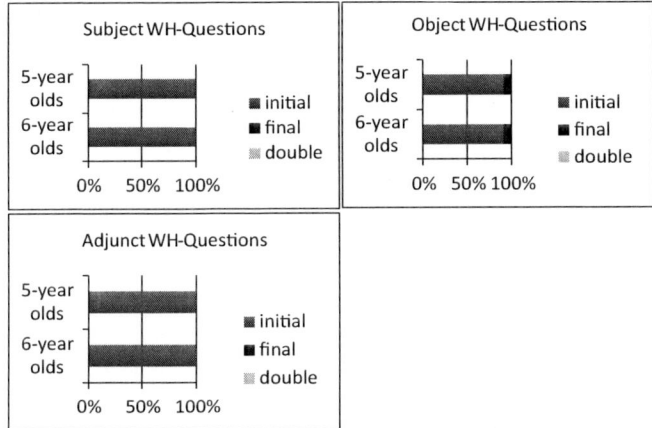

Figure 10.2 American kodas overwhelmingly favor WH-initial order for all types of WH-questions in ASL

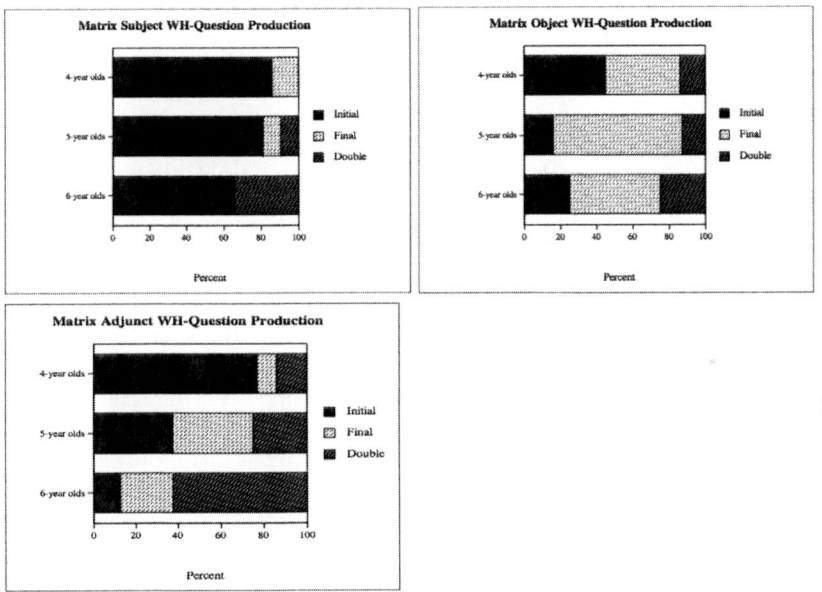

Figure 10.3 Varied order for WH-questions in ASL produced by Deaf 4–6-year-olds
Source: Reproduced with permission from Lillo-Martin (2000)

these children might have been quite capable of varied WH-question forms in ASL, but assumed that language tests are always for English, and therefore the WH-task we gave them must be targeting their English grammar (koda children are not typically tested on their ASL skills). In such a case, signed English could be a compensation strategy, offering a signed response to what the child assumes is an English task. Either way, from the perspective of language synthesis, signed English can be viewed as one extreme on the bilingual spectrum between ASL and English; simultaneous activation of the structures and vocabularies of both languages offers kodas the option of producing a variety of WH-question forms, including those consisting of ASL signs in an English word order. This explanation is compatible with the fact that several of the kodas in question also participated in our longitudinal studies as toddlers, and we know from our extended observations of them that they developed strong foundations in ASL, employing word order variety beyond what is available in English. Further analysis of our longitudinal and experimental WH-data is necessary to determine which of the above explanations of the WH-test results is correct, but either way, we again note the importance of considering kodas' knowledge of *both* ASL and English when analyzing their language production.

In addition to differences in word order choices, degree of exposure to ASL also appears to affect children's use of morphologically complex 'classifier constructions' and depictive structures in their elicited narratives. Depiction is a common linguistic strategy in ASL and other signed languages used to visually represent or 'show' an action or appearance rather than simply 'telling' it (Dudis, 2007; Liddell, 2003). For example, in Figure 10.4 a Deaf mother creates an ASL narrative about Elmo approaching Cookie Monster and giving him a kiss. Although it is possible in ASL to 'tell' this event through a sequence of lexical signs, parallel to what one would say in English (5), the mother instead depicts the event using 'classifier' handshapes that represent Elmo approaching Cookie Monster (frames a–b) then kissing him (frames c–e). The use of space and facial expressions effectively convey the relative position of the two entities, the size of the kiss and other additional information that is absent in (5).

(5)   ELMO KISS COOKIE-MONSTER
       'Elmo kissed Cookie Monster.'

Sign languages are particularly rich in depictive structures. They are widely considered hallmarks of skilled signing, so many Deaf parents are concerned when they note the limited use of depiction in their koda children's signing.

(a)   **(b)**   **(c)**   **(d)**   **(e)**

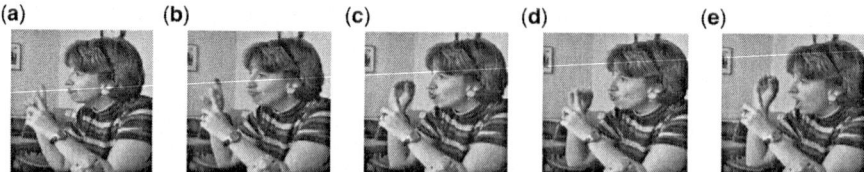

Figure 10.4 Depiction in ASL showing one upright figure approaching another and giving it a kiss.

Likewise, shifts in word order of the type described earlier for WH-questions may also be interpreted as an indication that their children's ASL competence is stagnating or even deteriorating as their English proficiency increases. These concerns have led to discussions with parents in our project on the importance of maintaining the home language, with the goal of maximizing their children's bilingualism (see section on Maximalizing Bilingualism below).

Multi-generation Deaf children with cochlear implants

Although the overwhelming majority of children with cochlear implants are born to hearing, non-signing parents, a small number of Deaf parents have opted for cochlear implants for their Deaf children. Cochlear implants are a very sensitive topic in the Deaf community, which traditionally views them as a major threat to its future existence. In our experience, the Deaf families who choose implants for their children do so for various, personal reasons, but they are similar in one important respect: they are culturally Deaf, and are thus committed to signing ASL with their children, in the hope that they will develop as bimodal bilinguals. Multi-generational Deaf children with cochlear implants thus differ from other implanted children by being exposed to a fully accessible natural language (in this case, ASL) from birth and throughout their childhood.

Given the well-documented importance of L1 exposure in the first year of life (see Morford & Mayberry, 2002 for an overview), the early and unfettered access to language that multi-generational Deaf children receive throughout the pre-implantation, activation and adjustment periods is a highly desirable benefit that is rarely available to implanted children. Indeed, recent research on this unusual group has demonstrated the important advantages of early sign language exposure in areas such as sign and speech perception (Giezen, 2011), speech intelligibility and comprehension (Hassanzadeh, 2012) and phonological memory (Quadros et al., 2012). These results stand in stark contrast to the comparatively large body of research reporting negative effects of signing on speech development among cochlear implanted children (e.g. Geers et al., 2002; Kirk et al., 2003; Svirsky et al., 2000). These studies define 'signing' children as those who are enrolled in 'total communication' (TC) school programs and/or use signed supported speech at home with their hearing parents. Such limited use of signs cannot be equated with a full and natural sign language such as ASL. Multi-generation Deaf children are thus a critical group for clarifying the role of early and sustained exposure to a full sign language in the acquisition of speech through a cochlear implant.

At the same time, multi-generation implanted Deaf children are also a logical comparison group for kodas in the study of bimodal development, offering unique insights into the effects of cochlear implantation on simultaneous development of spoken and signed languages. We have therefore included both groups in our research project. We have just recently begun analysis of the longitudinal and experimental data from our cochlear implanted participants, and so far they appear very similar to their koda counterparts in many respects. Both groups show English development that is within monolingual English norms, according to the results of our test battery (Davidson *et al.*, in press); both make frequent use of code blending, and are proficient in ASL, but with identifiable cross-linguistic influence from English in their word order choices once they reach school age (e.g. predominant use of WH-initial structures in our WH-test, as described earlier), triggering concerns among Deaf parents that their children's ASL development is lagging behind that of English. These are all very general preliminary patterns, of course, and much more analysis of the data is necessary before we can determine the true extent of similarities between bimodal bilingual development for kodas and implanted multi-generational Deaf children.

Maximizing Bilingualism

Parents who wish to raise their children bilingually face two competing demands. On the one hand, they want their children to fully function in the majority, surrounding language. In the case under discussion here, Deaf parents want their hearing children to speak, comprehend, read and write English. Achieving this goal means that the children need to interact with English speakers for a significant length of time. On the other hand, in order to develop and maintain competence in the home language, in our case ASL, sufficient input is also required, including opportunities to interact with a variety of ASL users at an increasingly sophisticated level.

Researchers studying bilingual language development have noted the role of input factors in each language for appropriate development and maintenance. We do not know of any such research specifically addressing these issues for bimodal bilinguals. For this reason, we will summarize some of the major points based on research with unimodal bilinguals, and then offer some speculations and ideas on how that research might translate for bimodal bilinguals.

It has been often been reasoned that, on average, children who are exposed to two languages will experience less input in each language as compared to monolingual children (Paradis & Genessee, 1996). Although this much input must be 'enough' for acquisition – indeed, children in many parts of the world manage to acquire three or more languages, indicating that even less input per language is sufficient for acquisition – there is evidence that the relative amount of exposure in each language is a strong predictor of *rate* of development (Gathercole & Thomas, 2009; Pearson *et al.*, 1997; and many others). Some of these studies find that these effects are greatest in early stages of acquisition, with groups tending to equalize at later ages, at least in areas where there is a high degree of bilingualism (e.g. grade 5; Oller & Eilers, 2002).

Unsworth (2013) reports that a more fine-grained measure of input quantity is a better predictor for certain linguistic characteristics. She estimated *cumulative* language exposure by having parents complete a detailed questionnaire about the language used by various input providers (parents, other adults at home, daycare providers, adults at school, etc.) currently and retrospectively for each year of the child's life. This measure was a significant predictor of the participant's appropriate use of gender in Dutch determiners for simultaneous Dutch/English bilinguals, ages 3–17.

Researchers have also looked further into the input factors affecting bilingual development. Place and Hoff (2011) studied the early development of Spanish and English by children living in southern Florida, a strongly bilingual community. Parents were asked to complete a diary recording the child's language environment for every 30-minute block of the day, over the course of seven days. Parents also reported their children's language development using the MacArthur–Bates Communicative Development Inventory (CDI) in both English and Spanish. The study found that three input properties were positive predictors of the children's English skills: 'the number of conversational partners with whom the child spoke only English, the number of different speakers from whom the child heard English, and percent of the child's English exposure that was provided by native speakers' (Place & Hoff, 2011: 1845).

Gathercole and Thomas's (2009) study arrived at some conclusions that may be particularly applicable for the case of bimodal bilinguals in the US. They examined bilingualism in Welsh and English in stable bilingual areas of Wales, including both children and adults. For Welsh, the minority language, they found a strong relationship to input factors at all stages, for measures including the development of vocabulary, grammatical gender and the identification of grammatical subjects. The strongest effects correlated with the language used in the home (Welsh only, English only, or both Welsh and English). A smaller effect was found for language used in school. In contrast, for English, the dominant language, input factors were relevant to early periods of language development, but differences across groups attenuated by mid-school years.

Given these results, as well as our own observations, we make the following suggestions regarding maximizing bilingualism for families with koda children. First, because of the dominance of English as the primary language of the larger community, koda children are highly likely to develop English fully and to consider themselves dominant in English as adults (Bishop *et al.*, 2006). Second, during development, bilingual children should be compared not with monolingual English speakers but with other bilinguals (Cantone *et al.*, 2008). There may be some areas in which bilingual English development progresses more slowly than for monolinguals, and some types of language mixing or language synthesis may be observed (as noted earlier in the chapter), but the children can be expected to display essentially age-appropriate English development by school age.

With regard to ASL, on the other hand, extra effort may be needed to promote and maintain the home language. Below is a list of input factors that have been noted in previous research regarding home language maintenance.

- *Quantity of input, particularly cumulative exposure.* Certain areas of the language may be dependent on the child's exposure to a threshold of quantity over a period of years. In the case of the Unsworth (2013) study, this was found for a morphological phenomenon with a high degree of idiosyncrasy.
- *Number of different speakers who use ASL with the child.* Psycholinguistic studies indicate that word recognition and word production benefit from experiencing multiple speakers, to aid recognition of phonetic variation (Singh, 2008). Sign language researchers also propose that word order variation within a single signer's production can aid Deaf children in 'exploration of linguistic possibilities' of the target sign language (Hoiting & Slobin, 2002: 3).
- *Number of conversational partners with whom the child uses only ASL.* Since koda children frequently switch to spoken language with hearing interlocutors, it may be important to expose the child to a wider range of Deaf signers beyond the immediate family.
- *Language used at school.* There is some evidence to suggest that use of the minority language at school aids in the child's development of this language. Although there are few opportunities for most koda children to use ASL at daycare or school, some programs and special schools provide a bilingual environment in both signed and spoken languages. Such bilingual school environments have been identified as a strong predictor of lexical competence in sign language for Deaf children (Tomasuolo *et al.*, 2010). Certainly, for parents of kodas hoping to maintain their children's use of ASL, programs at which children may use ASL with their peers may be highly valuable.

Based on our observations so far, certain linguistic areas may be more susceptible to effects of input factors than others. For example, the use of ASL-specific word orders that are different from corresponding orders of English, such as the WH-final and WH-doubled structures in ASL discussed earlier, may be particularly sensitive to the amount and variation of ASL input that the children receive. This is an area in which further empirical investigation is needed.

Integration into Clinical Practice

Given the traditional tendency for bilingual effects of koda language development to be mistaken for language disorders, the incidence of true language disorders in the koda population is probably much lower than currently assumed. We can look to studies of language disorders within the Deaf population for possible insight. Sign language researchers in the UK have developed and normed a battery of standardized tests of British Sign Language (BSL) that can now be used to identify Deaf children with potential specific language impairment (SLI) in that country. These children show significant language delays relative to their Deaf peers, despite having normal cognitive, social and motor abilities, and despite the fact that they come from signing, Deaf families that have provided them with high levels of BSL input. Using these tests, Mason *et al.* (2010) conclude that true cases of SLI within the British Deaf population occur with the same relatively low frequency as they do in the monolingual population (about 7%). Parallel investigations on SLI within Deaf populations in the US are currently being carried out by Quinto-Pozos *et al.* (see this volume).

Similarly, there is no evidence to suggest that the incidence of true language disorder among kodas should be any higher than it is in the general hearing population. Yet Lee (the second author of this chapter) notes that during his 20 years of professional service in the Washington, DC area, every Deaf family he encountered that engaged the DC public schools and some of the neighboring public school systems received special educational SLP services for their koda children. Such universal provision of services is unheard of for unimodal spoken language bilinguals, indicating again that SLPs and school officials perceive koda children as different from spoken bilinguals and inherently at higher risk for language delays.

It is essential that parents, teachers and clinicians take bilingualism into consideration before concluding that koda children are language disordered. Intervention should only be carried out on the basis of consistent evaluation of a koda child's English and ASL that shows marked delay in *both* languages, such as difficulty acquiring new language concepts, even with explicit and repeated exposure. In the following section, we discuss practices followed at the Gallaudet University HSC to ensure that koda children receive accurate diagnoses with regard to language delay or disorder.

Dynamic assessment of koda clients

For more than a generation, kodas have been served at the Gallaudet University HSC through speech and language evaluations assessing their spoken English. Deaf parents unable or uncertain of their ability to monitor the spoken English development of their koda children bring them for evaluation after someone has expressed concerns about language delays or more serious disorders. This prompting may come from hearing family members and/or school officials who notice aspects of koda language (discussed earlier) that appear to deviate from monolingual English development. Concerns about koda delay or disorder may also be prompted by koda behaviors reflecting Deaf cultural practices that are viewed as unacceptable in the mainstream hearing culture. For example, important attention-getting strategies for ASL that are acquired early by kodas involve a variety of visual (e.g. hand-waving in the addressee's line of vision), tactile (e.g. touching or tapping the addressee) and vibratory (e.g. stomping on the floor) techniques to draw the attention of a potential communication partner. These practices are cultural conventions observed across Deaf cultures, and many koda children continue to use them when they transition into hearing-dominant contexts such as public school. This often leads to conflicts and misunderstanding with public school staff, who follow a strict no-touching policy. Persistent use of attention-getting strategies that are viewed as inappropriate in hearing schools often leads to punitive measures against koda students, who may also be labeled as having behavioral or cognitive problems.

In general, while understanding of bilingual acquisition has improved in the US, this improvement has not extended to koda bilingual development, due to the fact that there has been little documentation of developmental patterns that are typical for koda children. From a clinical point of view, koda children are unique among bilinguals in that they must acquire language in two different modalities, visual/gestural and aural/oral. This dynamic presents diagnostic challenges for determining the presence or absence of a speech-language disorder, particularly with respect to phonology. The bimodal nature of koda language development, combined with parents who do not model a spoken language at home, plus the general unavailability of tools for assessing koda children's proficiency in their home language (ASL) and its effects on the child's English, make it challenging to accurately determine whether koda production patterns deviating from monolingual English norms indicate a language disorder or simply a bilingual difference. New norms specifically for koda English phonological development need to be developed through careful observation and documentation of koda language development that is informed by linguistic and cultural awareness on the part of the evaluator.

Lee (2008) discussed the development of more culturally and linguistic sensitive practices for assessing koda language, based on the following definition of dynamic assessment from ASHA:

> A method of conducting a language assessment which seeks to identify the skills that an individual child possesses as well as their learning potential. The dynamic assessment procedure emphasizes the learning process and accounts for the amount and nature of examiner investment. It is highly interactive and process-oriented. (http://www.asha.org/practice/multicultural/issues/Dynamic-Assessment.htm)

Dynamic assessment varies from traditional static testing by actively engaging the family, increasing the participation of the examiner, promoting modification in administration of test items and interpretation of scores, and being more fluid and responsive to the child/family. Techniques used at the Gallaudet University HSC include extensive interviews to precisely ascertain the age at which the koda was first exposed to ASL and English, parents' perceptions of the koda's ASL and English development compared to that of siblings and other peers, the language(s) used at home and at school/work, the amount and integrity of exposure to each language, the koda's preferred language with siblings, peers, parents, etc., progress made as an English Language Learner, if relevant, and a report of academic perfor-mance. Trial teaching has also been used to determine the koda's ability to acquire new linguistic information in a highly stimulating environment. More formally, the Response to Intervention (RTI) model (Haywood & Lidz, 2007) was utilized during the multi-year assessment journey to assess the language disorder of a koda child presented as a case study at ASHA (Lee, 2010). RTI is a process of establishing non-IEP interventions and mea-suring impact over time to assist in determining if a true language disorder exists and if more formal IEP-based services are required. These dynamic assessment techniques can be augmented with commercially available cri-terion- and norm-referenced tests, such as the PLS, the Clinical Evaluation of Language Fundamentals (CELF), the Rossetti Infant-Toddler Language scale (Rossetti, 2006, etc.), and the MacArthur–Bates CDI for English (Fenson *et al.*, 1993) and ASL (Anderson & Reilly, 2002), provided the examiner per-forms the evaluation in accordance with the ASHA Code of Ethics and the guidelines for evaluating English language learners:

> It should be noted that test scores would be invalid for testing a client who is not reflected in the normative group for the test's standardiza-tion sample, even if the test were administered as instructed. However, these tests can provide valuable descriptive information about a cli-ent's abilities and limitations in the language of the test. (http:/www.asha.org)

Accordingly, the Gallaudet HSC employs static testing for future compara-tive purposes only, and test scores are interpreted with extreme cau-tion. Working closely with the families of koda clients ensures that the assessment process takes into consideration relevant cultural and linguistic aspects of ASL and the Deaf community. It also helps minimize the histori-cally contentious relationship between Deaf families and speech therapy professionals and increases the family's willingness to share their percep-tions of their child's language development. Additionally, the Gallaudet HSC recognizes the importance of ASL proficiency among speech and language professionals for effective communication with Deaf families, as well as for a more comprehensive understanding of koda children's language abilities (some of which may have developed for ASL, but not yet for English).

Language stimulation groups

In addition to providing diagnostic services, the Gallaudet HSC has for many years provided spoken language stimulation groups for koda children, focused on developing English vocabulary, syntax and phonological awareness. These group sessions also provide important language-related feedback that Deaf families may not typically provide, such as feedback on koda children's speech intelligibility and explicit training in cultural practices that differ across Deaf and hearing communities (such as the attention-getting strategies mentioned earlier). Language stimulation occurs twice a week for approximately 50 minutes each session, in small groups of three to five children. A variety of discussion themes, age-appropriate books and table and motor activities encourage children to develop new English skills in experiential and natural ways. In particular, nursery rhymes, songs and rhyming books are incorporated to provide auditory experience for fostering phonological awareness skills.

Paul (2010) evaluated the effect on one koda child who attended the Gallaudet HSC English language stimulation groups described above between the ages of 2;4 and 2;8 (with a final data collection session at 3;0). She found that spoken English intervention had a positive impact on English development, reporting increases in the child's Mean Length of Utterance (MLU) (as measured by Brown, 1973 & Retherford, 1993), phonemic inventory and intelligibility. She also emphasized the crucial importance of ASL competence for clinicians working with koda children, noting the frequency with which she depended on her subject's use of ASL to understand otherwise unintelligible English utterances. Also, her subject displayed numerous lexical gaps in English, but was able to express these words in ASL, giving a more accurate picture of his vocabulary development than would be possible if the clinician assessing his language skills attended only to his English production.

As koda children's exposure to spoken language increases, many Deaf parents express concern that their koda children's ASL development begins to lag behind their English development. Additionally, some parents report with distress that their koda children begin communicating with them solely in spoken English, seriously hindering parent–child communication. These parental observations are consistent with reports by researchers at the annual ASHA conventions between 2009 and 2010 that although unimodal bilingual children respond positively to intervention in their second language, their first language (home language) tends to plateau or diminish in use and sophistication (personal communication at ASHA conventions). In response to these concerns, the Gallaudet HSC developed a pilot project involving two 50-minute sessions of ASL stimulation in addition to existing English stimulation sessions. Four children (three girls and one boy) between the ages of 18 and 24 months participated in the pilot project. The purpose of these ASL sessions was to increase the perceived value of ASL use among young kodas and enhance their ASL input by exposing them to a greater variety of signing adults. Whereas the English stimulation groups are traditionally facilitated by two hearing, SLP graduate students, the facilitators of the ASL group needed to be native or near-native users of ASL, with an understanding of language development in general and ASL development specifically. An understanding of child development, behavior management and practical experience working with young children was also important. Ultimately, two graduate students (in linguistics and Deaf education) and an undergraduate education student were selected to facilitate the ASL pilot sessions. All three were native or near-native ASL users; two were Deaf and one was a coda.

In terms of content, the ASL and English stimulation sessions often shared themes but did not attempt to mirror one another, reflecting the opinion that trying to force acquisition of the same linguistic concepts in both ASL and English at the same time would be artificial and unnecessary. To promote the expectation of ASL use and to ensure that the Deaf adults in the room (as well as Deaf parents, who often observed the sessions from an adjacent chamber) had direct access to communication, it was decided that facilitators would only use ASL during the ASL sessions. The hearing student in the room would not respond to spoken utterances by the koda children. Similarly, in the spoken language groups, emphasis was placed on spoken English to promote the children's use of that language. Kodas' ASL utterances were acknowledged by the clinicians but reflected back to the children in spoken English.

From the beginning of the pilot program, there were significant differences in spoken English use across the four children. The boy and the youngest girl were the least willing to use spoken English, while the two older girls used much more spoken English. Over the one-semester course of the project, facilitators expanded short utterances produced by the older, more verbal girls and modeled target forms for the their non-target utterances containing syntactic or morphological errors. These techniques evidenced a positive effect as judged by increased MLU and overall sophistication of utterances across sessions. The two younger children, who had started the semester very reluctant to speak, evidenced progress in the increased use of their voices and engagement in spoken English activities.

As for the ASL stimulation groups, these also appear to have been successful, as Deaf families reported an increase in their children's use and sophistication of ASL at home. Through observation of the ASL sessions, Deaf parents were exposed to a variety of explicit language stimulation techniques, and became familiar with themes and activities that they could reinforce with their children throughout the week. Additionally, the ASL facilitators documented the types of signs and sign combinations each child was using, and shared this information with parents. This helped parents see more clearly where their children's ASL seemed on target and where they might need additional stimulation. As mentioned earlier, variety in input is a key factor for supporting a vulnerable home language, and the ASL stimulation groups not only exposed koda participants to new signers beyond their parents, they also provided parents with techniques for increasing variety in the input at home. Overall, the Deaf families had a very positive reaction to the new paradigm for language stimulation that included both English and ASL sessions.

Concluding Remarks and Future Directions

The present volume focuses on disorder in the signed modality, making this (and the previous) chapter a bit of an exception to the overall theme of the other chapters. The koda children described in here are not, to our knowledge, language disordered in any way. While koda English (as well as koda ASL) displays non-target features in comparison to monolingual counterparts, we argue that these differences are an outcome of bimodal bilingualism rather than a language disorder. Studies of bimodal bilinguals are still relatively rare compared to those of more traditionally studied unimodal bilinguals, so it is still too early to define the developmental characteristics that are typical of koda children. Nevertheless, projects like the one described in this chapter, which track selected aspects of ASL and English development for multiple koda subjects, are already finding general patterns that could turn out to be widespread across koda populations, within the US and abroad. Chief among these patterns is the observation that young kodas from strong signing homes develop fluency in both English and ASL, but display cross-linguistic influence from ASL to English (particularly under 4;0 years) and English to ASL (particularly once children have entered school). While much more research is needed to clarify the nature and distribution of the cross-linguistic effects in our data, it is already abundantly clear that such effects occur in koda production, and must be taken seriously into consideration during clinical assessments of koda language development and disorder.

Acknowledgments

We are very grateful to the families who have participated in our research, for permitting us to observe their children's language development in all its rich complexity. Thanks also to our many research assistants and collaborators who join us in our investigations of bimodal bilingualism, particularly Dr Ronice de Quadros, the co-Principal Investigator for the Development of Bimodal Bilingualism project in Brazil. Funding for this work comes from the NIDCD of the National Institutes of Health [R01DC009263 to D.L-M. and D.C.P.]. The content is solely the responsibility of the authors and does not necessarily represent the official views of the National Institutes of Health.

Notes

(1) We acknowledge that 'monolingual' is not an appropriate label for the Deaf signing children who form the comparison group for our koda participants' ASL production. Although Deaf signing children in the US have varying exposure to and proficiency in English, they are most appropriately characterized as bilingual (Grosjean, 1992). However, their access to English is largely visual only, whereas kodas have unrestricted access to English, both visual and auditory. Our selection of Deaf children as the control group for koda ASL reflects a reasonable hypothesis that unrestricted access to English may lead to a higher degree of cross-linguistic influence from English to ASL than is typical for Deaf children.

(2) We consider code blending to be distinct from simultaneous communication or SimCom in that the former occurs spontaneously in mixed Deaf-hearing households, is generally accessible to all parties, and is used in low-stake, informal contexts, while the latter is essentially sign-supported English, and is noted for being inaccessible to Deaf addressees, particularly in high-stake contexts such as classroom lectures, meetings, etc. (Emmorey *et al.*, 2008).

References

Anderson, D. and Reilly, J. (2002) The MacArthur Communicative Development Inventory: Normative data for American Sign Language. *Journal of Deaf Studies and Deaf Education* 7, 83–106.

Bialystok E., Craik, F., Green, D. and Gollan, T. (2009) Bilingual minds. Psychological Science in the Public Interest 10 (3), 89–129.

Bishop, M. and Hicks, S. (2005) Orange eyes: Bimodal bilingualism in hearing adult users of American Sign Language. *Sign Language Studies* 5 (2). Washington, DC: Gallaudet University Press.

Bishop, M., Hicks, S., Bertone, A. and Sala, R. (2006) Capitalizing on simultaneity: Features of bimodal bilingualism in hearing Italian native signers. In C. Lucas (ed.) *Sociolinguistics in Deaf Communities, Vol. 12*. Washington, DC: Gallaudet University Press.

Brown, R. (1973) *A First Language: The Early Stages*. Cambridge, MA: Harvard University Press.

Cantone, K.F. (2007) *Code-switching in Bilingual Children*. Dordrecht: Springer.

Cantone, K., Müller, N., Schmitz, K. and Kupisch, T. (2008) Rethinking language dominance. *Linguistische Berichte* 215, 129–160.

Chen Pichler, D., Hochgesang, J., Lillo-Martin, D. and Quadros, R.M. (2010a) Conventions for sign and speech transcription of child bimodal bilingual corpora in ELAN. *Language, Interaction and Acquisition* 1, 11–40.

Chen Pichler, D., Quadros, R. and Lillo-Martin, D. (2010b) Effects of bimodal production on multi-cyclicity in early ASL and Libras. In J. Chandlee, K. Franich, K. Iserman and L. Keil (eds) *BUCLD 34 Proceedings Supplement*. See http://www.bu.edu/bucld/proceedings/supplement/vol34/.

Crasborn, O. and Sloetjes, H. (2008) Enhanced ELAN functionality for sign language corpora. In *Proceedings of LREC 2008, Sixth International Conference on Language Resources and Evaluation*.

Darcy, N.T. (1953) A review of the literature on the effects of bilingualism upon the measurement of intelligence. *Journal of Genetic Psychology* 82, 21–57.

Davidson, K., Lillo-Martin, D. and Chen Picher, D. (in press) Spoken English language measures of native signing children with cochlear implants. *Journal of Deaf Studies and Deaf Education.*

De Houwer, A. (2009) *Bilingual First Language Acquisition.* Bristol: Multilingual Matters.

Dudis, P. (2007) Types of depiction in ASL. Available at: http://www.gallaudet.edu/documents/academic/drl-dudis2007.pdf

Emmorey, K., Borinstein, H., Thompson, R. and Gollan, T. (2008) Bimodal bilingualism. *Bilingualism: Language and Cognition* 11, 43–61.

Fenson, L., Dale, P.S., Reznick, J.S., Thal, D., Bates, E., Hartung, J.P., Pethick, S. and Reilly, J.S. (1993) *The MacArthur Communicative Development Inventories: User's Guide and Technical Manual.* San Diego, CA: Singular Publishing Group.

Gathercole, V. and Thomas, E.M. (2009) Bilingual first-language development: Dominant language take-over, threatened minority language take-up. *Bilingualism: Language and Cognition* 12, 213–237.

Geers, A.E., Brenner, C., Nicholas, J.G., Uchanski, R., Tye-Murray, N. and Tobey, E.A. (2002) Rehabilitation factors contributing to implant benefit in children. *Annals of Otology, Rhinology and Laryngology* 111, 127–130.

Genesee, F. (1989) Early bilingual development: One language or two. *Journal of Child Language* 16, 161–179.

Giezen, M. (2011) Speech and sign perception in deaf children with cochlear implants. Doctoral dissertation, University of Amsterdam.

Grosjean, F. (1992) The bilingual and the bicultural person in the hearing and in the deaf world. *Sign Language Studies* 77, 307–320.

Grosjean, F. (2010) *Bilingual: Life and Reality.* Cambridge, MA: Harvard University Press.

Guerrera, K., Davidson, K. and Petroj, V. (2013) Language dominance: Evidence from whispering in bimodal bilingual children. Presented at Boston University Conference on Language Development, Boston, MA.

Hassanzadeh, S. (2012) Outcomes of cochlear implantation in deaf children of deaf parents: Comparative study. *Journal of Laryngology & Otology* 126, 989–994.

Haywood, H.C. and Lidz, C.S. (2007) *Dynamic Assessment in Practice: Clinical and Educational Applications.* New York: Cambridge University Press.

Hoiting, N. and Slobin, D. (2002) What a Deaf child needs to see: Advantages of a natural sign language over a sign system. In R. Schulmeister and H. Reinitzer (eds) *Progress in Sign Language Research. In Honor of Siegmund Prillwitz/Fortschritte in der Gebärdensprachforschung. Festschrift für Siegmund Prillwitz* (pp. 268–277). Hamburg: Signum.

Hulk, A. and Müller, N. (2000) Bilingual first language acquisition at the interface between syntax and pragmatics. *Bilingualism: Language and Cognition* 3 (3), 227–244.

Johnson, J., Watkins, R. and Rice, M. (1992) Bimodal bilingual language development in a hearing child of deaf parents. *Applied Psycholinguistics* 13 (1), 31–52.

Kirk, K.I., Miyamoto, R.T., Ying, E., Perdew, A.E. and Zuganelis, H. (2003) Cochlear implantation in young children: Effects of age at implantation and communication mode. *Volta Review* 102, 127–144.

Koulidobrova, H. (2012) When the Quiet Surfaces: 'Transfer' of Argument Omission in the Speech of ASL-English Bilinguals. Doctoral thesis, Department of Linguistics, University of Connecticut.

Lee, J. (2008) Assessment considerations with hearing children of deaf parents. Presented at the Annual Meeting of the American Speech-Language-Hearing Association (ASHA).

Lee, J. (2010) Diagnosis of language disorder with a bilingual child: A case study. Presented at the Annual Meeting of the American Speech-Language-Hearing Association (ASHA), Philadelphia, PA.

Liddell, S. (2003) *Grammar, Gesture and Meaning in American Sign Language.* Cambridge: Cambridge University Press.

Lillo-Martin, D. (2000) Aspects of the Syntax and Acquisition of WH-questions in American Sign Language. In K. Emmorey and H. Lane (eds) *The Signs of Language Revisited: An Anthology in Honor of Ursula Bellugi and Edward Klima*. Mahwah, NJ: Lawrence Erlbaum Associates, 401–414.

Lillo-Martin, D., de Quadros, R., Koulidobrova, H. and Chen Pichler, D. (2010) Bimodal bilingual cross-language influence in unexpected domains. In J. Costa, M. Lobo and F. Pratas (eds) *Language Acquisition and Development: Proceedings of GALA 2009*. Cambridge: Cambridge Scholars Publishing.

Lillo-Martin, D., Koulidobrova, H., Quadros, R. and Chen Pichler, D. (2012) Bilingual language synthesis: Evidence from WH-questions in bimodal bilinguals. *Proceedings of the 36th Annual Boston University Conference on Language Development* (pp. 302–314). Somerville, MA: Cascadilla Press.

Mallory, B.L., Zingle, H.W. and Schein, J.D. (1993) Intergenerational communication modes in deaf-parented families. *Sign Language Studies* 78, 73–92.

Mason, K., Rowley, K., Marshall, C.R., Atkinson, J.R., Herman, R., Woll, B. and Morgan, G. (2010) Identifying SLI in Deaf children acquiring British Sign Language: Implications for theory and practice. *British Journal of Developmental Psychology* 28, 33–49.

Morford, J. and Mayberry, R. (2000) A reexamination of 'early exposure' and its implications for language acquisition by eye. In C. Chamberlain, J. Morford and R. Mayberry (eds) *Language Acquisition by Eye*. Mahwah, NJ: Lawrence Erlbaum.

Oller, D.K. and Eilers, R.E. (eds) (2002) *Language and Literacy in Bilingual Children*. Clevedon: Multilingual Matters.

Padden, C. (1988 [1983]) *Interaction of Morphology and Syntax in American Sign Language*. Garland Outstanding Dissertations in Linguistics series. New York: Garland. (Originally distributed as PhD dissertation, University of California.)

Paradis, J. and Genesee, F. (1996) Syntactic acquisition in bilingual children. *Studies in Second Language Acquisition* 18, pp. 1–25.

Paul, E. (2010) Spoken language acquisition of a bimodal-bilingual 2-year-old: Outcome of language stimulation and influence of quantity of L2 input. Masters thesis, Department of Hearing, Speech and Language Sciences, Gallaudet University.

Pearson, B.Z., Fernández, S.C., Lewedeg, V. and Oller, D.K. (1997) The relation of input factors to lexical learning by bilingual infants. *Applied Psycholinguistics* 18, 41–58.

Petitto, L. A., Katerelos, M., Levy, B., Gauna, K., Tétrault, K. and Ferraro, V. (2001) Bilingual signed and spoken language acquisition from birth: Implications for the mechanisms underlying early bilingual language acquisition. *Journal of Child Language* 28, 453–496.

Pizer, G. (2008) Sign and speech in family interaction: Language choices of Deaf parents and their hearing children. Doctoral thesis, Department of Linguistics, University of Texas at Austin.

Place, S. and Hoff, E. (2011) Properties of dual language exposure that influence 2-year-olds' bilingual proficiency. *Child Development* 82 (6), 1834–1849.

Poplack, S. (1980) Sometimes I'll start a sentence in English y termino en Español: Toward a typology of code-switching. In J. Amastae and L. Elías-Olivares (eds) *Spanish in the United States: Sociolinguistic Aspects* (pp. 230–263). Cambridge: Cambridge University Press.

Quadros, R., Lillo-Martin, D. and Chen Pichler, D. (2010) Two languages but one computation: Code-blending in bimodal bilingual development. Presented at Theoretical Issues in Sign Language Research: Purdue University, Indiana.

Quadros, R., Rebello Cruz, C. and Lemos Pizzio, A. (2012) Memória fonológica em crianças bilíngues bimodais e crianças com implante coclear. *ReVEL* 10 (19).

Quadros, R., Lillo-Martin, D. and Chen Pichler, D. (2013) Early effects of bilingualism on WH-question structures: Insight from sign-speech bilingualism. *Proceedings of GALA 2011* (pp. 300–308). Newcastle upon Tyne: Cambridge Scholars Publishing.

Quadros R., Chen Pichler, D., Lillo-Martin, D., Cruz, D., Kozak, L.V., Palmer, J., Lemos Pizzio, A. and Reynolds, W. (in press) Methods in bimodal bilingualism research: Experimental studies. In E. Orfanidou, B. Woll and G. Morgan (eds) *The Blackwell Guide to Research Methods in Sign Language Studies*. Oxford: Blackwell.

Quinn, L. (2004) Code mixing in bilingual-bimodal children. Masters thesis, Department of Audiology and Speech Language Pathology, Gallaudet University.

Retherford, K. (1993) *Guide to Analysis of Language Transcripts* (2nd edn). Eau Claire, WI: Thinking Publications.

Romaine, S. (1999) Bilingual language development. In M. Barrett (ed.) *The Development of Language* (pp. 251–276). London: University College London Press.

Rossell, C. and Baker. K. (1996) The educational effectiveness of bilingual education. *Research in the Teaching of English* 30 (1), 7–74.

Rossetti, L. (2006) *The Rossetti Infant-Toddler Language Scale: A Measure of Communication and Interaction*. East Moline, IL: LinguiSystems.

Sachs, J., Bard, B. and Johnson, M.L. (1981) Language learning with restricted input: Case studies of two hearing children of deaf parents. *Applied Psycholinguistics* 2 (1), 33–54.

Schiff, N. and Ventry, I. (1976) Communication problems in hearing children of deaf parents. *Journal of Speech and Hearing Disorders* 41 (3), 348–358.

Singh, L. (2008) Influences of high and low variability on infant word recognition. *Cognition* 106, 833–870.

Svirsky, M.A., Robbins, A.M., Kirk, K.I., Pisoni, D.B. and Miyamoto, R.T. (2000) Language development in profoundly deaf children with cochlear implants. *Psychological Science* 11, 153–158.

Todd, P. (1971) A case of structural interference across sensory modalities in second-language learning. *Word* 27 (1–3), 102–118.

Tomasuolo, E., Fellini, L., Di Renzo, A. and Volterra, V. (2010) Assessing lexical production in deaf signing children with the Boston naming test. *Language, Interaction and Acquisition* 1, 110–128.

Unsworth, S. (2013) Assessing the role of current and cumulative exposure in simultaneous bilingual acquisition: The case of Dutch gender. *Bilingualism: Language and Cognition* 16 (1), 86–110. doi:10.1017/S1366728912000284.

Van den Bogaerde, B. (2000) Input and interaction in deaf families. PhD dissertation, University of Amsterdam. See http://wwwlot.let.uu.nl.

van den Bogaerde, B. and Baker, A. (2005) Code mixing in mother-child interaction in Deaf families. *Sign Language and Linguistics* 8, 153–176.

Index